U. K. Munzinger · J. G. Boldt · P. A. Keblish (Eds.)

Primary Knee Arthroplasty

Springer

Berlin
Heidelberg
New York
Hong Kong
London
Milan
Paris
Tokyo

U. K. Munzinger · J. G. Boldt
P. A. Keblish (Eds.)

PRIMARY
KNEE
ARTHROPLASTY

With 306 Figures in 567 Separate Illustrations
and 24 Tables

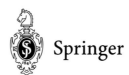

Springer

Urs K. Munzinger MD
Senior Consultant Orthopaedic Surgeon
Chief, Devision of Orthopaedic Surgery
Schulthess Klinik
Lengghalde 2
CH-8008 Zurich
Switzerland

Jens G. Boldt MD
Specialist Orthopaedic Surgeon
Orthopaedic Center Geilenkirchen
Am Weinberg 22
D-52511 Geilenkirchen
Germany

Peter A. Keblish MD
Professor of Clinical Orthopaedics
Orthopaedic Associates of Allentown
1243 South Cedar Crest Blvd.
Allentown, PA 18103
USA

ISBN 3-540-43065-2
Springer-Verlag Berlin Heidelberg New York

Library of Congress Cataloging-in-Publication Data
Primary knee arthroplasty / Urs K. Munzinger, Jens G. Boldt,
Peter A. Keblish, editors.
p. ; cm. Includes bibliographical references and index.
ISBN 3-540-43065-2 (alk. paper)
1. Knee–Surgery. 2. Total knee replacement. 3. Arthroplasty.
I. Munzinger, Urs K. II. Boldt, Jens G., 1963- III. Keblish, Peter A.
[DNLM: 1. Arthroplasty, Replacement, Knee–contraindica-
tions. 2. Arthroplasty, Replacement, Knee–methods. 3. Knee
Prosthesis–adverse effects. 4. Postoperative Complications–
prevention & control. WE 870 P952 2004]
RD561.P75 2004
617.5'82059–dc22

Springer-Verlag is a part of Springer Science + Business Media

springeronline.com

© Springer-Verlag Berlin Heidelberg 2004
Printed in Germany

The use of general descriptive names, registered names, trade-
marks, etc. in this publication does not imply, even in the
absence of a specific statement, that such names are exempt
from the relevant protective laws and regulations and therefore
free for general use.

Product liability: The publishers cannot guarantee the accuracy of any information about dosage and application contained in this book. In every individual case the user must
check such information by consulting the relevant literature.

Editor: Gabriele M. Schröder
Desk editor: Irmela Bohn
Cover design: F. Steinen, ᵉStudio Calamar, Spain
Product management and layout: B. Wieland, Heidelberg
Reproduction and typesetting: AM-productions, Wiesloch
Printing and bookbinding: Stürtz AG, Würzburg

24/3150 – 5 4 3 2 1 0
Printed on acid-free paper

Preface

Primary knee arthroplasty as a safe, accepted, predictable and reproducible procedure has a relatively short history. The first metallic prostheses were implanted as partial metallic or hinged metallic types in the 1960s. Subsequent developments and success with the use of bone cement in total hip replacements (Charnley, Mueller, and colleagues) helped stimulate improvements of technique and fixation in knee arthroplasty. Partial (UKA) and total knee (TKA) designs evolved in the 1970s, at times exceeding the advances in the technique (and instrumentation) required to allow for reproducible implantation.

Knee arthroplasty has gradually evolved over the past three decades to a high level of reproducibility that must be appreciated and acquired by all orthopaedic surgeons who perform arthroplasty or are learning to become accomplished arthroplasty surgeons. The basics of exact clinical examination as well as basic principles of surgical treatment are described competently and in utmost detail in K. Krackow's book (Mosby, 1990). We consider this a valuable contribution to the fundamentals of knee arthroplasty. Continuous improvement of soft tissue management, instrumentation, and surgical approaches will result in improved ligament balancing. Bone bed management with bone preservation/enhancement techniques, grafting, and alignment must enhance soft tissue management. Different philosophies regarding these issues exist; the ultimate and shared goal, however, is a stable, well-aligned arthroplasty that will provide the best longevity current materials can offer. Newer innovations such as navigation systems for bone/soft tissue balancing (and possibly robotics) offer a further dimension.

"Getting it right the first time" should be the motto of all total knee surgeons.

The authors and contributors to this text have had extensive interest/experience with total knee designs of the mobile bearing type over the past 20 plus years. Experience with these different designs and basic philosophies will be covered from different standpoints; these include bio-mechanical issues, relationships of patella-femoral tracking to femoral-tibial stability, and cement vs cementless fixation.

Short- or long-term complications after TKA are serious issues, which are addressed from a preventative and active treatment perspective. Chapters dealing with prosthetic loosening, osteolysis, arthrofibrosis, infection and the infected knee provide a current approach for the understanding and surgical management of these challenging problems.

Rehabilitation and physical therapy is an integral part of the preoperative and postoperative management of knee arthroplasty patients. Criterion-based programs which address general principles, as well as specific higher-level goals such as sport activities, are discussed in light of improvements in design, technique and materials.

In summary, this book is addressed to practicing knee replacement surgeons, residents/fellows in training as well as orthopaedic nurses, physiotherapists and others who have a special interest in knee arthroplasty. The many tips and advice will hopefully be informative and relevant to obtaining the best possible outcomes.

We wish to thank our editors at Springer-Verlag (Heidelberg) Gabriele Schröder and Irmela Bohn for their competent support and Carol Varma at Lehigh Valley Hospital (Allentown, Pennsylvania) for numerous illustrations.

List of Contributors

Banks, Scott A.
Orthopaedic Research Laboratory
Good Samaritan Medical Center
1309 N. Flagler Drive
West Palm Beach, FL 33401
USA

Beverland, David
Musgrave Park Hospital Northern Ireland
Stockman's Lane
Belfast BT9 7JB
Northern Ireland, GB

Bizzini, Mario
Schulthess Klinik
Lengghalde 2
CH-8008 Zurich
Switzerland

Boldt, Jens G.
Orthopaedic Center Geilenkirchen
Am Weinberg 22
D-52511 Geilenkirchen
Germany

Briard, Jean Louis
Clinique du Cèdre
F-76235 Bois Guillaume
France

Gyssler, Bernhard
Centerpulse Orthopedics Ltd.
P.O. Box 65
CH-8404 Winterthur
Switzerland

Henkel, Thomas R.
Andreasklinik Cham
Rigistr. 1
CH-6330 Cham
Switzerland

Keblish, Peter A.
Orthopaedic Associates of Allentown
1243 South Cedar Crest Blvd.
Allentown, PA 18103
USA

Kramers-de Quervain, Inès
Laboratorium für Biomechanik
ETH Zurich
Wagistr. 4, CH-8952 Schlieren
and
Schulthess Klinik
Lengghalde 2, CH-8008 Zurich
Switzerland

Munzinger, Urs K.
Schulthess Klinik
Lengghalde 2
CH-8008 Zurich
Switzerland

Rieker, Claude
Centerpulse Orthopedics
P.O. Box 65
CH-8404 Winterthur
Switzerland

Vogt, Markus
Zuger Kantonsspital
CH-6300 Zug
Switzerland

Windler, Markus
Centerpulse Orthopedics
P.O. Box 65
CH-8404 Winterthur
Switzerland

Wyss, Urs
Queen's University
McLaughlin Hall
Kingston, K7L 3N6
Ontario, Canada

Contents

Contents

CHAPTER 1

Urs K. Munzinger · Urs Wyss · Jens G. Boldt
Bernhard G. Gyssler · M. Windler
Inès Kramers-de Quervain · Christian B. Rieker
S. Banks · C. Reinschmidt · A. Stacoff
G. Luder · T. Staehelin

Basic Science, Design, and Materials

1.1 History and Development

Urs K. Munzinger

The knee is the major joint most commonly affected by osteoarthritis. Before the advent of knee replacement, conservative measures such as debridement, osteotomy and arthrodesis represented the basics of surgical management. Therefore, end-stage knee arthritis often led to a significant proportion of disabled patients. This was radically changed with the development of knee arthroplasty, which paralleled that of total hip arthroplasty in the 1970s.

Prior to 1971, examples of pioneer total knee replacements included mould arthroplasty of the femoral condyles and metal-on-metal hinge arthroplasties (Walldius and Shiers). The Guepar hinge arthroplasty represented an improvement in which the disadvantages of metal-on-metal hinges were overcome by the use of polyethylene bushings and a silastic extension stop (Fig. 1.1). However, most of these implants underwent early revision surgery, often requiring a knee joint arthrodesis. The polycentric total knee replacement developed by Gunston and Sheehan was the first low-friction arthroplasty, but its success was limited because of increased constraint (Fig. 1.2). The Freeman–Swanson TKA represented the concept of a condylar implant, which contributed to the importance of instrumentation and soft tissues in TKA (Fig. 1.3). In Germany and Switzerland, a new type of semiconstrained knee replacement was introduced by Blauth and the GSB group (Fig. 1.4), which had the advantage of a relatively standardized surgical technique, improved range of motion and ligament stability. Disadvantages included a high frequency of anterior knee pain, toxic synovitis (metallosis), and a high percentage of late infections.

In the USA, the polycentric TKA was modified, leading to the Geomedic implant, which was similar to the Freeman–Swanson device. The Geomedic implant, however, was highly constrained, causing high

Fig. 1.1. Guepar knee prosthesis

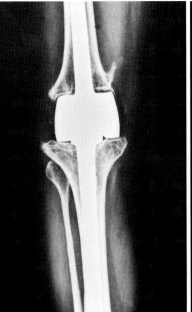
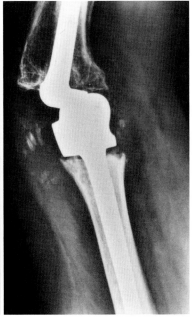

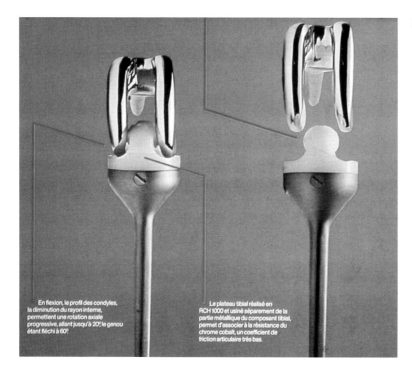

Fig. 1.2. Sheehan knee prosthesis

En flexion, le profil des condyles,
la diminution du rayon interne,
permettent une rotation axiale
progressive, allant jusqu'à 20°, le genou
étant fléchi à 60°.

Le plateau tibial réalisé en
RCH 1000 et usiné séparement de la
partie métallique du composant tibial,
permet d'associer à la résistance du
chrome cobalt, un coefficient de
friction articulaire très bas.

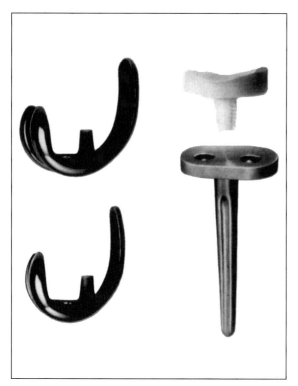

Fig. 1.3. Freeman condylar knee prosthesis

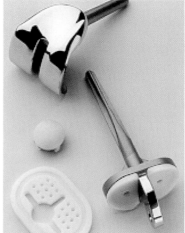

Fig. 1.4. GSB constraint knee prosthesis

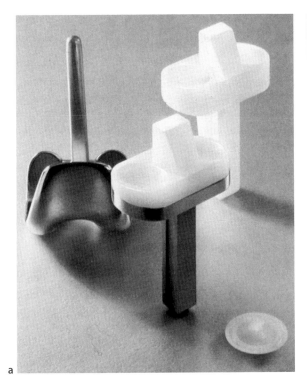

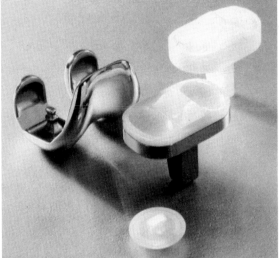

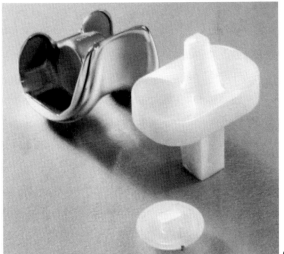

Fig. 1.5. Total condylar knee prosthesis

constraint forces at the tibial implant–bone interface, ultimately triggering aseptic loosening. Both devices were deficient with regard to patellofemoral articulation. The group at the Hospital of Special Surgery in New York improved the condylar prosthesis concept, offering the option of posterior cruciate ligament (PCL) sacrifice or substitution (Fig. 1.5). In Boston, a prosthesis with PCL retention enlarged the choice of implants and preferences. The first long-term results were acceptable. However, there were drawbacks when utilizing fixed bearing designs, particularly with regards to the patellofemoral joint, malalignment, wear and aseptic loosening.

In the 1980s, the debate on TKA focused on fixation (cemented, cementless, hybrid), metal backing of both tibial and patellar components, and round-on-flat articulations. Not all improvements led to better function and, as a result of increased longevity, high numbers of complications and revisions were reported.

In the late 1970s, O'Connor and Goodfellow designed the first mobile bearing unicondylar knee replacement (Oxford Unicompartmental Knee Arthroplasty) with a highly conforming articulation and freely moveable polyethylene bearing (Fig. 1.6). This new design combined decreased contact stresses and reduced constraint forces at the tibial implant–bone interface, two major factors for reducing wear and its associated problems, including osteolysis and loosening. This concept was further improved by Buechel and Pappas, who designed a total condylar low contact stress (LCS) mobile bearing knee prosthesis with specific appreciation to the patellofemoral articulation (Fig. 1.7).

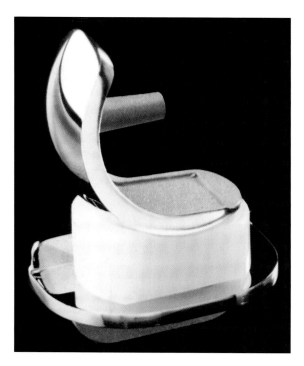

Fig. 1.6. Oxford mobile bearing unicondylar knee prosthesis

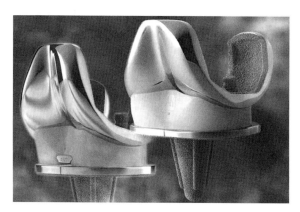

Fig. 1.7. Low contact stress mobile bearing knee prosthesis

Today, mobile bearing TKA have been successfully implanted for over 25 years, with excellent long-term records and clinical outcomes (95 % after 20 years for the Oxford knee and about 90 % after 20 years for the LCS knee). However, inlay dislocations have been reported in both knee systems. Most bearing failures with the LCS knee, particularly when utilizing meniscal bearings, were due to thin and poor polyethylene quality (gamma in air sterilization), often combined with prolonged shelf life (at times 7 years). Data in the recent literature suggest that mobile bearing knee prostheses, with a patella-friendly design, perfect tracking, well-aligned components and balanced soft tissues have an excellent long-term outcome and satisfactory function, allowing patients to continue with daily and sports activities.

In the future, surgical techniques for TKA will improve and there will be an increased appreciation of soft tissue balancing and proper component positioning, more accurate instrumentation and computer navigation, and improved component design. At present, one should be cautious about robotic technology in TKA because of recent soft tissue concerns and medicolegal implications.

Bibliography

Buechel FF Sr (2002) Long-term followup after mobile-bearing total knee replacement. Clin Orthop 404:40–50

Callaghan JJ (2001) Mobile-bearing knee replacement: clinical results: a review of the literature. Clin Orthop 392:221–225

Gschwend N, Drobny T (1992) A comparative study of two different knee systems in the same patient. Elsevier Science Publishers BV 359–364

Jordan LR, Dowd JE, Olivo JL, Voorhorst PE (2002) The clinical history of mobile-bearing patella components in total knee arthroplasty. Orthopedics 25 [Suppl 2]:s247–s250

Nelissen RG (2003) The impact of total joint replacement in rheumatoid arthritis. Best Pract Res Clin Rheumatol 17:831–846

Price AJ, Rees JL, Beard D, Juszczak E, Carter S, White S, de Steiger R, Dodd CA, Gibbons M, McLardy-Smith P, Goodfellow JW, Murray DW (2003) A mobile-bearing total knee prosthesis compared with a fixed-bearing prosthesis. A multicentre single-blind randomised controlled trial. J Bone Joint Surg Br 85:62–67

Ranawat CS (2002) History of total knee replacement. J South Orthop Assoc 11:218–226

Rand JA, Trousdale RT, Ilstrup DM, Harmsen WS (2003) Factors affecting the durability of primary total knee prostheses. J Bone Joint Surg Am 85A:259–265

Sorrells RB (2002) The clinical history and development of the low contact stress total knee arthroplasty. Orthopedics 25 [Suppl 2]:s207–s212

1.2 Biomechanics in Normal and Prosthetic Knees

Urs Wyss

Biomechanics of the Knee Joint and Total Joint Arthroplasty

The knee joint is the largest joint in the human body. It is mechanically more complicated than the ball-and-socket joint of the hip. It has three compartments, the two condylar femorotibial compartments and the patellofemoral compartment. The articulating areas of the femur, tibia and patella are made up of different thicknesses of articular cartilage. A system of menisci, internal and external ligaments, muscles and contoured bones allows for movement between the thigh and the calf during walking, managing stairs and all other types of activities. The range of motion (ROM) of healthy subjects is larger than what can be achieved with total knee arthroplasty (TKA). The available ROM of these joints has increased over the years, so that a patient with a well-functioning TKA can do most activities of daily living of Western societies. However, gaining high flexion beyond 120 degrees in TKA is still challenging for Eastern societies, who wish to perform activities such as kneeling, squatting and cross-legged sitting.

Biomechanics of the Knee Joint

In a simplified way the knee joint can be considered in the sagittal plane as a four-bar linkage formed by the anterior and posterior cruciate ligaments, the distal femur and proximal tibia, as described by Menschik in 1974. There is no fixed center of rotation at the knee joint. Instead, there is a combination of rotation and translation of the knee joint, as described by the Weber brothers in 1836. There is also movement in the frontal plane, which is restricted by the shape of the bones, the collateral ligaments and the muscles, as well as rotation between the femur and the tibia in the longitudinal direction. The menisci optimize the load transmission between the femur and the tibia, by adjusting their shape and providing the largest contact area possible during the full arc of motion. The biomechanics of cartilage, menisci, ligaments, muscles and bones have been researched extensively, and summarized by Van Mow (1990). Much of the work in knee biomechanics results from cadaver work and simulation studies, as it is impossible to instrument a healthy knee joint with implantable devices. Fluoroscopy technology has dramatically enhanced our knowledge of knee joint (and TKA) biomechanics in healthy as well as diseased knees. Equipment restrictions do not allow an assessment of all movements, but fluoroscopy technology is a very useful tool to look at translations and rotation during movement of the femur and tibia.

This chapter focuses on the range of motion and forces during various activities after TKA. Force data in TKA are required for finite element analysis studies, but also for fatigue testing of new or modified TKA. Most of the motion studies deal with walking or gait, the most common activity of daily living, followed by managing stairs, kneeling, squatting, cross-legged sitting and others.

Gait Analysis

Human locomotion has been studied for over a century. The Weber brothers in 1836 were among the first to study gait. Braune and Fischer in 1895 were the pioneers of motion studies using elaborate photographic and analytical techniques. They carried out research to optimize equipment for the German infantry and many of their techniques are still used today. The availability of sophisticated equipment and computers, however, has allowed the analysis of data in a few minutes instead of the months and years it took Braune and Fischer. Morrison and Winter reported gait studies in the late 1970s, looking at joint angles, joint forces, joint moments, energy and power during locomotion (Morrison 1968, Winter 1979). Their efforts focused mainly on the mechanism of how we walk, and how walking is controlled. In a limited way the findings of gait research have been used in the process of developing new TKA, but the potential for a much wider use of gait research still exists. There are many systems used today to track motion data from video-based and magnetic to optoelectronic devices that record flashing infrared LEDs placed over anatomic landmarks. Gait analysis has been used to provide three-dimensional information about joint rotations, bone-on-bone forces and moments during walking and managing stairs, which are the most important activities of daily living for the lower extremity. It is important to be aware of the accuracy of gait analysis data, so that it can be used appropriately. Validation of systems, such as described by Deluzio et al. (1993), or direct range of motion comparisons with pins inserted in bones, have shown that it is possible to generate data with errors of less than 10 %. Force and moment data during short periods of initial foot contact might be exposed to larger errors due to the smoothing effects of the motion tracking data, before kinetic analysis is possible. Skin movements over bone are another source of errors. This error is less critical during the stance phase of gait, when there is less movement than during the swing phase, with more movement between the soft tissue and the underlying bone. Another limitation of most gait data is that it represents net moments and net bone-on-bone forces. The influence of co-contraction is neglected and could only be overcome by the addition of electromyographic (EMG) data to get closer to the real bone-on-bone forces.

Knee Joint Rotations

Data about range of motion are important when designing artificial knee joints. Placement of the TKA in the bone, soft tissue constraints and limited muscle function are further reasons for reduced ROM. The kinematics of level walking and managing stairs of a healthy group of 35 subjects are presented. The mean age of the group was 24.4 years with a standard deviation of 3.2 years. A smaller group of elderly normal subjects was also analyzed, but the mean curves were almost identical, except for a larger standard deviation. Some elderly normal subjects had radiographic signs of osteoarthritis that was already interfering with their gait; however, they were unaware of the beginning of osteoarthritis. Figure 1.8 shows the conventions used to give directions of joint angles, forces and moments. The curves presented in Fig. 1.9 show the normalized data for one walking cycle or stride, and one managing stairs cycle. Time is eliminated by expressing the data as a percentage of a gait cycle from 0 to 100%. The curves show that the range for adduction–abduction and internal–external rotation is between 5 and 10 degrees, but with considerable variation among subjects, as indicated by the standard deviation bands. It also shows that for managing stairs, almost 90 degrees of flexion are required, while for walking, about 60 degrees of flexion are sufficient.

Eastern cultures require increased range of motion, particularly high flexion for cross-legged sitting, kneeling, squatting, getting in and out of a car, and sitting. The maximum knee flexion angles for these types of activities of daily living are shown in Table 1.1 for an elderly Chinese population with a mean age of 56 years and a mean body mass of 58 kg.

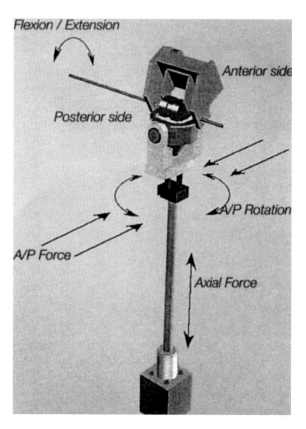

Fig. 1.8. Sign convention for rotations, forces and moments. Distal-proximal (DP), posterior-anterior (PA), and lateral-medial (LM) indicate the positive directions. The curved arrows around the DP, PA and LM axes indicate the direction of positive rotation and moments

Table 1.1. Maximum knee flexion angles

Activity	Degrees
Kneeling heels up	145
Kneeling with plantar flexion	146
Squatting heels flat	134
Squatting heels up	147
Sitting cross-legged	134
Sitting on small stool	122
Getting into a minibus	102

Tibiofemoral rotation was measured for these activities, showing values up to 30 degrees associated with 10 degrees of adduction. It should be appreciated that these activities require higher rotation than during walking and managing stairs.

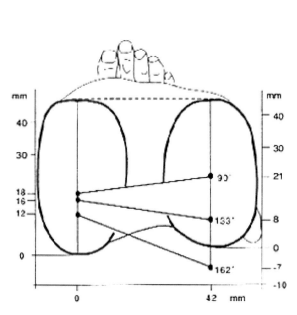

Fig. 1.9. Three knee rotations during level walking from initial foot contact, and during managing stairs from toe-off to toe-off

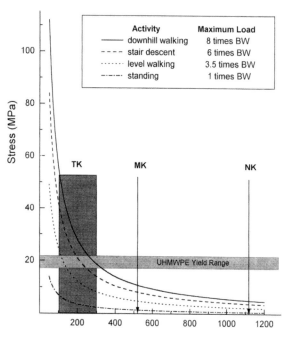

Fig. 1.10. Net bone-on-bone forces at the patellofemoral joint normalized to body mass during level walking (*top*) and during managing stairs (*bottom*)

Knee Joint Forces

Net knee forces do not account for torque or moment generated within the knee joint, thereby neglecting the muscle forces required to produce the moments. Only bone-on-bone forces can be used to determine the strength of an implant and the type of fixation required. It is important to remember that the actual bone-on-bone forces are larger during phases of the motion with muscle contraction. EMG set-up is required for determination of co-contraction and actual bone-on-bone forces.

Peak values of tibiofemoral bone-on-bone forces during level walking occur shortly after initial foot contact and during push-off of the walking cycle. Forces range from two to five times body weight. Forces during swing phase are much lower, with one to two times body weight before initial foot contact. Knee joint shear forces (posterior-anterior and lateral-medial) peak at similar points during the gait cycle as the distal-proximal forces, with peak values of about half body weight for the posterior-anterior forces and only about a tenth body weight for the lateral-medial forces at the same locations. It is logical that the lateral-medial forces are lowest, as they are in

the frontal plane and not in the plane of movement, or the sagittal plane.

The magnitude of net bone-on-bone forces at the tibiofemoral joint during managing stairs is similar to that during walking. The peak for the distal-proximal forces, however, occurs in the phase when the body is pushed up the stairs with the knee in about 50 degrees of flexion, as compared to the peaks during level walking with less than 10 degrees of knee flexion. The peak in the distal-proximal forces during managing stairs must be considered when designing artificial knee prostheses.

The patellofemoral joint is an integral part of the knee joint and must be considered when designing knee prostheses. Figure 1.10 shows the net bone-on-bone forces during level walking and managing stairs normalized to body weight. The forces were set to zero during phases where the moment indicates net knee flexor activity. There is a net bone-on-bone force of two to three times body weight during push-up phase with the knee at about 50 degrees flexion, similar to the peak distal-proximal forces at the tibiofemoral joint.

Knee Joint Moment

The net knee joint moments are also a useful indicator for the design of artificial knee joints, as the moments must be balanced with muscle action. The net flexor moment balanced by the extensor muscles is several times larger during managing stairs than during level walking, which is obvious as the center of gravity has to be pushed upwards by each step. Prodromos et al. (1985) reported the adduction moment in the assessment of high tibial osteotomies, but their findings were not conclusive. They indicated that changes in gait pattern could mask the alignment correction achieved during surgery. Weidenhielm et al. (1992) concluded that the adduction moments were reduced when TKA were correctly aligned during implantation, thus stressing the importance of perfect implant size and alignment.

Total Knee Arthroplasty

Total knee replacement surgery was first performed by Gluck more than 100 years ago. The few implants that were performed had to be removed after a few months, mainly because of inadequate sterilization techniques, both of the implant and during surgery. It was not until the 1950s that TKA was more widely used. Several hundred different designs have been developed over the past 50 years, of which only a few typical ones are mentioned to illustrate the evolution in the designs. The first TKA were constraint, such as the Walldius and Shiers knees, and were press-fit implanted as bone cement was not available. They lasted several years, and loosened because of significant constraint and poor fixation technique. Furthermore, the rigid axis led to metal wear and metallosis. The recognition that a fixed axis should be avoided led to the development of condylar replacements such as the Gunston hemiarthroplasty and others. The GSB knee prosthesis represented a stemmed fixation with a guided axis. One of the earlier surface replacements was the Freeman–Swanson knee prosthesis, developed in 1973, which could be used when the ligaments were still in good condition. These types of knee joints have evolved over the past 30 years but are still conceptually similar. The introduction of mobile bearing knees, such as the low contact stress and self-aligning prostheses, appeared to increase joint mobility, reduce wear, decrease constraint forces and lead to longer outcomes. Other knee systems such as the NK I and II, with solutions for cruciate sparing and cruciate sacrificing types, cemented, cementless

and revision systems became available, and were used extensively. The INNEX system (rotating platform mobile bearing TKA) was introduced recently and early results are reported in Sect. 3.6. It includes an ultracongruent femoral design for posterior cruciate ligament sacrifice.

Unicompartmental knee systems have gained a recent renaissance, particularly for medial compartment disease. Many of the currently used TKA are designed for cementless fixation, relying on good primary fixation and subsequent bone ingrowth into porous structures.

Most modern TKA serve the purpose of relieving pain, restoring function, and allowing a return to normal daily and recreational activities. Sound biomechanics, implant design, and patellofemoral tracking are the most crucial factors for successful outcomes. In contrast, polyethylene wear appears to play a lesser role in TKA compared with total hip arthroplasty.

Bibliography

Andriacchi TP, Galante JO, Fermier RW (1982) The influence of total knee-replacement design on walking and stair-climbing. J Bone Joint Surg Am 64:1328–1335

Banks SA, Hodge WA (1996) Accurate measurement of three-dimensional knee replacement kinematics using single-plane fluoroscopy. IEEE Trans Biomed Eng 43:638–649

Bloebaum RD, Bachus KN, Jensen JW, Scott DF, Hofmann AA (1998) Porous-coated metal-backed patellar components in total knee replacements. J Bone Joint Surg Am 80:518–528

Bourne RB, Whitewood CN (2002) The role of rotating platform total knee replacements: design considerations, kinematics, and clinical results. J Knee Surg Fall 15:247–253

Braune W, Fischer O (1895) Der Gang des Menschen, 1. Teil. Versuche am unbelasteten und belasteten Menschen. Abhandl D Math-Phys Kl K Sächs Gesellsch Wissensch

Chapman-Sheath PJ, Bruce WJ, Chung WK, Morberg P, Gillies RM, Walsh WR (2003) In vitro assessment of proximal polyethylene contact surface areas and stresses in mobile bearing knees. Med Eng Phys 25:437–443

Cheng CK, Huang CH, Liau JJ, Huang CH (2003) The influence of surgical malalignment on the contact pressures of fixed and mobile bearing knee prostheses – a biomechanical study. Clin Biomech (Bristol, Avon) 18:231–236

Costigan PA, Wyss UP, Deluzio KJ, Li J (1992) Semiautomatic three-dimensional knee motion assessment system. Med Biol Eng Comput 30:343–350

Deluzio KJ, Wyss UP, Li J, Costigan PA (1993) A procedure to validate three-dimensional motion assessment systems. J Biomech 26:753–759

Dennis DA, Komistek RD, Mahfouz MR (2003) In vivo fluoroscopic analysis of fixed-bearing total knee replacements. Clin Orthop 410:114–130

Draganich LF, Piotrowski GA, Martell J, Pottenger LA (2002) The effects of early rollback in total knee arthroplasty on stair stepping. J Arthroplasty 17:723–730

Freeman MA, Swanson SAV, Todd RC (1973) Total replacement of the knee using the Freeman-Swanson knee prosthesis. Clin Orthop Relat Res 94:153–170

Gunston PH (1979) Polycentric knee arthroplasty. J Arthroplasty 2:1–9

Hofmann AA, Evanich JD, Ferguson RP, Camargo MP (2001) Ten- to 14-year clinical followup for the cementless Natural Knee system. Clin Orthop 388:85–94

Kaper BP, Smith PN, Bourne RB, Rorabeck CH, Robertson D (1999) Medium term results of a mobile bearing total knee replacement. Clin Orthop Relat Res 367:201–209

Ladouceur DT (2000) Three-dimensional kinematics of seven activities of daily living commonly found in Asia. M Sc thesis, Queen's University, Kingston, Canada

Lafortune MA, Cavanagh PR, Sommer HJ, Kalenak A (1992) Three-dimensional kinematics of the human knee during walking. J Biomech 25:347–357

Menschik A (1974) Mechanik des Kniegelenkes, Teil 1. Z Orthop 112:481–495

Morrison JB (1968) Bioengineering analysis of force actions transmitted by the knee joint. Bio Med Eng 3:164–170

Mow Van C (1990) Biomechanics of arthrodial joints. Springer, Berlin Heidelberg New York

Mulholland SJ, Wyss UP (2001) Activities of daily living in non-Western cultures: range of motion requirements for hip and knee joint implants. Int J Rehab Res 24:191–198

Prodromos CC, Andriacchi TP, Galante JO (1985) A relationship between gait and clinical changes following high tibial osteotomy. J Bone Joint Surg Am 67:1188–1193

Ranawat CS (2002) History of total knee replacement. J South Orthop Assoc 11:218–226

Romagnoli S (1996) The unicompartmental knee prosthesis and the rotatory gonarthrosis kinematic. In: Insall JN, Scott WN, Scuderi GR (eds) Current concepts in primary and revision total knee arthroplasty. Lippincott-Raven, Philadelphia

Stiehl JB, Komistek RD, Dennis DA, Keblish PA (2001) Kinematics of the patellofemoral joint in total knee arthroplasty. J Arthroplasty 16:706–714

Taylor M, Barrett DS (2003) Explicit finite element simulation of eccentric loading in total knee replacement. Clin Orthop 414:162–171

Weber W, Weber E (1836) Mechanik der Gehwerkzeuge. Dieterichsche Buchhandlung, Göttingen

Weidenhielm L, Svensson OK, Broström LA (1992) Change in adduction moment about the knee after high tibial osteotomy and prosthetic replacement in osteoarthritis of the knee. Clin Biomech 7:91–96

Winter DA (1979) Biomechanics of human movement. Wiley, New York

Wyss UP, Costigan PA (1995) Gait analysis: a biomechanical tool in the development of artificial joints. In: Morscher EW (ed) Endoprosthetics. Springer, Berlin Heidelberg New York, pp 103–115

1.3 Mobile Bearing Knee Prostheses

Jens G. Boldt, Urs K. Munzinger

The ultimate goal in total knee arthroplasty (TKA), whether with fixed or mobile bearings, is a well-functioning implant providing patient satisfaction and a survivorship of more than 90% after 15–20 years. Parameters include increased congruency in the full arc of motion in frontal, sagittal, and coronal planes, decreased contact stress of the polyethylene bearing and finally decreased constraint forces at the implant–bone interface. Moveable bearings in TKA are beneficial in the conflict between articulating congruency versus constraint forces on the polyethylene, thereby reducing polyethylene wear debris, which is the ultimate reason for late failures. The use of moveable bearings in TKA allows the achievement of articulating congruency without increasing the joint forces at the interface between prosthetic components and the bearing. However, complications that may occur, particularly in the mobile bearing TKA, include spinout and soft tissue impingement. Exacting surgical technique as well as limitation of the bearing mobility may considerably reduce these complications. Long-term outcome data suggest that mobile bearing TKA appear to have an equal or longer life when compared with fixed bearing devices.

In the early 1970s, Buechel and Pappas designed the New Jersey low contact stress (LCS) arthroplasty, one with two meniscal bearings and one with a rotating platform bearing. In recent years, a variety of systems with different kinematic principles have been introduced (Figs. 1.11–1.21). The lateral compartment

Fig. 1.11.
SAL, Centerpulse, Switzerland

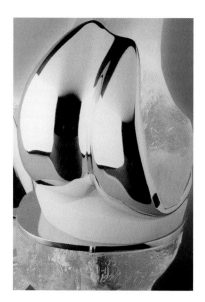

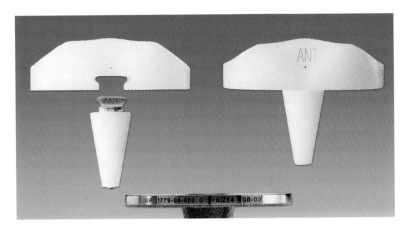

Fig. 1.12. LCS ap-glide and rotating platform, DePuy, USA

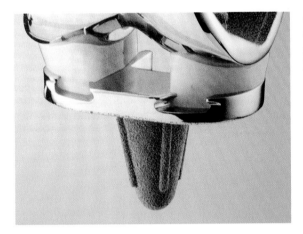

Fig. 1.13. LCS meniscal bearing, DePuy, USA

of the knee joint has to manage a considerable incongruency of the articulating surfaces in both flexion and extension. The mobility of both medial and lateral menisci guarantees an almost perfect congruency of the entire arc of motion in an anatomical situation.

The role of the cruciate ligaments is still controversial. In 1904, Zuppinger proposed that certain ligaments in the knee joint were tight at all times and that they acted as "guiding ligaments" to control the movement of the knee. He also proposed that the cruciate ligaments acted as two elements in a rigid four-bar kinematic chain, causing the femur to move bodily back across the top of the tibia during knee joint flexion. In 1917, Strasser illustrated the concept of the four-bar chain in his book, but in the text argued that the mechanism could not be present, as both cruciate ligaments were not both tight at all times. This subject was not discussed in the literature for decades. Between 1965 and 1975, various authors demonstrat-

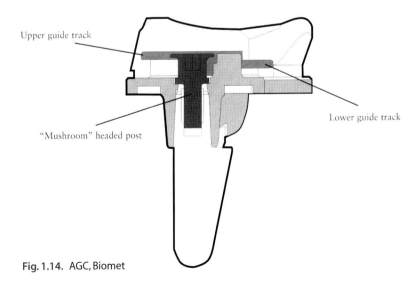

Upper guide track

Lower guide track

"Mushroom" headed post

Fig. 1.14. AGC, Biomet

Fig. 1.15. Interax, Howmedica

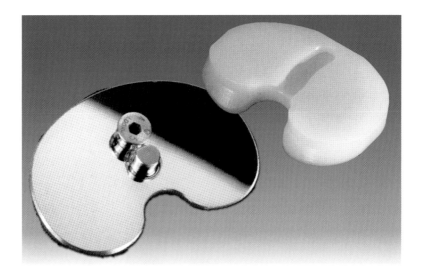

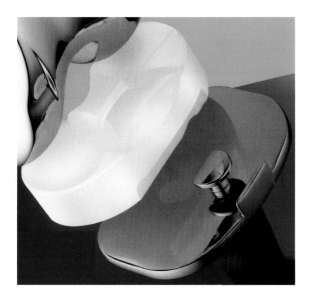

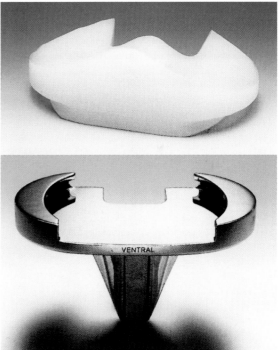

Fig. 1.16. MBK, Zimmer, USA

Fig. 1.17. Minns MB, Corin

ed that rollback exists, using knee joints of cadavers with rigid cruciate ligaments. Designing prosthetic components that simulate normal physiological motion and stability of a knee joint is highly challenging. These problems are addressed by using posterior cruciate ligament (PCL) retaining components or posterior stabilized components with a cam-and-post mechanism when the PCL is sacrificed. Latter mechanisms prevent posterior slope of the tibia in

flexion without "hinging" in extension in particular. Another disadvantage is that back in TKA causes decreased congruency of the polyethylene bearing and therefore increased contact stress, leading to higher wear.

Using both magnetic resonance imaging and anatomical dissection, Freeman demonstrated that the PCL is relaxed from 5 to 60 degrees. As the PCL becomes tight at 60 degrees, it appears to act on the

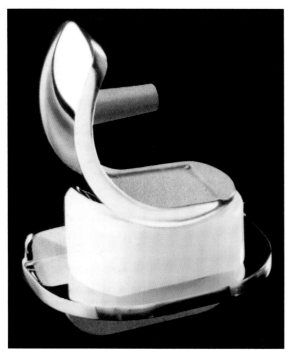

Fig. 1.18. Oxford, Unicompartmental II, Biomet

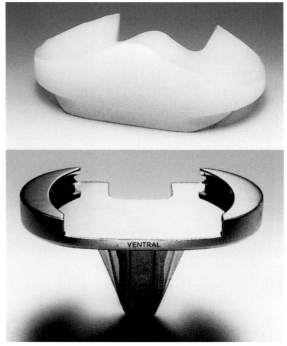

Fig. 1.20. TACK, Waldemar Link

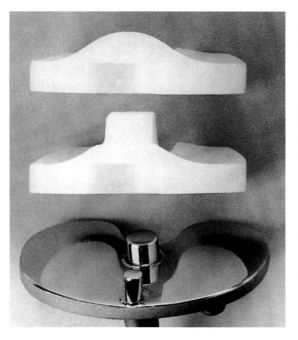

Fig. 1.19. Rotaglide Corin

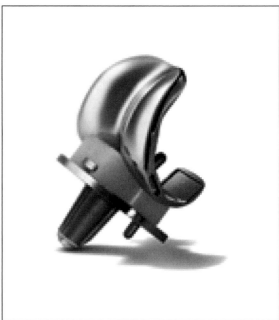

Fig. 1.21. INNEX ap-glide TKA, Centerpulse, Switzerland

femur, tending to displace its femoral attachment posteriorly with further flexion. As this is impossible naturally, the PCL tends to restrict rollback to 4 mm in 10–45 degrees flexion.

In summary, simultaneous rollback of both femoral condyles does not occur as the knee flexes. The unloaded medial femoral condyle does not move anteroposteriorly with flexion, but the lateral femoral condyle does roll back according to tibial internal rotation. The vast majority of TKA prosthetic surface designs are non-conforming and less congruent in flexion, therefore leading to increased contact stress of the polyethylene. The introduction of additional moveable bearings in TKA allows for motion of the bearings on the tibial plateau following the femoral condyles in flexion and extension. This is logical, as moveable bearings may adapt to a more anatomical situation.

Furthermore, moveable bearings in TKA are a possible solution to the conflict between articulating congruency versus constraint forces acting on the polyethylene, as reported by Buechel et al. (2001), thereby reducing polyethylene wear debris, which is the ultimate reason for late failures. The use of moveable bearings in TKA allows the achievement of articulating congruency without increasing the joint forces at the interface between prosthetic components and bearing. Goodfellow and O'Connor were the first to use the principle of mobile bearings, and did so by introducing a unicompartmental arthroplasty with maximum congruency and low constrained forces. In fixed bearings TKA, this problem is compromised by the use of partial congruency.

Characteristics of the Available Mobile Bearing Arthroplasties

One or Two Mobile Bearings?

Some companies offer two separate meniscal bearings: one for the medial and one for the lateral compartment, i.e. Oxford Modular (Biomet), LCS (DePuy), and Minns (Corin). All other companies provide one rotating bearing for both medial and lateral compartments.

Limited and Unlimited Mobility of Moveable Bearings?

The mobility of bearings can be limited by special set-ups of the tibial plateau. The Oxford TKA is designed with a vertical metal bar at the tibial eminentia, which limits excessive movements of the bearings. Most TKA designs prevent mobility of bearings in one or more directions. The guidance (of bearings) is realized by various elements: (i) straight or bend gauge as part of the tibial plateau acts as a guide for polyethylene bearing components. Mediolateral movements are restricted, whereas anteroposterior movements are possible. Femorotibial rotation (in the longitudinal axis) is achieved by opposite forward and backward movement of the meniscal bearings (LCS, Minns); (ii) partial and peripheral restraining edge for guidance of the polyethylene, i.e. TACK (Link); (iii) rotating platform with a conical or cylindrical peg, which is excavated in the tibial cone, i.e. LCS, INNEX (Sulzer), TRAC (Biomet); (iv) a separate mobile guide arm, which is located in the tibial cone (LCS, INNEX), allows for rotation of the bearing in a horizontal plane and anteroposterior translation (apglide); (v) a mounted and fixed peg on the tibial plateau combined with a cavity in the polyethylene bearing may allow for a 4–5 mm limited rotation and/or anteroposterior translation, i.e. SAL (Sulzer), TRK (Cremascoli), TRI-CCC (SME), Oxford 3c (Biomet), AGC Duo-Articular (Biomet); (vi) two vertical elements that limit both anteroposterior translation and rotation of the bearing are utilized in the Rotaglide (Corin) and MBK (Zimmer). In an asymmetrical array the amount of translation can be increased in the lateral compartment. The Interax (Howmedica) TKA is designed with a limited rotation of 36 degrees, and a curved gouge on the lower surface of the polyethylene bearing combined with an asymmetrical contact surface allows for increased translation of the lateral compartment compared with the medial.

Femorotibial Congruency and Contact Area

The ultimate goals of mobile bearings in TKA are: (1) increased congruency in the full arc of motion in frontal, sagittal, and coronal planes; (2) decreased contact stress of the polyethylene bearing; and (3) decreased constraint forces at the implant–bone interface. In the sagittal plane, a maximum congruency is achieved by a constant radius of the femoral component, i.e. Oxford, Mims, and Rotaglide. The MBK prosthesis contains a combination of two different radii. Most prostheses that are congruent in the sagittal plane (in extension) show a decreased congruency in flexion (LCS, SAL, TRAC). The congruency in the frontal plane is as important as in the sagittal plane, as shown by Bartel.

During daily activities, the forces acting on the normal knee joint are 1.3–1.8 times body weight and during stair climbing or rising from a flexed position up to five times body weight, according to Kuster (1997). The load is distributed over an area of 750–1150 mm². The contact stress of the surfaces in a normal knee joint is less than 5 MPa. Most knee prostheses with fixed bearings have a contact area of 100–300 mm² with a resulting contact stress of up to 60 Mpa; however, the maximal resistance of modern polyethylene is less than 21 MPa. Therefore, the longevity of the polyethylene bearing is significantly reduced if the contact stress exceeds 20 MPa. A contact area of at least 400 mm² from 0 to 60 degrees flexion is required to avoid contact stress of 20 MPa. The contact area can be calculated by the method of finite element analysis or measured with contact stress films. The LCS, SAL, and Rotaglide prostheses have a contact area of 600–700 mm² in extension. The MBK prosthesis has a contact area of 800–1000 mm². Posterior stabilized-type prostheses have an increased contact area due to the central stabilizing peg (TRAC, LCS-PS, TRI-CCC, Rotaglide PS).

Total knee arthroplasties with mobile bearings show an increased contact area and therefore a reduced contact stress (delaminating, link destruction) of the polyethylene. However, contact stress in flexion varies depending on implant geometry, load and both active and passive stability of the knee joint. Reduced contact stress leads to reduced destruction of the polyethylene, particularly in the first 2 mm of the surface (von Mieses stress).

Other important intrinsic and extrinsic parameters that should be considered are: (1) quality and endurance of polyethylene; (2) sterilization technique (gamma irradiated, ethylene oxide, etc.); (3) shelf life of polyethylene (prevention of oxidation and link destruction); (4) consistency and smoothness of metal on polyethylene articulating surfaces; (5) articulating behavior of femorotibial joint in three dimensions under load (lift off, shear forces, peak loads, active and passive stability, etc.).

Bicruciate Retaining, Posterior Stabilized, or Bicruciate Sacrifice Designs?

The LCS and Oxford components can be implanted with retention of both anterior and posterior cruciate ligaments (ACL/PCL). In cases where the anteroposterior stability is not supported or provided by both cruciate ligaments, the stability has to be obtained by the appropriate geometry of the articulating components with or without a posterior-stabilizing peg. The retention of the PCL in TKA alone does not guarantee normal kinematics, even in cases where optimal surgical technique has been carried out. Canton and Goutallier proved that the function and anatomy of the PCL is abnormal when the ACL is absent. A secondary progressive insufficiency of the PCL often leads to clinically relevant ligamentous instability (progressive ligamentous instability, PLI). Alternatively, the missing PCL function may be more or less compensated by the anterior lip of the rotating platform bearing. Another approach can be seen in implants with a central intercondylar polyethylene peg, which prevents posterior movement of the tibia in flexion (posterior stabilized).

Advantages of Mobile Bearing TKA

Mobile bearings, when implanted perfectly, may lead to improved long-term clinical results because of: (1) improved articulating congruency and kinematics; (2) reduced contact stress; (3) reduced constraint forces at the implant–bone interface; and (4) improved patellofemoral tracking due to a more anatomically normal tibial and femoral rotation.

Kinematic Behavior of TKA

The kinematics of the knee joint have been evaluated in vivo in some studies using metal pins for orientation in both the tibia and the femur. A tibial rotation of 8–13 degrees in flexion and extension has been confirmed, although Lafortune was unable to prove an occlusion in full extension. Non-fluoroscopic results of studies that evaluate the kinematics of the replaced knee include cadaver studies, non-weight-bearing radiography, gait analysis, goniometry, and photogrammetry. However, these techniques are static and do not consider muscle forces, weight bearing, or attachment to ligaments.

Studies on Cadaver Knees

Schlepkow compared the kinematics of the LCS meniscal bearing TKA with fixed TKA (Tricon M). The LCS prosthesis demonstrated an automatic rotation in flexion and extension, whereas the Tricon M showed no rotation. Eckhoff analyzed the rotation in flexion of cadaver knees with and without prostheses, looking at the Duracon and AGC prostheses. The cadaver knees presented automatic axial rotation of 9 degrees in flexion and extension, whereas no rotation was observed after both prostheses were inserted.

In Vivo Studies

El Nahass investigated and measured 25 patients with Kinematik II TKA using an electronic goniometer and discovered an automatic rotation of 5–10 degrees in walking, sitting down, getting up, and climbing stairs. Using an electronic goniometer, Terajma was unable to prove rotation during walking. Tarnowski (1998) analyzed the kinematics of the knee joint with the help of an optoelectronic system with four photo cameras and reported an automatic rotation of 4.7 degrees of the normal knee, 2.9 degrees rotation in a TKA case with retained PCL, and 1.5 degrees rotation in a TKA case with a posterior stabilized implant. Nilson investigated LCS and Miller Galante TKA with the use of roentgen stereophotogrammetry and found 0.5 degrees rotation in flexion with the LCS TKA and 3.5 degrees rotation with the Miller Galante TKA. No difference in either rotation or dorsal translation could be detected in comparing the Freeman–Samuelson (fixed bearing) with the Freeman SAL (mobile bearing) TKA. Dennis et al. (1997) analyzed automatic rotation during knee flexion with fluoroscopy and found very variable amounts of rotation. However, anterior translation of the femur in flexion could be detected. Stiehl et al. (1995) investigated LCS TKA cases with a rotating platform under fluoroscopy and measured internal rotation in flexion with a mean of 0.5 degrees in seven patients, no rotation in another five cases, and a maximum of 6.2 degrees external rotation in a further seven cases. Translation of the condyles occurred highly variably. Furthermore,

a decoaptation (lift off) of one compartment could be seen in more than 50 % of the cases, which implicates full load and stress to the opposite compartment.

Parameters Influencing Automatic Rotation

In TKA there are no clinical signs such as asymmetry of the femoral condyles and the tibial plateau, nor are there normal functioning cruciate ligaments with adapting tension during flexion and extension, as they are sacrificed in most TKA. The vast majority of TKA are designed for symmetrical articulating surfaces. Almost all authors sacrifice the ACL and in most cases the PCL. Remaining parameters are the passive tension of the capsulo-ligamentary complex, the active knee muscles, and coordination capability. Gait analysis studies after TKA note a reduced gait speed and gait length, a reduced knee flexion, as well as a reduced amplitude in range of motion. Kramers-de Quervain et al. (1997) studied gait analysis post-bilateral TKA, comparing semiconstrained GSB TKA with fixed bearing versus LCS with mobile bearing. No significant difference was noted.

Behavior of Mobile Bearings In Vivo

Bradly et al. (1987) reported dorsal translation of the Oxford bearings in flexion with 4.4 mm at the lateral side and 6.0 mm at the medial side. Stiehl (1996) demonstrated mobility of the meniscal bearing (LCS) in 50 % of the cases after 54 months. Lemoine discovered a mean mobility of the meniscal bearings of 5 mm (range 0–10 mm) in 35 LCS TKA. Nilson reported only minimal bearing mobility in both LCS and SAL TKA. Other recently reported studies conclude mobility of mobile bearing inserts even 10 years after surgery.

Mobile Bearings and Patellofemoral Tracking

Factors that improve patellofemoral tracking (independent of resurfacing) in the development of TKA include: (1) a more "patella-friendly" anatomical femoral design with an optimum trochlea groove in flexion and extension; (2) soft tissue release procedure for reduction of lateral patellar subluxation or dislocation; (3) rotational positioning of the femoral component parallel to the femorotibial flexion gap, or parallel to the transepicondylar axis; and (4) increased attention to a balanced capsule and ligament situation in both flexion and extension. All these parameters help to minimize patellofemoral problems. Mobile bearings in TKA may be of additional benefit in cases where the tibial plateau has not been implanted in a perfect rotational position; however, meniscal bearings have no influence regarding femoral component malpositioning.

Long-term Outcomes

The introduction of meniscal bearings in TKA allowed for increased congruent components, reduced contact stress at the metal-bearing interface and decreased constraint forces at the bone–implant interface, provided that the mobility of the bearings was minimally limited. Therefore, meniscal bearings appear to have an advantage and theoretically have an increased survivorship. Buechel et al. (2002) reported his personal LCS series in a number of follow-up studies, including an 83% survival rate for meniscal bearings after 16 years, 97.7% for cemented rotating platform, and 98.3% for cementless rotating platform after 18 years. Jordan et al. (1997) reported a 94.6% LCS survival rate after 8 years. Sorrels (2002) described LCS survival of 88% at 14 years. Callaghan (2001) studied 114 cemented LCS knees with 100% survival at 11 years follow-up. The clinical performance of the LCS remains exemplary based on long-term studies. Long-term data over 20 years are only available for the LCS and Oxford systems, with equal or superior results to condylar systems with fixed bearings.

Wear Reduction

Measurement of polyethylene debris in vivo is difficult in practice. Available parameters include linear penetration resulting from cold flow, delaminating, tear, oxidation, and surface rub off. Collier et al. (1991) investigated 122 specimens and found that very congruent systems showed the least changes in the polyethylene compared with less congruent components. Mobile bearing polyethylene components had no delamination or tears. Polyethylene particles are larger in diameter (less critical for particulate synovitis) compared with total hip wear particles. This led to the opinion that wear is less of a problem in TKA, provided that all components are perfectly implanted, with optimal soft tissue balancing.

In TKA with fixed bearings, where less congruent components are used, one can see an increased an-

teroposterior translation regardless of whether or not the PCL is retained. The amount of polyethylene debris is increased even more in cases of additional ligamentous instability. In TKA with mobile bearings, the motion of the femoral condyles is limited to gliding with no anteroposterior translation or rotation, as the latter occurs between the bearings and the polished tibial plateau. However, this theory remains critical, as Stiehl et al. (1995) demonstrated decoaptation (lift off) in fluoroscopic investigations of mobile bearing TKA.

The problem of long-term polyethylene destruction and debris remains, due to adherence and abrasion, particularly since mobile bearings provide two (upper and lower) surfaces compared with fixed bearings. Argenson calculated a polyethylene wear of 0.025 mm/year for the Oxford prosthesis. Berger et al. (1995) found similar wear rates in cases where highly congruent fixed bearings were used. In a comparative study, Cornwall et al. (1998) reported delaminating in 20/28 (71.4%) fixed bearing TKA, compared to 1/7 (14.3%) mobile bearing TKA. In the Schulthess Clinic, 41 out of more than 2,500 mobile bearing TKA were revised as a result of progressive ligamentous instability; they all revealed tears and delaminating of the polyethylene bearings. Another complication that could be specifically related to the ap-glide mobile bearing was impingement and partial necrosis of the Hoffa fat pad. These cases underwent successful excision of fat pad and polyethylene exchange to rotating platform polyethylene.

Specific Complications in Mobile Bearing TKA

Because of the nature of the designs, mobile bearings may cause considerable problems, including: (1) spinout or subluxation of meniscal bearings, both anteroposterior and mediolateral; (2) semi spinout (subluxation) of rotating platform of one compartment, usually posteriorly; (3) impingement of the anterior knee compartment (particularly when the fat pad is not or is only partially excised, or when an ap-glide bearing migrates anteriorly in flexion; (4) possible increased likelihood of PLI development, due to enhanced anteroposterior translation compared with fixed bearings; and (5) decreased mass of polyethylene in meniscal bearings with less than 10 mm height.

In the Schulthess Clinic, there was one mediolateral meniscal bearing subluxation out of 821 (0.12%) and one complete spinout of both meniscal bearings of 1,850 cases (0.12%). Of the 1,862 rotating platform bearing TKA, 11 (0.6%) had subluxation due to PLI or trauma and required revision surgery. In most cases this problem could be solved with an exchange of the mobile bearing. From the 236 ap-glide rotating platform TKA, seven (3.0%) cases complained of anterior knee pain and underwent secondary fat pad excision surgery.

The utilization of mobile bearings in TKA allows for increased overall congruency in both the sagittal and the frontal planes without increased constraint forces and interference with physiological knee joint kinematics. The current designs of mobile bearing TKA follow a common principle but show differences in the (1) absolute size of the congruent surfaces (ranging from 600 to 1,200 mm^2 in extension and a decreased surface at 60–90 degrees of flexion); (2) extent of bearing mobility for rotation and translation; (3) function and design of moveable elements including meniscal bearings, rotating platforms, ap-glide pegs and bars, as well as bearing symmetry; (4) possibility for retention of either ACL, PCL or both; (5) curvature of the articulating tibiofemoral bearing, which may be considerably flat to ultracongruent (deep dish) or posterior stabilized; (6) patellofemoral geometry; (7) posterior slope of the tibial cut; and (8) type of fixation, including cemented and uncemented components with or without additional screws.

The concept of mobile bearing TKA appears to permit close to normal knee joint kinematics; however, its clinical advantages are yet to be proven. Excellent long-term results are reported with follow-ups of up to 10–20 years, but most studies analyzing mobile bearing TKA have not investigated long-term outcomes. Parameters that are influential and beneficial for longevity of the prosthesis in situ include reduced contact stress, decreased constraint forces at the bone–implant interfaces, increased thickness of the polyethylene bearing in rotating platform designs, as well as diminished "von Mieses" forces inside the polyethylene. The existence of two articulating surfaces (femoral condyles and tibial plateau) of the mobile bearing polyethylene does not appear to increase the amount of wear particles. Axial malalignment, both physiological and technical, can be corrected by spontaneous rotation of the bearing, thus reducing polyethylene stress and wear. Increased mobility of the bearing and favorable rotational positioning of the femoral component may also contribute to the improved patellofemoral tracking throughout the full range of motion.

Functional outcome studies carried out at the Schulthess Clinic in Zurich, Switzerland, in which fixed bearing TKA were compared with mobile bearing TKA, demonstrated improved gait pattern in patients with mobile bearing TKA, particularly with regards to the achievement of normal gait velocity. However, additional complications may occur in mobile bearing TKA compared with fixed TKA, such as dislocation, spinout, or fracture of the polyethylene, as well as soft tissue entrapments (i.e. fat pad). Nevertheless, exact operating technique as well as limitation of the bearing mobility may considerably reduce these complications.

Moveable bearings in TKA are a possible solution to the conflict between articulating congruency versus constraint forces acting on the polyethylene, thereby reducing polyethylene wear debris, which is the ultimate reason for late failures. The use of moveable bearings in TKA allows the achievement of articulating congruency without increasing the joint forces at the interface between prosthetic components and bearing. There is clinical and radiographic evidence that mobile bearings are equal or superior to fixed bearings regarding long-term survivorship. Patella resurfacing, particularly metal-backed design, meniscal bearings and PCL-sparing designs seem to jeopardize successful long-term results. ACL and PCL sacrificing rotating platform designs perform best, with 90% plus survivorship at 20 years.

In conclusion, the use of mobile bearings appears to provide advantages compared with fixed bearing devices. Long-term success of their implementation has been proven in numerous excellent studies.

Bibliography

Banks SA, Markovich GD, Hodge WA (1997) In vivo kinematics of cruciate retaining and substituting knee arthroplasties. J Arthroplasty 12:297–304

Berger RA, Seel MJ, Crossett LS, Rubash HE (1995) The role of component malrotation in tibial polyethylene wear and failure after TKA. Orthop Trans 19:527

Bizzini M, Boldt J, Munzinger U, Drobny T (2003) Rehabilitation guidelines after total knee arthroplasty. Orthopade 32(6):527–534

Boldt JG, Munzinger UK, Zanetti M, Hodler J (2004) Arthrofibrosis associated with total knee arthroplasty: gray-scale and power Doppler sonographic findings. AJR Am J Roentgenol 182(2):337–340

Boldt J, Munzinger U, Keblish P (2004) Comparison of isokinetic strength in resurfaced and retained patellae in bilateral TKA. J Arthroplasty 19(2):264

Bourne RB, Whitewood CN (2002) The role of rotating platform total knee replacements: design considerations, kinematics, and clinical results. J Knee Surg 15:247–253

Bourne RB, Masonis J, Anthony M (2003) An analysis of rotating-platform total knee replacements. Clin Orthop 410:173–180

Bradly J, Goodfellow JW, Oconnor J (1987) Radiographic study of bearing movement in unicompartmental Oxford knee replacement. JBJS 69B:598–601

Buechel FF Sr (2002) Long-term followup after mobile-bearing total knee replacement. Clin Orthop 404:40–50

Buechel FF (2003) Recurrent LCS rotating platform dislocation in revision total knee replacement: mechanism, management, and report of two cases. Orthopedics 26:647–649

Buechel FF Sr, Buechel FF Jr, Pappas MJ, D'Alessio J (2001) Twenty-year evaluation of meniscal bearing and rotating platform knee replacements. Clin Orthop 388:41–50

Buechel FF Sr, Buechel FF Jr, Pappas MJ, Dalessio J (2002) Twenty-year evaluation of the New Jersey LCS Rotating Platform Knee Replacement. J Knee Surg 15:84–89

Buechel FF Sr, Buechel FF Jr, Pappas MJ (2003) Ten-year evaluation of cementless Buechel-Pappas meniscal bearing total ankle replacement. Foot Ankle Int 24:462–472

Callaghan JJ (2001) Mobile-bearing knee replacement: clinical results: a review of the literature. Clin Orthop 392:221–225

Collier JP, Major MB, McNamara JL, Surprenant JA, Jensen RE (1991) Analysis of the failure of 122 polyethylene inserts from uncemented tibial components. Clin Orthop 273:232–242

Cornwall GB, Rudan J, Bryant JT, Deluzio KJ, Simurda MA, Sorbie C (1998) The distribution of surface degradation mechanisms in TKA. A comparison of fixed bearings versus mobile bearing designs. JBJS 80B [Suppl]:I-37

Dennis DA, Komistek RD, Walker SA, Anderson DT (1997) In vivo analysis of tibiofemoral rotation: does screw home rotation occur after TKA? Trans Orthop Res Soc 23:386

Dorr LD (2002) Contrary view: wear is not an issue. Clin Orthop 404:96–99

Gill GS, Joshi AB, Mills DM (1999) Total condylar knee arthroplasty. 16- to 21-year results. Clin Orthop 367:210–215

Jordan LR, Olivio JL, Voorhoorst PE (1997) Survival analysis of cementless meniscal bearing total knee arthroplasty. Clin Orthop 338:119–123

Jordan LR, Dowd JE, Olivo JL, Voorhorst PE (2002) The clinical history of mobile-bearing patella components in total knee arthroplasty. Orthopedics 25 [Suppl 2]:s247–s250

Kijm H, Pelker PR, Lynch JK, Gibson DH, Irving JF (1995) Radiographic analysis of the "rollback" phenomenon in posterior cruciate retaining total knee arthroplasty. AAOS 19:1170

Kramers-de Quervain IA, Stüssi E, Müller R, Drobny T, Munzinger U, Gschwend N (1997) Quantitative gait analysis after bi-lateral TKA with two different systems within each subject. J Arthroplasty 12:168–179

Kuster MS, Wood GA, Stachowiak GW, Gächter A (1997) Joint load considerations in total knee replacement. JBJS 79B: 109–113

Moilanen T, Freemann MAR (1995) The case for resection of the posterior cruciate ligament. J Arthroplasty 10:564–567

Poilvache PL, Insall JN, Scuderi GR, Font-Rodriguez DE (1996) Rotational landmarks and sizing of the distal femur in total knee arthroplasty. Clin Orthop 331:35–46

Polyzoides AJ (1996) The Rotaglide total knee arthroplasty. Prosthesis, design and early results. J Arthroplasty 11:453–459

Price AJ, Rees JL, Beard D, Juszczak E, Carter S, White S, de Steiger R, Dodd CA, Gibbons M, McLardy-Smith P, Goodfellow JW, Murray DW (2003) A mobile-bearing total knee prosthesis compared with a fixed-bearing prosthesis. A multicentre single-blind randomised controlled trial. J Bone Joint Surg Br 85:62–67

Ranawat CS (2002) History of total knee replacement. J South Orthop Assoc 11:218–226

Rand JA, Trousdale RT, Ilstrup DM, Harmsen WS (2003) Factors affecting the durability of primary total knee prostheses. J Bone Joint Surg Am 85A:259–265

Sathavisan S, Walker PS (1998) Optimisation of meniscal knee design to eliminate the stresses which cause delamination wear. JBJS 80B [Suppl I]:37

Schunck J, Jerosch J (2003) Knee arthroplasty. Mobile- and fixed-bearing design. Orthopade 32:477–483

Sorrells RB (2002) The clinical history and development of the low contact stress total knee arthroplasty. Orthopedics 25 [Suppl 2]:s207–s212

Stiehl JB (1996) Comparison of long-term results with cruciate substituting or sparing mobile bearing cementless total knee arthroplasty. Orthop Trans 20:928

Stiehl JB, Abbott B (1995) A morphological analysis of the transepicondylar axis and the relationship of the mechanical axis of the leg. J Arthroplasty 10:785–789

Stiel JB, Cheverny PM (1996) Femoral rotational alignment using the tibial shaft axis in total knee arthroplasty. Clin Orthop 331:47–55

Stiehl JB, Komistek RD, Dennis DA, Paxson RD, Hoff WA (1995) Fluoroscopic analysis of kinematics after posterior cruciate retaining arthroplasty. JBJS 77B:884–889

Tarnowski LE, Andriacchi TP, Berger RA, Galante JO, Rosenberg AG (1998) Three dimensional motion of cruciate retaining and cruciate stabilized knees during walking. Trans Orthop Res Soc 23:804

Vertullo CJ, Easley ME, Scott WN, Insall JN (2001) Mobile bearings in primary knee arthroplasty. J Am Acad Orthop Surg 9:355–364

Wasielewski RC (2002) The causes of insert backside wear in total knee arthroplasty. Clin Orthop 404:232–246

1.4 Developing a Mobile Bearing Knee Prosthesis

Bernhard G. Gyssler

This chapter describes the development of the IN-NEX knee system, focusing on design and engineering aspects. Common instrumentation should be available for indications from intact posterior cruciate ligament (PCL) to collateral instability. In the late 1980s and early 1990s, the biomechanical direction came primarily from surgeon authors, orthopedic consultants and university institutes, and finally, in 1993, from A. Bähler, U. Munzinger, T. Drobny, H. Frei, and the knee engineering group at Sulzer Medical Technology. From prototypes to serial production was a long journey, involving materials, manufacturing, testing, inspection, purchasing and planning specialists.

Schulthess Clinic Specification

The Schulthess Clinic knee specification has the following requirements.

Design requirements: (1) mobile bearing knee with better kinematics than low contact stress; (2) modular capabilities, but manageable scope (size and diversity); (3) anatomical patellar flange for the natural non-replaced patella, with good tracking, but also without overstraining the patella; (4) asymmetric (anatomical) femoral component design to replicate the kinematics, including the lever arm of the quadriceps muscle group; (5) tibial component suitable for asymmetric loading. Material requirements: ultra-high molecular weight polyethylene (UHMWPE) or better, with good resistance to loading. Fixation: cementless and cementing. Stabilization: (1) simple, stems, ribs, fins; (2) femoral component with modular stem for revisions; (3) tibial component with short central stem, conical in shape to compress the spongy cancellous bone and with lateral wings or four short peripheral pegs, possibly a double cone; (4) surface structure for biological fixation, such as porous coating, Sulmesh, hydroxyapatite (HA) coating. Sizing: five sizes of femoral components, at least five sizes of tibial components, which could be combined freely. Instrumentation and surgical procedure: user friendly, as simple as possible (Sects. 4.1, 4.2).

These requirements led to development of a modular mobile bearing knee system covering three basic indications: (1) intact PCL, cruciate retaining (CR), type I; (2) insufficient PCL, posterior sacrificing (PS), type II; (3) loss of collateral stability, semiconstrained (SC), type III.

This required a common femoral component for modular augments, a stabilizing box to convert a type I femoral component into a type II or III femoral component, mobile bearings for each of the three types, guide pins for all three types, a tibial plateau for all three types, anchoring stems and spacers for bone defects. With monobloc femoral design, the medial and lateral mobile condyles are equidistant and in the same relative position to one another. Furthermore, anteroposterior translation as well as rotation was desired. The CR post has a curved shape to reduced medial translation, with an increased lateral translation. This corresponds to the kinematics of the physiological knee.

The femoral component and mobile bearings were based on spherical condyles, to ensure conforming congruity throughout the range of motion (Figs. 1.22, 1.23). Beyond 20 degrees of flexion, all femoral designs have an approximated circle shape in common. Sagittal plane kinematics of a knee joint can be broken down into a combination of rotation and translation, whereby the two types of motion are split onto two joint levels by the menisci. Kinematics are not determined by joint shape, but are controlled by soft tissues (Wright).

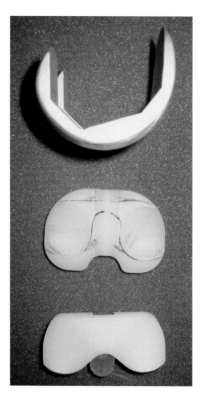

Fig. 1.22. Femoral and mobile condyles with spherical profile

When describing the relative femorotibial motion without translation, the femur is rotating and on the tibia with a fixed pivot center. Similarly, the contact point between femur and tibia condyles remains stationary, assuming the condyle is perfectly spherical and concentric. If this is not the case, the contact point can move, despite a fixed pivot remaining. A change in radius can effect a large shift in the point of contact without translation. These features were the basis for the design of this new device.

A study by Engelbrecht (1984) showed that the posterior femoral condyle outlines are very similar, independent of femoral size. The concentration of the tangents at the points of contact at 0 and 90 degrees flexion are highest, especially the medial condyle. Since the roll-to-slide ratio in the first 20 degrees of flexion is about 1:2, Mueller (1982) concluded that the center of the rotation, independent of radius, experiences practically no translation. This also explains why hinged prostheses function well, provided the center of rotation has been wisely chosen.

The large distance from the femorotibial point of contact to the femoral tangent at the patellar ligament indicated an increased anterior femoral radius of approximately 20 degrees of flexion. To assess the

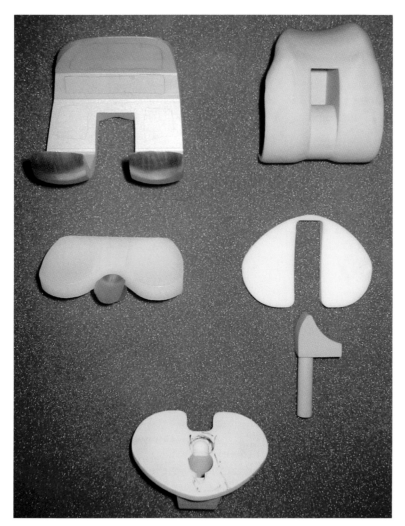

Fig. 1.23. First models of type I and II femoral components

merits of the different femoral sagittal profiles, the rectangular transformation method was applied. Based on the point-of-contact data from the literature, a theoretical femur was flexed through its range of motion; four points, arranged in a rectangle, were observed at intervals of 30 degrees and their paths plotted. This was considered to be the ideal knee. Different femoral sagittal profiles were positioned on mobile bearing condylar forms at intervals of 30 degrees flexion and new positions of the four points plotted. Finally, a curve was drawn through the sequence of points. Some profiles showed jagged paths. The best-fit sagittal profile was selected and models were created by a computer-aided designer. Femoral size M and tibial size 3 were elected. The mobile bearing inserts had to conform with the femoral components and be available in different thicknesses. A 6 degrees slope was built into the tibial alignment instrumentation and in the femoral distal cut. The optimal tibial component contour was determined on various radiographs to ensure sufficient cortical support. Designs of the femoral box and SC guide pin are related to the GSB constrained knee.

Manufacturing

Cobalt chrome (CoCr) castings were chosen for the femoral and tibial components, since implant components require good stiffness at the interface to the cement/bone. Wrought-forged CoCr guide pins were the adapted technology from hip metal couplings, while oxygen-less packaged UHMWPE was the state-of-the-art material for the mobile bearings. The mobile bearing upper surface of the tibial component required a low roughness and a near-perfect flatness. The tibial components are lapped to high specifications. Femoral component articulating surfaces are profile ground and polished to a low roughness and high profile accuracy.

INNEX Cruciate Retaining

INNEX CR is designed for primary PCL retention and anterior cruciate ligament sacrifice, no varus/valgus constraints, and allows for free axial rotation and anteroposterior translation. Sufficient anterior and posterior design of the mobile bearing inserts limits tibiofemoral dislocation.

INNEX Posterior Stabilized

The PS is designed for bicruciate sacrifice with a cam-post mechanism. The prosthesis has no varus/valgus constraints, allows free axial rotation and limited anteroposterior translation. It requires a larger number of instruments.

Preclinical Testing

The PS has a stable metal-on-metal post in the tibial cam, with proximal engagement and without polyethylene wear. The post made of wrought-forged CoCr showed little wear effect and higher "self-polishing" after 3 million cycles (Stallforth Ungethüm knee testing machine and Stanmore knee simulator). Both the PS femoral and the PS tibial component underwent dynamically loaded physiological tests set up with modular stems. Test results were good for the tibial and femoral components without modular stem attached, but not with stems. This led to a change of PS modularity and SC box designs, and required a stronger tibia post.

Physiological femoral and tibial components were tested with 4,000 Newton sinusoidal loads against a restraining force on the patellar groove, the femoral condyles, as well as unsupported medial and tibial plateaus. The femoral stem was tested utilizing the SC femoral with the stiffest stems and largest offset under 2,500 Newton sinusoidal load at a slightly flexed position and 5 degrees varus position. Finite element analysis (FEA) was used to assess areas of excessive stress. On the tibial component, both FEA and physiological testing showed a particular design challenge of all tibial components, particularly the PCR version, which requires well-rounded corners to reduce stresses.

Further mechanical tests assess the risk of dislocation. These were carried out by Seth Greenwald at Mount Sinai Laboratory, Columbus, Ohio, and in-house. For contact pressure, Fuji film tests were performed. Other investigations included taper, material, impaction, and pull-out tests.

Clinical Studies

In 1996, the first knee component was implanted. Initial experience highlighted that instrumentation was a crucial factor, as was implant refinements (sharp corners) and bone sparing. The conical-shaped PS box made it more difficult to prepare the femur. An open proximal box offered particulate access. Instruments are modular and dedicated.

Cementless Fixation

The INNEX Total Knee System offers both cemented and cementless implant options. Previous surface finishing included titanium mesh, CoCr mesh, full titanium components, titanium coating, HA coating, cancellous structured titanium (CSTi), and plasma spray process (Sulzer Metco). Most interfaces demonstrated ingrowth potential. CSTi worked with the Natural Knee (Intermedics Orthopedics Inc., Allopro) allows for porous coating and bone paste, and was chosen for INNEX. CSTi is "welded" onto CoCr components and fills cement pockets, so that the same casting can be used for cemented and cementless versions. A multicenter clinical study investigated femoral components for hybrid use and other practical issues, including fat pad impingement, manufacturing changes from peeling to milling mobile bearings, and different casting heat treatment.

Patellar Component

The INNEX is designed for patella resurfacing or retaining and represents a cemented congruent dome-shaped UHMWPE button. It is well stabilized by the lateral anterior condyle of the femoral flange and comes in four sizes.

INNEX Ultracongruent Only Rotating

Clinical experiences demonstrated that ultracongruent offers similar stability to the PS design, with the advantages of less bone removal and fewer instrumentation steps. The INNEX CR and ultracongruent only rotating (UCOR) are the devices preferred by most surgeons in Europe (Figs. 1.24, 1.25). The rotating platform has a metal pin fitted into the tibial component, allowing for free rotation without translation.

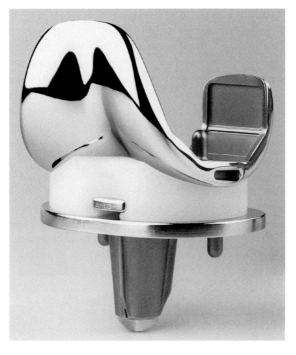

Fig. 1.24. INNEX CR

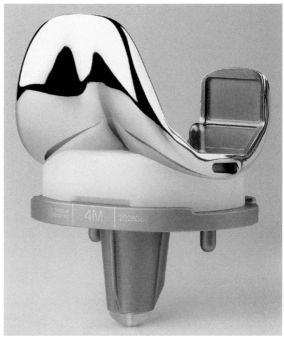

Fig. 1.26. INNEX Fix CR

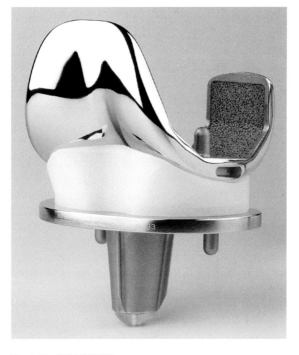

Fig. 1.25. INNEX UCOR

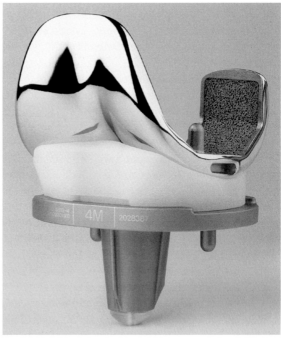

Fig. 1.27. INNEX Fix UC

Fig. 1.28. INNEX SC, tibial offset stems and angled femoral stem

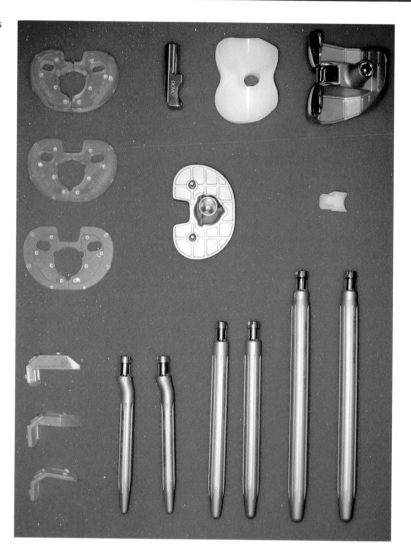

INNEX Fix

In 1998, Allopro decided to merge INNEX and Allo-flex (N. Böhler, Linz and W. Schwägerl, Vienna) into INNEX Fix, keeping the shape of both femoral and tibial components, but with an increased tibial component sizing option (11 instead of 8) (Figs. 1.26, 1.27).

INNEX SC

The indication for INNEX SC is a joint with insufficient collateral stability, missing collateral ligaments, severe varus/valgus misalignment, or bone defects. A standard SC prosthesis is always implanted with stems and is interchangeable with other INNEX implants (Fig. 1.28). In the SC system, a large guide pin enables the prosthesis to resist varus/valgus forces. In extension, the femoral condyles are positioned concentrically in the inlay and the congruence offers resistance to rotation with the femur moving posteriorly in flexion. Since the guide pin can rotate and the radii are no longer congruent in flexion, a limited amount of rotation is possible.

Continuing Development and Product Support

Cross-linked polyethylenes (Durasul) show improved wear patterns in vitro and are currently in development for the UCOR model. The INNEX knee system contains about 220 implants and 280 instruments, representing modularity, compatibility, custom prostheses, and computer-aided surgery. Midterm results are reported in Sect. 3.6.

Acknowledgements. I thank André Bähler, Heribert Frei, Dr U. Munzinger, Dr T. Drobny, Prof. N. Böhler and Prof. W. Schwägerl.

1.5 Metal Alloys and Polyethylenes

M. Windler

Knee prostheses are manufactured from different materials, including CoCrMo alloys, titanium alloys and ultra-high molecular weight polyethylene with or without cross-linking. The metal alloys can be formed by means of precision casting or forging. Compression-moulded polyethylenes are commonly used for tibial bearings. The final shape of the metals and the polyethylene is obtained through machining or, if necessary, by means of grinding, grit blasting or other surfacing techniques. These processing stages have a considerable influence on the properties (strength, wear, aging) of individual prosthetic components. Polyethylene components that have been gamma sterilized under atmospheric oxygen or that have rested on the shelf are subject to aging. The oxygen diffuses into the surface of these components and makes it brittle. Under mechanical load, this leads to cracks and surface delaminations. Since the material suffers less damage when it is sterilized in a nitrogen atmosphere, this process is now regarded as "state of the art" with conventional polyethylene.

For some years, there have been reports on so-called highly cross-linked polyethylenes. The chain structure of the polyethylene can be cross-linked by means of different processes: gamma irradiation, electron beams, or a melting process. In vitro experiments show that the material only ages to a minimum degree and is very resistant to wear. However, long-term clinical results of this new generation of polyethylene are not yet available.

Metallic Materials

Metal alloys such as titanium and/or CoCrMo alloys are preferred for knee endoprostheses. Ti-6Al-4 V and Ti-6Al-7Nb alloys are the most commonly utilized titanium alloys for orthopedic applications. Due to its poor mechanical properties, pure titanium is not considered suitable as a construction material, but is employed for surface structures (osseointegration). With the CoCrMo alloys, we have to differentiate between three types in which chemical compositions are almost identical, but mechanical and tribological properties differ to a major extent.

CoCrMo Casting Alloys

The CoCrMo casting alloys are utilized for femoral and tibial components. The components are manufactured according to the precision investment casting process. The expandable patterns are made from wax and surrounded with a ceramic mass. The wax pattern is melted and molten metal is then poured into the empty ceramic shell. This process is employed primarily for the manufacture of geometrically complicated components. Efforts are made to improve the mechanical properties of the cast blanks by means of downstream process-engineering methods: hot isostatic pressing process to heat seal possible closed porosities or heat treatments to homogenize the crystal structure.

The improvements are difficult to verify scientifically; because of normal variation in mechanical properties between casting charges, they are mostly greater than the improvement obtained after treatment. The raw castings are inspected by radiography to determine internal defects (cavities), and liquid penetration inspection is used to detect surface defects such as cracks. Due to the carbon content of

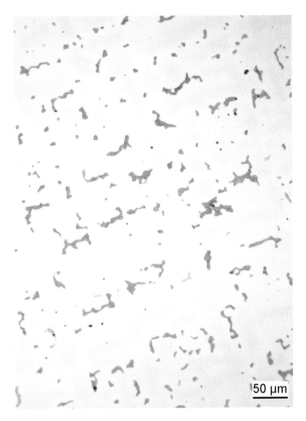

Fig. 1.29. Microstructure of CoCrMo casting alloy with large grain sizes and carbides

about 0.2%, the microstructure of the CoCrMo casting alloy is primarily carbide precipitations, which are embedded in a coarse-grained, austenitic matrix structure. These carbide precipitations are responsible for the excellent wear resistance of CoCrMo casting alloy (Fig. 1.29).

CoCrMo Wrought Alloys

Components are made directly from this alloy type by means of machining, or it serves as parent material for thermomechanical forming (forging). A distinction should be made between "low" and "high" carbon material, although the mechanical properties are similar (Table 1.2). The high carbon material is preferred for tribological applications, e.g. for metal-on-metal coupling (METASUL) for hip endoprostheses because of wear resistance. Except in cases of an annealed condition (Table 1.3), the mechanical properties of this alloy type are approximately twice those of CoCrMo casting alloy (Figs. 1.30, 1.31).

Titanium Alloys

Titanium alloys differ between pure titanium and technical alloys. Because of its poor mechanical properties, pure titanium is not recommended as a material for knee prostheses. However, surface structures to promote osseointegration can be made from pure titanium (Tables 1.4 and 1.5).

Ti-6Al-4 V and Ti-6Al-7Nb Alloys

Among technically known titanium alloys, the Ti-6Al-4 V and, since 1985, the Ti-6Al-7Nb alloys have been used for knee prostheses (Fig. 1.32). Vanadium was replaced with niobium to eliminate the possible toxic effect of soluble vanadium alloying elements and thus improve biocompatibility. Although there have been reports that soluble vanadium alloying elements exhibit toxic effects, no toxic reactions after use of Ti-6Al-4 V alloy have been reported so far. Ti-6Al-4 V alloy has been used clinically for more

Table 1.2. Chemical composition of CoCrMo alloys

Element	CoCrMo casting alloy ISO 5832-4	CoCrMo wrought alloy ISO 5832-12
Carbon	Max. 0.35%	Max. 0.35%[a]
Chromium	26.5–30.0%	26.0–30.0%
Molybdenum	4.5–7.0%	5.0–7.0%
Iron	Max. 1.0%	Max. 0.75%
Manganese	Max. 1.0%	Max. 1.0%
Nickel	Max. 1.0%	Max. 1.0%
Silicone	Max. 1.0%	Max. 1.0%
Nitrogen	Not specified	Max. 0.25%
Cobalt	Balance	Balance

[a] Low carbon CoCrMo: C 0.05–0.08%; high carbon CoCrMo: 0.2–0.25%

Table 1.3. Mechanical properties of CoCrMo alloys

Condition	Standard	Yield strength (MPa)	Tensile strength (MPa)	Elongation at break (%)	Fatigue strength (MPa)
Casting	ISO 5832-4	Min. 450	Min. 665	Min. 8	300
Wrought, annealed	ISO 5832-12	Min. 550	Min. 750	Min. 16	NA
Wrought, forged	ISO 5832-12	Min. 827	Min. 1172	Min. 12	600

NA not analyzed

Fig. 1.30. Microstructure of a low carbon CoCrMo wrought alloy with no carbides, mode differential interference contrast

Fig. 1.31. Microstructure of a high carbon CoCrMo wrought alloy with fine carbide distribution, mode differential interference contrast

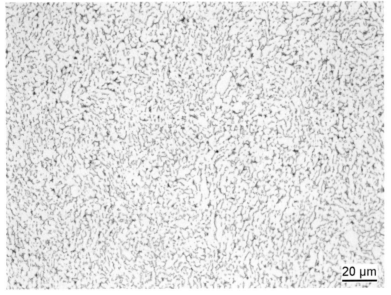

Fig. 1.32. Microstructure of Ti-6Al-7Nb wrought alloy with globular a+b structure

Table 1.4. Chemical composition of titanium alloys

Element	Ti-6Al-4 V alloy ISO 5832-3	Ti-6Al-7Nb alloy ISO 5832-11
Aluminium	5.5–6.75%	5.5–6.5%
Vanadium	3.5–4.5%	Not specified
Niobium	Not specified	6.5–7.5%
Tantalum	Not specified	Max. 0.5%
Iron	Max. 0.3%	Max. 0.25%
Oxygen	Max. 0.2%	Max. 0.2%
Carbon	Max. 0.08%	Max. 0.08%
Nitrogen	Max. 0.05%	Max. 0.05%
Hydrogen	0.015%	Max. 0.009%
Titanium	Balance	Balance

Table 1.6. Fatigue strength of Ti-6Al-7Nb alloy at 10 million cycles, load ratio R=−1.0, in air (95% failure probability and 50% confidence)

Condition	Fatigue strength (Mpa)
Forged and polished	600
Forged and grit-blasted R_a=1–2 μm	550
Forged and corundum-grit blasted R_a=4–6 μm	450
Forged and Tribosul-ODH and polished	340
Wrought and CSTi-coated	200
Wrought and laser-marked	190
Wrought and laser-marked (optimized)	450

Table 1.5. Mechanical properties of titanium alloys

Condition	Standard	Yield strength (MPa)	Tensile strength (MPa)	Elongation at break (%)	Fatigue strength (MPa)
Ti-6Al-4 V, wrought	ISO 5832-3	Min. 780	Min. 860	Min. 10	550
Ti-6Al-7Nb, wrought	ISO 5832-11	Min. 800	Min. 900	Min. 10	550

than three decades. The fatigue strength of titanium alloys is affected by manufacturing conditions, microstructures, and surface conditions. Table 1.6 shows the fatigue strengths of the alloy Ti-6Al-7Nb in rotating bending stress after different final treatments (thermomechanical and surface finish). These values originate from in-house tests with up to 10 million cycles and R = −1.0 load ratio. Applications in knee prostheses include: femoral components with surface treatment, tibial metal-backed implants, and stems.

Untreated titanium or titanium alloys are unsuitable for articulation with polyethylene because of their poor tribological properties. Different techniques are emphasized to improve these poor tribological characteristics: diffusion hardening with nitrogen or oxygen ions (disadvantage: decreased fatigue limit), ion implantation (disadvantage: maximum penetration depth 0.5 m), and hard coating techniques (disadvantage: insufficient adhesive strengths in the presence of wear particles).

CSTi Surface Application

This coating is pure titanium powder mixed with a polymer pore-former and filled into prepared implant pockets (Fig. 1.33). Sintering is conducted under vacuum to protect the titanium against oxidation, a process during which titanium particles combine with one another and the base material (CoCrMo casting or titanium alloy). The pore size of CSTi surfaces (Sulzer Orthopedics, Austin, TX, USA) is 500 micrometers, with a porosity volume of 55%. Bloebaum et al. (1997) reported an average appositional bone index of 73% on eight tibial components analyzed post-mortem, with an in-situ time from 3 to 84 months.

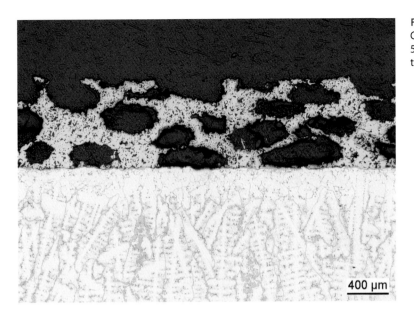

400 µm

Fig. 1.33. Cross-section of a sintered CSTi porous coating, average pore size 500 µm and porosity volume 55%. Matrix CoCrMo casting alloy

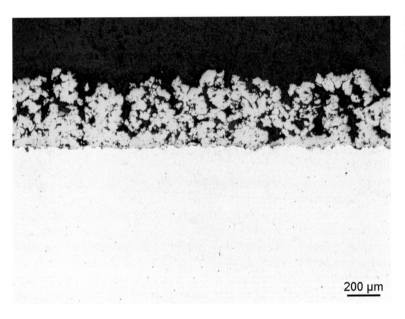

200 µm

Fig. 1.34. Cross-section of a vacuum plasma-sprayed titanium coating with a pore size of up to 100 µm. Matrix CoCr wrought alloy

Plasma Spraying

Prosthetic surfaces are plasma sprayed with titanium under vacuum to enhance osseointegration. The current state of the art is to spray pure titanium powder, which is then fused by the plasma flame and applied to the substrate surface at high speed. The individual particles adhere mechanically to the surface, which is usually grit-blasted beforehand. The large number of adjustable parameters make it possible to produce coatings with variations in thickness and porosity. The coating thickness varies from 200 to 500 micrometers, the pore size from 20 to 200 micrometers and the porosity volume from 15 to 40% (Fig. 1.34).

Polymers and Polyethylene

Since the introduction of polyethylene in orthopedics at the beginning of the 1960s, this material has prevailed as the articulation partner for hip and knee prostheses. Although international standards exist (ISO 5834-1 and -2), various qualities of polyethylene are available. Most commonly known are sheets manufactured in the so-called direct compression moulding process. Polyethylene is a semi-crystalline plastic with amorphous and crystalline regions. All unfinished products have a crystallinity of about 55–60%. The most common sterilization method for polyethylene components employs gamma rays from a cobalt

Fig. 1.35. Cross-section of a polyethylene tibial component, which had been shelf stored for 10 years and gamma sterilized in air. Oxidation maximum is about 1 mm below the surface

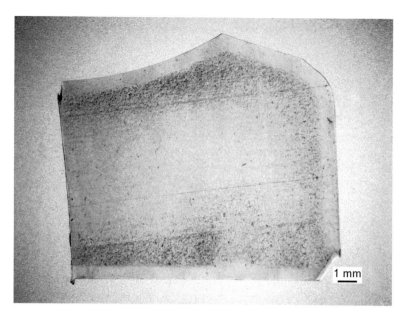

1 mm

source with a dosage range of 25–40 kGy. Due to high energy introduced by the radiation, free radicals are produced within the polyethylene, leading to molecular chain breaks, a process known to cause further chemical reactions (aging). An inert atmosphere must be ensured for protecting radiation-activated polyethylene components during further storage (shelf life). An inert gas, a vacuum, or a process that chemically binds oxygen in the packaging (O_2-less), can be used as an alternative to nitrogen.

Aging

The physical, mechanical and chemical properties of polyethylene change with time. This aging behavior is described as oxidative degradation, and occurs from outside-in. Numerous studies have shown that free radicals dominate, leading to oxidation of the material when gamma sterilization in air is utilized. Remaining molecular fragments in low cross-linking of polymer chains is the dominating factor in a pure nitrogen atmosphere, significantly depressing oxidation effects. Polyethylene sterilized in air ages immediately after being sterilized in packages. Air oxygen diffuses into the polyethylene and reacts with free radicals. Blood also delivers oxygen, which can age gamma-sterilized polyethylene inside a joint. Oxidative degradation causes mechanical properties at the surface (0.5–2 mm below the surface) to deteriorate. These changes, known as "white bands", can be seen in polished microtomed wafers (Fig. 1.35) made from explanted acetabular cups and tibial components. An

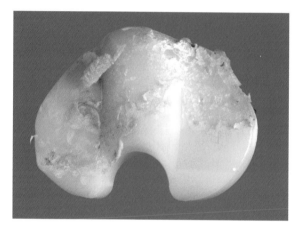

Fig. 1.36. Delaminated polyethylene tibial component after 1.5 years in vivo, which had been gamma sterilized in air

additional factor is mechanical loading resulting from normal articulation, which induces maximal stress peaks just below the surface. The superposition of these two processes – mechanical loading and degradation – causes detachment of polyethylene surface layers. Such delaminations are often lightly yellow-coloured, exhibiting additional cracks in the articulation surface and are frayed at the edge (Fig. 1.36). Sulzer Orthopedics Ltd (Winterthur, Switzerland) introduced gamma sterilization in a nitrogen atmosphere in 1991 with SULENE polyethylene for tibial components (GUR1020, compression moulding, $-N_2$). Alternative methods of sterilization such as ethylene oxide (EtO) were introduced later in orthopedics. This method does not change the polyethylene structure; however, EtO gas is toxic and all components need to be degassed afterwards.

Highly Cross-Linked Polyethylenes

Polyethylene chains can be cross-linked by high-energy gamma or electron irradiations. The process of inducing breaks in polyethylene chains followed by chemical reactions of free radicals has already been described. Damaging long-term effects of oxidation can be prevented via additional heat treatment after irradiation. Laboratory tests of these new materials were conducted exclusively with hip prostheses some 5 years ago. Wear resistance increased significantly with this process. Oonishi et al. (1998) reported positive clinical tribological experiences with polyethylene cups irradiated with 100 Mrad. The linear wear rate, articulating against either a metal or alumina head, was 0.04 mm per year, which is six-fold less than with conventional polyethylenes. Likewise, Wroblewski et al. (1999) reported very low clinical linear wear rates of 0.022 mm/year for cross-linked polyethylene (Marathon, DePuy, Warsaw, USA) in combination with a 22.2 mm diameter alumina head.

In collaboration with the Massachusetts General Hospital and the Massachusetts Institute of Technology, a highly cross-linked polyethylene (DURASUL, Sulzer Orthopedics) was developed. These components are sterilized with EtO and wear tests with 5 million cycles were performed with an AMTI knee simulator (Advanced Mechanical Technology Inc.), showing articulation surfaces with scratches but no gravimetric wear (NK II knee prosthesis). Control components (O_2-less/aged), however, exhibited distinct signs of wear and also showed damage such as "pitting", subsurface cracks and delaminations after 1 million cycles. Hip prostheses wear spherically in comparison to knee prostheses (translational, impact), which makes highly cross-linked polyethylene more suitable for hip than for knee prostheses. In addition, wear is less important in total knee arthroplasty than in total hip arthroplasty. However, long-term clinical studies are needed to prove the superiority of highly cross-linked polyethylene.

Bibliography

Bloebaum RD et al (1997) Post-mortem analysis of consecutively retrieved asymmetric porous-coated tibial components. J Arthroplasty 12:920–929

Blunn GW et al (1991) The dominance of cyclic sliding in producing wear in total knee replacements. Clin Orthop 253–260

Buchanan RA et al (1987) Ion implantation of surgical Ti-6Al-4 V for improved resistance to wear-accelerated corrosion. J Biomed Mater Res 21:355–366

Costa L et al (1998) Oxidation in orthopaedic UHMWPE sterilized by gamma-radiation and ethylene oxide. Biomaterials 19:659–668

Dobbs HS et al (1983) Heat treatment of cast Co-Cr-Mo for orthopaedic implant use. J Mat Sci 18:391–401

Goldman M et al (1998) The influence of sterilization technique and ageing on the structure and morphology of medical-grade ultrahigh molecular weight polyethylene. J Mat Sci Mat Med 207–212

Gomez-Barrena E et al (1998) Role of polyethylene oxidation and consolidation defects in cup performance. Clin Orthop 105–117

Imam MA et al (1996) Titanium alloys as implant materials. In: Browns SA, Lemons JE (eds) Medical application of titanium and its alloy. ASTM STP 1272. American Society for Testing Materials, pp 3–16

Kral MV et al (1993) Erosion resistance of diamond coatings. Wear 166:7–16

Kurtz SM et al (1999) Advances in the processing, sterilization, and cross-linkage of ultra-high molecular weight polyethylene for total joint arthroplasty. Biomaterials 20:1659–1688

Muratoglu OK et al (1999) Unified wear model for highly cross-linked ultra-high molecular weight polyethylenes (UHMWPE). Biomaterials 20:1463–1470

Muratoglu OK et al (2001) Markedly improved adhesive wear and delamination resistance with a high cross-linked UHMWPE for use in total knee arthoplasty, 47th annual meeting ORS San Francisco, California, p 1009

Oonishi H et al (1998) Retrieved total hip prostheses, part I. The effect of cup thickness, head size and fusion defects on wear. J Mat Sci Mat Med 9:393–401

Rieker CB et al (1998) Clinical wear performance of metal-on-metal hip arthroplasties. In: Jacobs JJ, Craig TL (eds) Total joint replacement. ASTM STP 1346. American Society for Testing Materials, pp 144–156

Semlitsch M et al (1986) Development of a vital, high-strength titanium-aluminium-niobium alloy for surgical implants. In: Christel P, Meunier A, Lee AJC (eds) Biological and biomechanical performance of biomaterials. Elsevier, Amsterdam, pp 69–74

Semlitsch M et al (1995) 15 years' experience with the Ti-6Al-7Nb alloy for joint prostheses (15 Jahre Erfahrung mit Ti-6AL-7Nb-Legierung für Gelenkprothesen). Biomed Technik (Berlin) 40:347–355

Simmons CA et al (1999) Osseointegration of sintered porous-surfaced and plasma spray-coated implants: an animal model study of early post implantation healing response and mechanical stability. J Biomed Mat Res 47:127–138

Streicher RM et al (1996) Metal-on metal articulation for artificial hip joints: laboratory study and clinical results. Proc Inst Mech Eng 210:223–232

Wroblewski BM et al (1999) Low-friction arthroplasty of the hip using alumina ceramic and cross-linked polyethylene. A ten-year follow-up report. J Bone Joint Surg Br 81:54–55

1.6 Gait Analysis in Knees and Total Knee Arthroplasty

Inès Kramers-de Quervain

Gait and movement analysis techniques are widely used to study the normal behavior and the altered function of various pathologies of the locomotor system. The techniques of comprehensive gait and movement analysis are well suited for outcome research thanks to the possibility of quantifying the functional performance. The methods are also used for individual evaluations and treatment planning in subjects with complex locomotor pathologies.

Methodology of Instrumented Gait and Movement Analysis

There are various devices to measure different aspects of gait and other activities. Some are used in isolation, while others are used in combination in gait laboratories. It is crucial for clinicians and researchers to be familiar with the limitations of the different technologies if these are used for outcome research or treatment decision making. The simple isolated tools usually yield global parameters of function, whereas the comprehensive assessments allow insight into movement strategies.

Simple, easy-to-handle tools such as force plates, gait mats, pressure-measuring insoles, video cameras and velocity-measuring devices can be used within a clinical setting or physiotherapy department. They give information such as gait velocity and stride parameters, pressure, and ground reaction forces. These tools allow for monitoring global outcome, but do not reveal the pathomechanism of abnormal function (Table 1.7).

The comprehensive techniques are used in gait laboratories with simultaneous assessment of different technologies to collect kinematics, kinetic and electromyographic data. Because of the labor-intensive and time-consuming nature of these techniques,

Table 1.7. Comparison of simple and comprehensive gait analysis tools

Simple tools	Comprehensive analysis techniques
Isolated use of measuring tools:	Simultaneous assessment of:
Velocity measuring devices systems, ultrasound systems, film analysis	Kinematics: 3D motion analysis: opto-electronic or computerized 3D video
Gait mats, footswitches	Dynamic electromyography
1D or 3D force plates	Kinetics: 3D force plates
Force cells integrated in treadmills	
Pedabarography (plates or insoles)	
Plain video recordings	
Large number of individuals	Limited number of individuals
Yields:	Yields:
Gait velocity	Global parameters
Time–distance parameters	Quantified movement strategies
Ground reaction forces	Disclosure of key problems
Dynamic podograms	Inverse dynamic approach
Overview of motion	
Global parameters of function	Function and movement strategies
Outcome studies on large numbers	Specific outcomes on selected subjects
Individual testing	Pathomechanisms
Documentation of functional status	Individual testing
Limited individual treatment planning	Documentation of functional status
	Disclosure of key problems
	Comprehensive individual treatment planning

the reported studies usually involve only a limited number of subjects. The comprehensive techniques allow the computation of the global parameters as well as joint and segment kinematics, joint kinetics and information of the dynamic activity of several muscles and muscle groups.

Gait Analysis Techniques in Total Joint Replacements

In "History and fundamentals of gait analysis," Paul (1998) reported the increasing importance of biomechanical and orthopedic research, with development of refined measurement techniques. Andriacchi (1997) described the use of gait analysis as a basis for establishing functional design criteria based on in vivo loading and as a means for obtaining objective information on patient function. Table 1.8 lists the various questions that can be addressed by gait analysis techniques.

Functional outcome studies focus on the overall level of performance, such as:

1. How close does the functional performance match that of healthy people?
2. Are individuals with joint replacements able to keep up with their peers?
3. Which motion strategies are used for level walking and for more demanding tasks such as stair ambulation?
4. What are the functional deficits?
5. Which compensatory strategies are necessary to achieve functional goals?
6. Do certain surgical techniques or system designs have functional advantages over the others?

Local knee biomechanics research addresses the in vivo loading of the joint and the implants, such as estimating the forces acting on the knee during different functional tasks. Might they compromise the survival of the implant? By measuring external forces and kinematics data, the forces acting on the knee are estimated (inverse dynamic approach). However, there is quite a controversy about the methodological approach to estimate these forces accurately.

Pitfalls of Gait Analysis Techniques in Total Joint Replacement

We have to keep in mind that the performance of a locomotion task is not only a function of the replaced knee joint, but also depends on the integrity of the whole kinematics chain. Concomitant pathologies,

which are common in people with arthroplasty, have a great influence on the global functional outcome. This compromises the functional comparison of different designs in different individuals. As the majority of subjects receiving an arthroplasty have concomitant pathologies, proper case selection for functional gait studies is very difficult. Simon et al. (1983) reported that out of 1,126 total knee arthroplasties performed during the pioneering period from 1973 to 1978, only 20 patients fulfilled the inclusion criteria of unilateral disease and the absence of other gait-affecting pathologies and only 12 consented to participate in the study. Another pitfall of using gait analysis techniques for local knee biomechanics is seen in the inaccuracy of load estimations and kinematics assessments using surface markers and inverse dynamic modeling. More accurate in vivo load measurements are achieved by instrumented implants, such as those performed at the hip joint by Heller et al. (2001). Detailed in vivo knee kinematics is preferably studied by using fluoroscopy methods, as described by Banks et al. (1997) and Dennis et al. (2001) or by stereophotogrammetry, as described by Uvehammer et al. (2000). Table 1.9 gives an overview of pitfalls of gait analysis techniques in the research of total joint replacements.

Limb Alignment, Wear and Loosening

Studies by Andriacchi et al. (1997) stress the importance of limb alignment for the load distribution between the medial and the lateral compartments. Because of the adduction moment during gait, the authors state that the knees in varus alignment are more likely to have a substantial load imbalance, which may explain the problem of tibial component loosening in the early designs. Hilding et al. (1999) confirmed that individual gait patterns and subsequent differences in joint loading affect tibial component fixation. The prognosis of fixation in patients with total knee arthroplasty was classified as either good or poor based on migration results over 4–8 years using roentgen stereophotogrammetry. In the gait analysis assessment, the poor prognosis group (14 cases) walked with a predominantly flexing moment and higher moment peaks in the sagittal plane compared with the good prognosis group (14 cases), in which moments were abnormally small. Wimmer and Andriacchi (1997) demonstrated that substantial shear forces could be generated during sliding and rolling motion, which may be important factors generating wear debris.

Table 1.8. Questions addressed by comprehensive motion analysis techniques

Functional outcome research Assessment of the overall performance:	Local knee biomechanics research Assessment of in vivo loading:
Quantification of functional tasks	Wear of the bearing surface
Motion strategies	Mechanical implant failure
Functional deficits	Implant loosening
Compensatory mechanisms	Implant dislocation

Table 1.9. Pitfalls of gait analysis techniques in the research of total joint replacement

Functional outcome research	Local knee biomechanics research
Concomitant pathologies lead to:	In vivo loads and kinematics can only be estimated using surface markers and measurements of external forces
Large number of variables	
Influence neighboring and contralateral joints	

Global Functional Outcome

Several studies report that normal function is not achieved in the majority of patients after total joint replacement. Andriacchi et al. (1997) found that abnormalities such as shorter than normal stride length, reduced mid-stance knee flexion and abnormal patterns of external flexion–extension moment patterns were common, even in asymptomatic patients with excellent clinical results in a total of 26 subjects implanted with five different designs. Simon et al. (1983) reported gait analysis results of 12 patients with a semiconstrained design. Although gait velocity was comparable to a control group, the arthroplasty subjects spent approximately 30% more time in double-limb stance and had prolonged cycle times.

Dorr et al. (1988) found a stiff-legged gait pattern during stance on both sides in 11 subjects with bilateral arthroplasties. Wilson et al. (1996) studied 16 patients implanted with a posterior-stabilized prosthesis. The spacio-temporal gait parameters and isokinetic strength testing were comparable to an age-matched control group. The knee range of motion during level walking and stair descent was significantly decreased in the arthroplasty group, with no difference in knee motion during stair ascent. In a stepwise multiple regression analysis with 22 gait variables, Lee et al. (1999) showed not only that the velocity of gait after total knee arthroplasty is lower than in normal controls, but also that gait patterns are different.

However, Kelman et al. (1989) reported that a posterior cruciate ligament sparing design in eight subjects may function in an equivalent fashion to a contralateral normal limb during stair ascent and descent. Motion and force plate analysis reveal highly symmetric gait patterns. Sagittal angles were greater than previously reported for the total condylar prosthesis and were nearly equal to those recorded for the age-matched normal population. A recent study performed at our laboratory demonstrated that excellent functionality may be accomplished in individuals implanted with a mobile bearing design who did not present with concomitant pathologies. Six healthy control subjects and 12 subjects with a low contact stress mobile bearing arthroplasty (six subjects with a rotating platform, posterior cruciate ligament sacrificing, and six with meniscal bearings, posterior cruciate ligament retaining) were tested 2–5 years after surgery. The study revealed that the arthroplasty subjects were able to walk at a comparable speed to healthy individuals using a normal and symmetrical timing of the gait phases and a comparable range of knee motion. During more demanding tasks, such as stair ambulation, however, minor deficits and adaptations were seen in this highly functional group, such as a reduced cadence and increased trunk and pelvic motion, which were considered to be adaptation strategies.

Comparison of Different Designs and Implant Techniques

Gait analysis techniques have been widely used to compare the outcome of different designs, either by comparing the designs within bilaterally operated individuals, between individuals, or between different studies. Andriacchi et al. (1982) reported that stair climbing proved to be more discriminative between different designs than level walking. He found that patients who were treated with the least constrained cruciate retaining design have a more normal gait during stair climbing than those with more constraining cruciate sacrificing designs. He also reported a significant functional difference during stair climbing with regard to the tracking of the patella, depending on the shape of the femoral trochlea. Dorr et al. (1988) studied the gait pattern of 11 patients with bilateral paired posterior cruciate retaining and cruciate sacrificing total knee arthroplasties. He too found an advantage of the cruciate retaining design. On level walking, the cruciate sacrificed knees had increased flexion and varus moments with increased muscle activity of quadriceps and biceps femoris. On stairs they substituted soleus muscle activity for knee stability. However, patients with both designs had a stiff-legged gait during stance phase. Kelman et al. (1989) reported that successful cruciate ligament sparing total knee arthroplasty functions in an equivalent fashion to a contralateral normal limb during stair ascent and descent and that sagittal angles were nearly equal to those recorded for the age-matched normal population. Wilson et al. (1996) reported that the gait pattern of 16 patients implanted with a posterior-stabilized (posterior cruciate substituting) design was comparable to that of previously reported cruciate retaining prostheses and superior to that of cruciate sacrificing prostheses. Bolanos et al. (1998) found that cruciate retaining and posterior-stabilized total knee prostheses perform equally well during level gait and stair climbing in 14 bilaterally operated patients. Pollo et al. (2000) addressed the issue of whether resurfacing the patella during routine total knee arthroplasty is necessary. He found no significant differences in the biomechanics of walking, stair climbing, or chair rising between patients after total knee arthroplasty with and without a resurfaced patella.

A study conducted in our laboratory comparing an unconstrained and a semiconstrained design in five bilaterally operated subjects revealed a reduced gait velocity, an undynamic gait with slow loading, reduced modulation of the vertical forces and poor fore/aft shears bilaterally. Sagittal plane knee motion during gait was reduced in all subjects, with trunk and pelvic compensation patterns for foot clearance. Although the stride parameters were quite symmetric, there was a marked asymmetry of the motion pattern, with a side-to-side difference of peak knee flexion during stance and swing phase of up to 15 degrees. While peak knee flexion during swing phase was better on the unconstrained side, the pattern during stance phase was not clearly related to the type of prosthesis. Increased stance knee flexion was possible in both designs, whereas a hyperextension pattern occurred only on the side of the semiconstrained design (in two individuals). Muscle activity around the knee was prolonged bilaterally, with activity modulation related to the motion pattern. In a later study using the same gait analysis techniques, 12 unilaterally operated subjects who were implanted with an unconstrained mobile bearing design demonstrated a physiological gait performance comparable to healthy control subjects. Thus, we assume that the bilateral knee replacement and a semiconstrained design on one side accounted for part of the bilaterally compromised function in the previous study group.

Compensatory Strategies

The comprehensive gait analysis techniques are well suited to study compensatory mechanisms to various gait pathologies. In our laboratory, a study was performed to assess adaptation strategies during stair

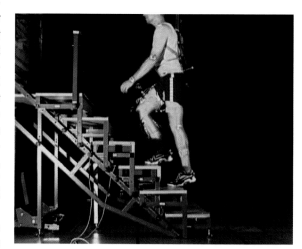

Fig. 1.37. Laboratory staircase, equipped with two Kistler force plates. Subject mounted with markers and electromyography electrodes during a stair-climbing analysis

Fig. 1.38. Dynamic peak knee flexion during gait and stair ambulation. Knee flexion clearly remains below the passive limit in the restricted knees. No further increase of flexion is seen in this group with increasing stair inclination, i.e. the flexion capacity is not utilized

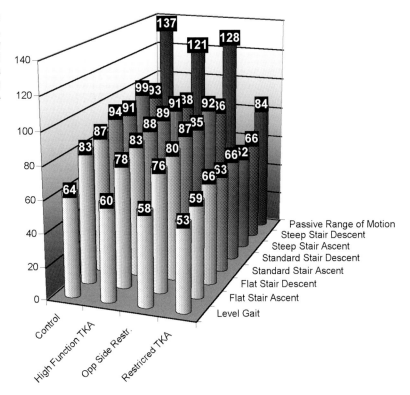

Table 1.10. Peak knee flexion after total knee arthroplasty (TKA)

	Control	Highly functional TKA	Opposite side restricted TKA	Restricted TKA
Passive range of movement	137 sd 5	121 sd 5	128 sd 7	84 sd 8
Level gait	63 sd 2	60 sd 1	58 sd 6	53 sd 8
Flat stair ascent	83 sd 4	78 sd 6	76 sd 5	59 sd 7
Flat stair descent	87 sd 4	83 sd 2	80 sd 2	66 sd 7
Standard stair ascent	93 sd 5	85 sd 12	87 sd 5	63 sd 8
Standard stair descent	91 sd 5	89 sd 5	85 sd 2	66 sd 10
Steep stair ascent	99 sd 4	90 sd 5	92 sd 4	62 sd 13
Steep stair descent	93 sd 4	88 sd 6	86 sd 3	66 sd 10

ambulation in subjects with restricted knee motion after total knee arthroplasty (Fig. 1.37). The gait pattern of four subjects with passive knee motion below 90 degrees of flexion was compared with four age- and sex-matched subjects having an excellent arthroplasty result, and with six healthy control subjects.

During gait and stair ambulation, the limit of passive knee flexion was never reached in the subjects with restricted knees (Fig. 1.38, Table 1.10). It leveled out in these subjects with increasing stair inclination, whereas a further increase of flexion was seen in the other groups. Interestingly, the dynamic knee motion remained 17 degrees below the passive limit on average in the restricted knees. Even during level gait, when the passive range of motion should allow a normal pattern, peak flexion lacked 6–10 degrees. During stair ambulation, the subjects with the restricted knees did not increase their knee flexion with increasing stair inclination, although the passive capacity would have allowed more flexion. Rather, they stressed out the compensation strategies with increasing pelvic and trunk motion in the frontal and transverse plane and an adaptation of the motion pattern on the contralateral side (Fig. 1.39).

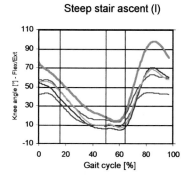

Steep stair ascent (I)

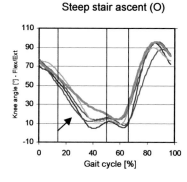

Steep stair ascent (O)

Fig. 1.39. Curves of knee flexion of the implant side (*I*) and the opposite side (*O*) of four individuals with restricted-knee total knee arthroplasty, compared with a median curve of healthy control subjects (curve with the highest degree of flexion). The *arrows* mark the premature extension in stair ascent and the delayed flexion in stair descent in the contralateral knees. This is a contralateral adaptation strategy to the reduced flexion of the knee with total knee arthroplasty

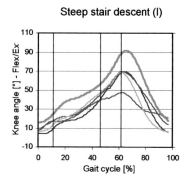

Steep stair descent (I)

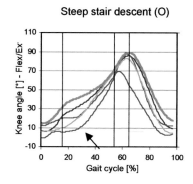

Steep stair descent (O)

There are various devices to measure different aspects of gait and other activities. It is crucial for clinicians and researchers to be familiar with the limitations of the different gait analysis technologies if these are used for outcome research or treatment decision making. The simple isolated tools used in a clinical setting usually yield global parameters of function, whereas the comprehensive simultaneous assessments used in gait analysis laboratories allow insight into movement strategies. The reported studies demonstrate the value of quantifying functional tasks for outcome research. Motion strategies and compensation mechanisms can be recognized and described. The functional advantages of a design or a surgical technique may be illuminated. However, data must be interpreted with extreme care, as the performance of locomotor tasks is strongly influenced by concomitant pathologies.

Bibliography

Andriacchi TP, Galante JO, Fermier RW (1982) The influence of total knee-replacement design on walking and stair-climbing. J Bone Joint Surg 64A:1328–1335

Andriacchi TP, Hurwitz DE (1997) Gait biomechanics and the evolution of total joint replacement. Gait Posture 5:256–264

Andriacchi TP, Yoder D, Conley A, Rosenberg A, Sum J, Galante JO (1997) Patellofemoral design influences function following total knee arthroplasty. J Arthroplasty 12:243–249

Banks SA, Markovich GD, Hodge WA (1997) The mechanics of knee replacements during gait. In vivo fluoroscopic analysis of two designs. Am J Knee Surg 10:261–267

Benedetti MG, Bonato P, Catani F, D'Alessio T, Knaflitz M, Marcacci M, Simoncini L (1999) Myoelectric activation pattern during gait in total knee replacement: relationship with kinematics, kinetics, and clinical outcome. IEEE Trans Rehabil Eng 7:140–149

Berman AT, Zarro VJ, Bosacco SJ, Israelite C (1987) Quantitative gait analysis after unilateral or bilateral total knee replacement. J Bone Joint Surg Am 69:1340–1345

Bolanos AA, Colizza WA, McCann PD, Gotlin RS, Wootten ME, Kahn BA, Insall JN (1998) A comparison of isokinetic strength testing and gait analysis in patients with posterior cruciate-retaining and substituting knee arthroplasties. J Arthroplasty 13:906–915

Dennis DA, Komistek RD, Walker SA, Cheal EJ, Stiehl JB (2001) Femoral condylar lift-off in vivo in total knee arthroplasty. J Bone Joint Surg Br 83:33–39

Dorr LD, Ochsner JL, Gronley J, Perry J (1988) Functional comparison of posterior cruciate-retained versus cruciate-sacrificed total knee arthroplasty. Clin Orthop Relat Res 236:36–43

Heller MO, Bergman G, Deuretzbacher G, Dürselen L, Pohl M, Claes L, Haas NP, Duda GN (2001) Musculo-skeletal loading conditions at the hip during walking and stair climbing. J Biomech 34:883–893

Hilding MB, Ryd L, Toksvig-Larsen S, Mann A, Stenstrom A (1999) Gait affects tibial component fixation. J Arthroplasty 14:589–593

Kelman GJ, Biden EN, Wyatt MP, Ritter MA, Colwell CW Jr (1989) Gait laboratory analysis of a posterior cruciate-sparing total knee arthroplasty in stair ascent and descent. Clin Orthop 248:21–25; discussion 25–26

Kramers-de Quervain IA, Stüssi E, Müller R, Drobny T, Munzinger U, Gschwend N (1997) Quantitative gait analysis after bilateral total knee replacement with two different systems within each subject. J Arthroplasty 12:168–179

Kramers-de Quervain IA, Reinschmidt C, Munzinger U, Stüssi E (1999) Pattern of stair ambulation in highly functional individuals after total knee joint replacement. XVIIth ISB Congress Calgary, p 299

Kramers-de Quervain IA, Tunesi R, Luder G, Stüssi E, Stacoff A (2001) Pattern of stair ambulation in individuals with restricted knee motion after total knee arthroplasty in comparison to highly functional arthroplasty subjects and to a healthy control group (Scherb Award). Proceedings of the 18th ISB Congress Congress, Zürich, p 366

Lee TH, Tsuchida T, Kitahara H, Moriya H (1999) Gait analysis before and after unilateral total knee arthroplasty. Study using a linear regression model of normal controls – women without arthropathy. J Orthop Sci 4:13–21

Pagnano MW, Cushner FD, Scott WN (1998) Role of the posterior cruciate ligament in total knee arthroplasty. J Am Acad Orthop Surg 6:176–187

Paul JP (1998) History and fundamentals of gait analysis. Biomed Mater Eng 8:123–135

Pollo FE, Jackson RW, Koeter S, Ansari S, Motley GS, Rathjen KW (2000) Walking, chair rising, and stair climbing after total knee arthroplasty: patellar resurfacing versus nonresurfacing. Am J Knee Surg 13:103–108; discussion 108–109

Simon SR, Trieshmann HW, Burdett RG, Ewald FC, Sledge CB (1983) Quantitative gait analysis after total knee arthroplasty for monarticular degenerative arthritis. J Bone Joint Surg Am 65:605–613

Uvehammer J, Karrholm J, Brandsson S, Herberts P, Carlsson L, Karlsson J, Regner L (2000) In vivo kinematics of total knee arthroplasty: flat compared with concave tibial joint surface. J Orthop Res 18:856–864

Wilson SA, McCann PD, Gotlin RS, Ramakrishnan HK, Wooten ME, Insall JN (1996) Comprehensive gait analysis in posterior-stabilized knee arthroplasty. J Arthroplasty 11:359–367

Wimmer MA, Andriacchi TP (1997) Tractive forces during rolling motion of the knee: implications for wear in total knee replacement. J Biomech 30:131–137

1.7 Tribology in Total Knee Arthroplasty
Christian B. Rieker

Tribology describes the interactions of sliding surfaces and includes three main subjects: friction, wear and lubrication. In orthopedics, the goals of tribology are to minimize wear and friction and to optimize lubrication. Both wear and friction may jeopardize clinical results of orthopedic implants. The implications of wear particles on implant loosening have been well documented since the 1970s by Willert et al. Increased friction creates shear forces at the implant (cement)–bone interface causing implant loosening. This type of failure was seen in the 1960s and 1970s with metal-on-metal hip total prostheses that had an equatorial bearing.

Types of Wear in Total Knee Arthroplasty

The four types of wear are:
1. Fatigue wear (Figs. 1.40, 1.41)
2. Abrasive wear (Fig. 1.42)
3. Adhesive wear (Figs. 1.43, 1.44)
4. Third-body wear (Fig. 1.45)

Fatigue Wear

Fatigue wear (delamination) occurs when the stresses in the polyethylene insert are larger than its fatigue limit, which is approximately 20 Mpa (Fig. 1.46). When stresses are above this limit, micro-cracks will occur below the polyethylene surface and these will ultimately lead to delamination. This phenomenon is accelerated when polyethylene inserts are oxidized due to gamma sterilization in air (Fig. 1.47).

To minimize fatigue wear or delamination in total knee arthroplasty, the level of stresses in polyethylenes should be kept to a minimum by increasing the thickness (not less than 8 mm) and increasing the femorotibial insert congruency, allowing for more uniform stress distribution. The low contact stress mobile bearing knee prosthesis (DePuy, Warsaw, USA) was developed in the 1970s to overcome this problem and is still used successfully without design changes at the articular interface. With a highly conforming rotational mobile bearing insert, this device represents an optimal combination of minimal contact stress and minimal constraint forces. Mobile bearing knee prostheses have two articulation surfaces and backside wear has been of concern; however, clinical outcome and retrieval studies did not

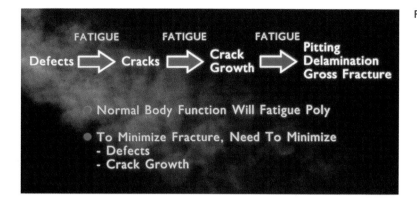

Fig. 1.40. Fatigue wear algorithm

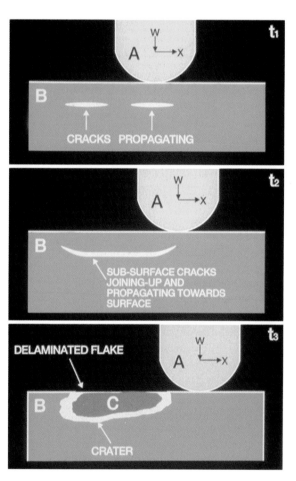

Fig. 1.41. Fatigue wear and pitting

Abrasive and Adhesive Wear

Abrasive wear occurs when hard particles penetrate into the polyethylene, creating scratches in the direction of relative motion. Hard particles are entrapped on the femoral component (carbides) or derive from polymethylmetracylate cement. Load-controlled knee simulators impose forces on knee prostheses corresponding to in vivo forces resulting from forces, implant design, and soft tissues. Advantages include the use of different prostheses, mobile and fixed bearings. A standard (ISO 14243-1) is available. Displacement-controlled knee simulators impose displacement on knee implants corresponding to relative motions within the total knee prosthesis depending on its geometry. It is recommended that fluoroscopic studies are performed for collection of specific motions. Standardized tests for fixed bearing knee prostheses are defined in ISO 14243-3.

Various studies showed that abrasive and adhesive wear is of lesser concern in total knee arthroplasty than in total hip arthroplasty. One study compared fixed with mobile bearing total knee arthroplasty in simulators, showing a 3.5-fold increased abrasive wear in mobile bearings; however, other studies demonstrated the opposite. In general, abrasive wear is of lesser concern in congruent knee designs, but was a problem in flat-on-flat or edge-loading knee designs. Knee simulator wear rates are as follows:

1. Insall Burstein, Stanmore knee simulator 2.6 mm³ per 3 Mio cycles
2. Kinemax, Durham knee simulator 3.2 mm³ per 3 Mio cycles
3. Kinematic, Durham knee simulator 4.0 mm³ per 3 Mio cycles
4. Duracon, MTS knee simulator 16.4 mm³ per 3 Mio cycles

show increased wear particles. Delamination is further reduced in modern ultra-high molecular weight polyethylene (UHMWPE) materials that are gamma in gas sterilized or highly cross-linked (see Sect. 1.5).

Fig. 1.42. Example of abrasive wear

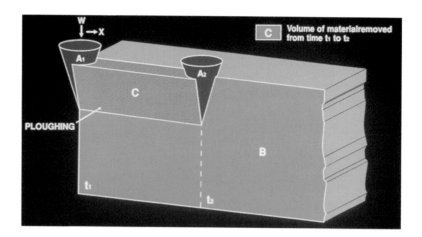

Fig. 1.43. Adhesive wear is a localized surface damage associated with local solid-state welding (adhesion) between sliding surfaces

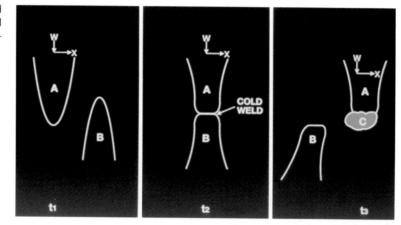

Fig. 1.44. Scratch wear in ceramics and other materials

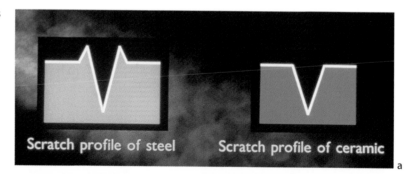

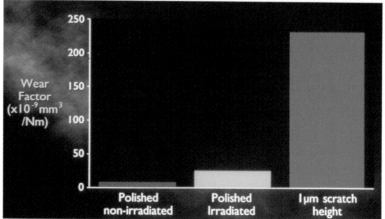

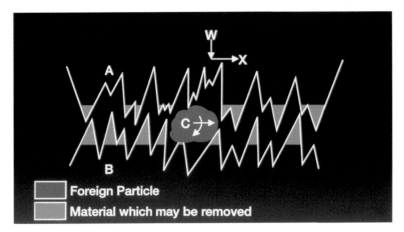

Fig. 1.45. Third-body wear

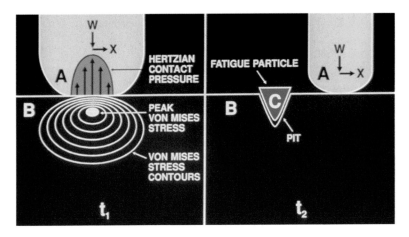

Fig. 1.46. Distribution of contact pressure within the polyethylene bearing

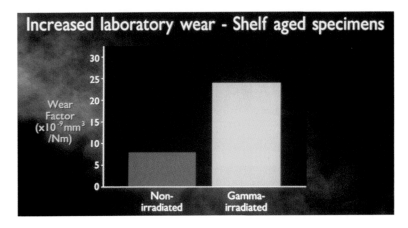

Fig. 1.47. Effect of gamma irradiation in air sterilization process on polyethylene durability

5. AGC, Loma Linda knee simulator 20.1 mm³ per 3 Mio cycles
6. NexGen CR, AMTI 29.8 mm³ per 3 Mio cycles

Wear rates for total hip prostheses are in the region of 50 mm³ per 3 Mio cycles. Highly cross-linked polyethylenes are designed to minimize abrasive wear, but are more brittle. Whether these less optimal properties of highly cross-linked polyethylenes may cause mechanical problems in total knee arthroplasty is difficult to say and has to be answered by clinical studies. Long-term outcomes of well-implanted fixed bearing total knee arthroplasty and mobile bearing total knee arthroplasty with conventional gamma in gas sterilized UHMWPE inserts show that wear does not appear to be the major limiting factor for failures.

Bibliography

Calonius O, Saikko V (2002) Analysis of polyethylene particles produced in different wear conditions in vitro. Clin Orthop 399:219–230

Chapman-Sheath PJ, Bruce WJ, Chung WK, Morberg P, Gillies RM, Walsh WR (2003) In vitro assessment of proximal polyethylene contact surface areas and stresses in mobile bearing knees. Med Eng Phys 25:437–443

Dorr LD (2002) Contrary view: wear is not an issue. Clin Orthop 404:96–99

Heimke G, Leyen S, Willmann G (2002) Knee arthroplasty: recently developed ceramics offer new solutions. Biomaterials 23:1539–1551

Majewski M, Weining G, Friederich NF (2002) Posterior femoral impingement causing polyethylene failure in total knee arthroplasty. J Arthroplasty 17:524–526

Puertolas JA, Larrea A, Gomez-Barrena E (2001) Fracture behavior of UHMWPE in non-implanted, shelf-aged knee prostheses after gamma irradiation in air. Biomaterials 22:2107–2114

Rand JA, Trousdale RT, Ilstrup DM, Harmsen WS (2003) Factors affecting the durability of primary total knee prostheses. J Bone Joint Surg Am 85A:259–265

Taylor M, Barrett DS (2003) Explicit finite element simulation of eccentric loading in total knee replacement. Clin Orthop 414:162–171

Walker PS, Haider H (2003) Characterizing the motion of total knee replacements in laboratory tests. Clin Orthop 410:54–68

Wasielewski RC (2002) The causes of insert backside wear in total knee arthroplasty. Clin Orthop 404:232–246

1.8 In Vivo Motions of Mobile Bearing Total Knee Arthroplasty

S. Banks, C. Reinschmidt, A. Stacoff, G. Luder, I. Kramers-de Quervain, T. Staehelin, U. Munzinger

Mobile bearing total knee arthroplasty (MB-TKA) was developed from the desire to provide conforming articulations for low contact stress while allowing relatively unrestricted motion of the joint. The rotational freedom of the articulation also provides a self-aligning characteristic, i.e. the bearing has the ability to align according to the individual forces and anatomical conditions. The self-aligning characteristic may also enhance the surgeon's ability to position the tibial baseplate for maximum bone coverage. The unconstrained motion ability of MB-TKA may also help to enhance fixation through the reduction of the interface stresses between the tibial baseplate. These potentially beneficial properties have made MB-TKA an increasingly popular implant choice worldwide. Until very recently, there have been two common approaches to MB-TKA: posterior cruciate ligament retaining designs that provide for translation and rotation of the mobile bearing (CR type), and posterior cruciate sacrificing designs that provide for rotation-only motion of the mobile bearing (ultracongruent only rotating, UCOR).

Several authors have reported their in vivo and in vitro comparisons of the CR and UCOR types of MB-TKA. Stiehl et al. (1997) reported that patients with CR type MB-TKA showed higher postoperative range of motion (ROM) than patients with UCOR type MB-TKA, but that these CR patients also had higher ROM preoperatively. Lewandowski et al. (1997) used a mechanical loading rig and cadaveric limbs implanted with both MB-TKA types to demonstrate that the CR type has quadriceps efficiency similar to the normal knee, while the UCOR type has significantly reduced quadriceps efficiency. Using a different mechanical test set-up, D'Lima et al. (2000) tested high- and low-conformity versions of both CR and UCOR types, and found that these variations in articular design did not adversely affect knee kinematics for the conditions tested. In studies of CR type MB-TKA, it has been demonstrated that the femur often slides anterior with knee flexion, a pattern attributed to the loss of the anterior cruciate ligament and menisci.

The purpose of this study was to determine if there are differences in knee kinematics between CR and UCOR knee replacements during a variety of weight-bearing activities including gait, stair and two deep flexion tasks. Twelve subjects with uniarticular osteoarthritis treated by MB-TKA participated in this study, which was approved by the Ethics Committee. Six subjects (six knees) received CR type MB-TKA (INNEX CR, Sulzer Orthopedics Ltd) and six subjects (six knees) received UCOR type MB-TKA (INNEX UCOR). All subjects had excellent clinical and functional outcomes at their 1-year postoperative clinic assessment. There were no statistically significant differences in age, height, weight, tibial slope, or postoperative time between the two groups (Table 1.11).

Subjects performed four weight-bearing activities: one-legged kneeling, lunge, step-up/down, and treadmill gait (Fig. 1.48). For the one-legged kneeling activity, subjects placed their shin on a padded, knee-height box, and were asked to bend to maximum flexion. For the lunge, subjects placed their foot on a 25 cm riser and were asked to bend to maximum comfortable flexion. One to three seconds of fluoroscopy video was acquired once the subject reached their maximally flexed position.

For the single-leg step-up/down activity, the subjects placed their foot on a 25 cm riser. They were instructed to lift themselves up and down on the riser repeatedly, not swinging through with the opposite

Table 1.11. Patient characteristics for six CR and six UCOR knees

Parameter	CR	UCOR	p value
Age (years)	67±6	71±8	0.389
Weight (kg)	73±14	84±11	0.178
Height (m)	1.73±0.09	1.75±0.09	0.758
Tibial posterior slope (degrees)	8±5	6±3	0.331
Postoperative time (months)	13±2	12±2	0.483

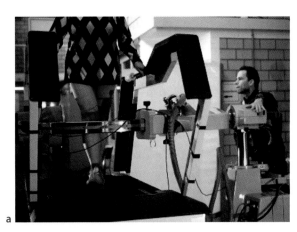

a

Fig. 1.48 a–d. Movements performed during fluoroscopic imaging. a Treadmill gait at approximately 1 m/s. b Single-leg stepping up and down on a 25 cm riser. c Maximum weight-bearing flexion with foot on a 25 cm riser ("lunge"). d One-legged kneeling to maximum flexion with the shank resting on a knee-height padded box

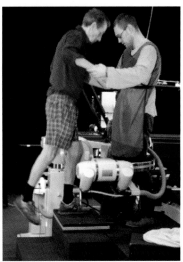
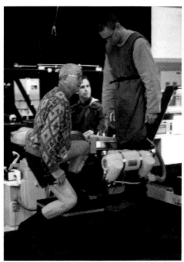
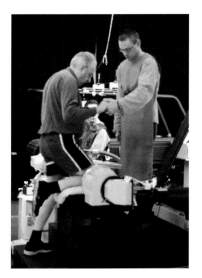

b–d

leg. Subjects were encouraged to reach a fully extended knee position before reversing direction. Fluoroscopy images were recorded at ten frames per second as the subject performed at least four cycles of the step activity at a self-selected pace.

The gait activity was performed on a motorized treadmill in order to accommodate fluoroscopic imaging. Subjects were allowed to walk on the treadmill until comfortable with its operation, and were en-

couraged to walk at a comfortable pace. The target speed was 1 m/s. Subjects were explicitly encouraged to extend their knees fully at heel-strike and to avoid a shuffling pattern of gait. Subjects were allowed to use the treadmill's handrails with only a light touch; they were not allowed to bear weight or lean on the handrails. The fluoroscopy unit was aligned to acquire knee images during the "front-half" of the gait cycle (late swing though early stance) and video was

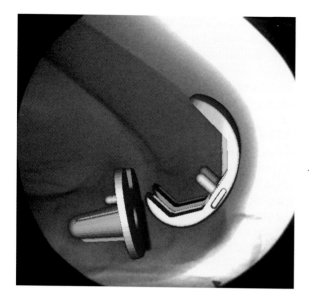

Fig. 1.49. Subjects' knees were imaged using fluoroscopy during weight-bearing activities. Models of the arthroplasty components were projected into the image and the shapes were matched to determine the three-dimensional position and orientation of the femoral and tibial components

recorded at 30 frames per second for a minimum of four gait cycles. As the subject continued to walk at a consistent speed, the fluoroscopy unit was positioned to record the "back-half" of the gait cycle (late stance through early swing) for at least four cycles.

Fluoroscopic images were obtained using a modified portable c-arm fluoroscopy unit (OEC 9000, GE-OEC). The system camera was removed and replaced with an electronically shuttered black and white CCD video camera to permit sharp images of fast-moving knees. The shutter speed of the camera was adjusted between 2 and 18 ms depending upon the speed of the activity. The NTSC video signal was recorded onto digital videotape.

The three-dimensional (3D) position and orientation of the implant components were determined using model-based shape-matching techniques, including previously reported techniques, manual matching, and image space optimization routines (Fig. 1.49). The fluoroscopic images were digitized and corrected for static optical distortion. The optical geometry of the fluoroscopy system (principal distance, principal point) was determined from images of a calibration target. The implant surface model was projected onto the geometry-corrected image, and its 3D pose was iteratively adjusted to match its silhouette with the silhouette of the subject's TKA components. The results of this shape-matching process have standard errors of approximately 0.5–1.0

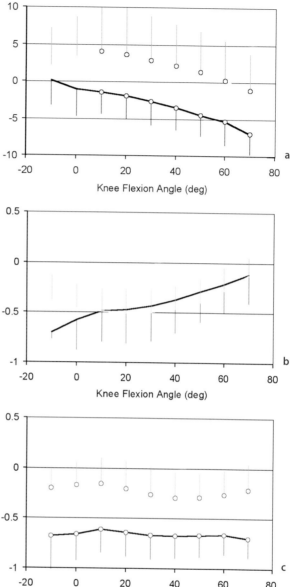

Fig. 1.50a–c. Knee kinematics during step-up/down activity. *Open circles* indicate flexion ranges where there was a significant difference between the CR and UCOR groups. a Both groups showed tibial internal rotation with knee flexion. The UCOR group showed a significant bias toward tibial external rotation over the flexion range. b The CR group showed linear anterior sliding of the medial condyle with flexion. The UCOR group showed posterior translation from −10° to 20° flexion, and then anterior sliding from 30° to 70° flexion. c Neither the CR nor the UCOR group showed significant translation of the lateral condyle during the step activity. The UCOR group showed significantly more anterior lateral condyle position over the range of flexion

degrees for rotations and 0.5–1.0 mm for translations in the sagittal plane.

Joint kinematics were determined from the 3D pose of each TKA component using the convention of Tupling and Pierrynowski (1987). The locations of condylar contact were estimated as the lowest point on each femoral condyle relative to the transverse plane of the tibial baseplate. The reported knee kinematics describe the relative motions of the femoral component and tibial baseplate; the mobile bearing insert was not visible on the x-ray images and could not be tracked without additional metallic markers.

The kneeling and lunge data were compared using t-tests. For the stair and gait data, an average curve for each knee (patient) was created from four trials of data. These average curves were then combined to create group averages. Statistical comparisons for the gait and step data were performed using a two-factor, repeated-measures analysis of variance with post-hoc pairwise comparisons (Tukey's honestly significant difference). The level of significance was set at $p \leq 0.05$.

There was no difference between CR and UCOR knees in maximum knee flexion during the lunge and kneeling activities (Table 1.12). The CR knees showed 5 degrees more tibial internal rotation in the kneeling position than the UCOR knees ($p<0.05$). The kneeling activity produced approximately 10 degrees more flexion than the lunge activity ($p<0.05$). For the kneeling activity, there was an average 9 degrees difference between knee flexion measured using a goniometer compared to the simultaneous measurement using fluoroscopy (paired t-test, $p<0.05$). Maximum flexion during kneeling was the same as the passive ROM and active ROM when measured using a goniometer ($p>0.05$).

Both CR and UCOR knees showed 5–7 degrees tibial internal rotation with flexion during the step activity (Fig. 1.50). From 10 to 70 degrees flexion, the UCOR knees showed an approximately 5 degrees bias toward tibial external rotation compared to the CR knees ($p<0.05$). The CR knees showed anterior translation of the medial condyle from extension to flexion during the step activity. The UCOR knees showed posterior medial condyle translation from –10 to 20 degrees flexion, and then anterior translation from 40 to 70 degrees flexion. Medial condyle locations were not significantly different over the flexion range, nor were the total translations from extension to flexion. Lateral condyle locations for the UCOR knees were significantly more anterior over the entire flexion range of the step activity (Fig. 1.50). For both groups, the lateral condyle showed less translation from extension to flexion than the medial condyle ($p<0.05$).

Similar to the step activity, the UCOR knees showed a bias toward a more externally rotated tibial position over the entire gait cycle (Fig. 1.51). Two of the CR patients were reluctant to extend their knees fully at heel-strike (because of unfamiliarity with using a treadmill), shifting the group flexion curve upward in early stance. However, there were no statistically significant differences between the flexion curves for the two groups, and both group averages showed hyperextension in late stance. From heel-strike to mid-stance, the CR knees showed a posterior translation of both condyles of approximately 5 mm (Fig. 1.51). On average, the UCOR knees showed little condylar translation from heel-strike to mid-stance. Both CR and UCOR knees exhibited some anterior femoral translation during swing phase.

Table 1.12. Range of motion and knee kinematics for non-weight-bearing and weight-bearing activities in six CR and six UCOR knees

	Parameter	CR	UCOR	p value
Knee angles measured with goniometer	Passive ROM (degrees)	120±9	123±9	0.659
	Active ROM (degrees)	119±10	123±9	0.557
	Kneeling flexion (degrees)	122±8	126±13	0.613
Kneeling measured fluoroscopically	Flexion (degrees)	112±16	115±10	0.677
	Tibial external rotation (degrees)	–6±5	–1±3	0.048
	Femoral anteroposterior translation (mm)	–6.0±3.4	–2.5±3.2	0.096
Lunge measured fluoroscopically	Flexion (degrees)	103±15	104±10	0.952
	Tibial external rotation (degrees)	–7±4	–3±4	0.116
	Femoral anteroposterior translation (mm)	–5.2±2.7	–3.0±1.8	0.126

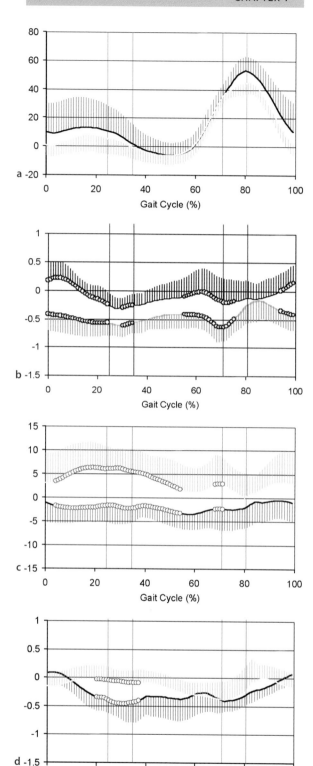

Fig. 1.51 a–d. Knee kinematics during treadmill walking at approximately 1 m/s. The *open circles* indicate phases where there is a statistically significant difference between the CR and UCOR groups. Two pairs of vertical lines indicate the phases of gait where the contralateral knee obscures the TKA (25–35% and 71–81%), leaving a gap that is filled by interpolation. a Knee flexion angles over the gait cycle. There were no statistically significant differences between the CR and UCOR groups. Both groups showed hyperextension of the TKA components in late stance phase. Several individuals in the CR group were reluctant to extend their knee fully at heel-strike, shifting the CR mean upward during early stance. b Tibial external rotation over the gait cycle. There was a significant bias toward tibial external rotation during stance in the UCOR group. c Anteroposterior location of medial condylar "contact" over the gait cycle. d Anteroposterior location of lateral condylar "contact" over the gait cycle. Both condyles in the CR group slide posterior during early and mid-stance phase, and anterior during swing. The UCOR group shows relatively little translation during stance phase, but both condyles slide forward during early swing

The goal of this study was to determine if there were differences in knee mechanics in matched groups of patients with two variations of a mobile bearing TKA. Differences in axial rotations and tibio-femoral translations were observed. For the most part, these differences were consistent with the constraints of the two design variations.

The fluoroscopy-based measurements report the angles and relative positions of the arthroplasty components. Thus, flexion angles and axial rotations are subject to bias from the implant positioning, which is influenced by anatomy and surgical alignment. The flexion angle during kneeling was observed to be about 10 degrees greater, when measured by a physiotherapist with a goniometer, than the fluoroscopy-based measures. This could be attributed mainly to the posterior tibial slope (Table 1.11) and the anterior bow of the femur, which bias the TKA components in hyperextension relative to the anatomical flexion angle. This is particularly important during gait, when the knee is normally extended at heel-strike and late stance. Five of twelve knees showed hyperextension (maximum: 10 degrees) of the TKA components at heel-strike and nine of twelve knees showed hyperextension (maximum: 20 degrees) in late stance. This degree of hyperextension is well accommodated in most cruciate retaining TKA designs, but can lead to anterior impingement and tibial post damage in many posterior stabilized TKA designs.

The UCOR knees showed approximately 5 degrees tibial external rotation compared to the CR knees in all activities. This could simply reflect a surgical bias in the axial alignment of the TKA components, although this seems unlikely, as the same surgeons were implanting both types of MB-TKA. This rotation might also result from sectioning the posterior cruciate ligament, or from adopting a central tibiofemoral anterior/posterior position by the rotating-only bearing. Clearly, this interesting observation needs further exploration.

The amount of anteroposterior translation was consistent with the constraints of the two mobile bearing designs. The CR knees, which had a mobile bearing free to rotate and translate, showed anteroposterior translation across the range of flexion. The UCOR knees, which had a rotating-only mobile bearing, showed condylar translations mostly at flexion angles above 30 degrees, where the femur is no longer fully congruent with the mobile bearing. Condylar translations were generally greater on the medial side. This is consistent with other reports of kinematics and wear patterns in fixed and mobile bearing TKA, and is probably related to the loss of the anterior cruciate ligament and the normal anteroposterior constraints of the knee. The greater amount of translation on the medial side indicates an average pivot point lateral to the midline, which is opposite to what has been reported for the normal knee.

Despite observing some interesting differences in knee kinematics, there were no discernible clinical or functional differences between these two groups of MB-TKA. This outcome might be the result of selection bias, and groups showing a wider spectrum of functional abilities or limitations may demonstrate a different result. These same subjects are now participating in a formal gait analysis study with motion capture, force platforms and electromyography to determine if the differences in knee mechanics influence body mechanics during gait and stair climbing. In this series of well-functioning patients, either approach to providing bearing mobility appears to offer the low contact stress and self-aligning properties desired of a mobile bearing TKA.

Bibliography

Banks SA (1992) Model based 3D kinematic estimation from 2D perspective silhouettes: application with total knee prostheses. PhD dissertation, Massachusetts Institute of Technology, Cambridge, MA

Banks SA, Hodge WA (1996) Accurate measurement of three-dimensional knee replacement kinematics using single-plane fluoroscopy. IEEE Trans Biomed Eng 43:638–649

Banks SA, Markovich GD, Hodge WA (1997) In vivo kinematics of cruciate-retaining and substituting knee arthroplasties. J Arthroplasty 12:297–304

Banks SA, Markovich GD, Hodge WA (1997) The mechanics of knee replacements during gait: in vivo fluoroscopic analysis of two designs. Am J Knee Surg 10:261–267

Banks SA, Harman MK, Hodge WA, Markovich GD, Kester M (1997) Kinematics of the medial unicondylar knee replacement. In: Cartier P, Epinette JA, Deschamps G, Hernigou P (eds) Unicompartmental knee arthroplasty. Expansion Scientifique Francaise, Paris, pp 27–31

Callaghan JJ, Squire MW, Goetz DD, Sullivan PM, Johnston RC (2000) Cemented rotating-platform total knee replacement. A nine to twelve-year follow-up study. J Bone Joint Surg 82:705–711

D'Lima DD, Trice M, Urquhat AG, Colwell CW (2000) Comparison between the kinematics of fixed and rotating bearing knee prostheses. Clin Orthop 380:151–157

Gillis A, Furman B, Schmieg J, Bhattacharyya S, Li S (2001) The effect of post impingement in posterior stabilized total knee replacements on femoral rotation and damaged area as determined from analysis of retrieved tibial inserts. Trans Orthop Res Soc 47

Lewandowski P, Askew M, Lin D, Hurst F, Melby A (1997) Kinematics of posterior cruciate ligament-retaining and -sacrificing mobile bearing total knee arthroplasties. An in vitro comparison of the New Jersey LCS meniscal bearing and rotating platform prostheses. J Arthroplasty 12:777–784

Nilsson KG, Karrholm J, Gadegaard P (1991) Abnormal kinematics of the artificial knee. Roentgen stereophotogrammetric analysis of 10 Miller-Galante and five New Jersey LCS knees. Acta Orthop Scand 62:440–446

Noble PC, Vagner G, Conditt M (2001) The role of the cam mechanism in posterior stabilized TKR: an analysis of 75 retrieved components. Trans Orthop Res Soc 47

Stiehl JB, Komistek RD, Dennis DA, Paxson RD, Hoff WA (1995) Fluoroscopic analysis of kinematics after posterior-cruciate-retaining knee arthroplasty. J Bone Joint Surg 77B:884–889

Stiehl JB, Dennis DA, Komistek RD, Keblish PA (1997) In vivo kinematic analysis of a mobile bearing total knee prothesis. Clin Orthop 345:60–66

Stiehl JB, Voorhorst PE, Keblish P, Sorrells RB (1997) Comparison of range of motion after posterior cruciate ligament retention or sacrifice with a mobile bearing total knee arthroplasty. Am J Knee Surg 10:216–220

Stiehl J, Dennis D, Komistek R, Crane H (1999) In vivo determination of condylar lift-off and screw-home in a mobile bearing total knee arthroplasty. J Arthroplasty 14:293–299

Stiehl J, Komistek R, Dennis D (1999) Detrimental kinematics of a flat on flat total condylar knee arthroplasty. Clin Orthop 365:139–148

Todo S, Kadoya Y, Moilanen T, Kobayashi A, Yamano Y, Iwaki H, Freeman M (1999) Anteroposterior and rotational movement of femur during knee flexion. Clin Orthop 362:162–170

Tupling S, Pierrynowski M (1987) Use of Cardan angles to locate rigid bodies in three-dimensional space. Med Biol Eng Comput 25:527–532

CHAPTER 2

Urs K. Munzinger · Peter A. Keblish
Jens G. Boldt · Alan C. Merchant

Knee Arthroplasty

2.1 Indications and Alternatives
Urs K. Munzinger

Indications and Assessment

This chapter focuses on patient evaluation, potential outcomes, and various treatment options for patients with knee pain and disability. It is based on Krackow's paper (1990) on indications and assessment. A well-performed total knee arthroplasty (TKA) in a properly selected patient should result in a 95% plus satisfaction range and must last for 20 years in more than 80% of patients in order to meet current standards. A poorly planned and executed arthroplasty, no matter how properly the patient was selected, will result in an unhappy patient. Similarly, a technically well-performed arthroplasty on the wrong patient can lead to patient dissatisfaction, significant complications, and potentially medicolegal litigation. The thrust is to select the patient appropriately and to perform the operation perfectly.

Patient History

The indications for TKA might be listed as knee pain, mechanical instability, and limited range of knee motion. From a practical standpoint, uncontrolled knee pain is the predominant indication for knee surgery. Functional instability, where alteration of joint surfaces has resulted in a knee that is incapable of providing weight bearing or function is the second most common indication. Decreased motion (arthrofibrosis), ankylosis, and cosmesis (usually females with less than incapacitating pain) are rare indications for TKA. Medical history must include pain, not only in general terms of severity, but also with its concomitants of requisite pain medication, use of weight-bearing assistive devices, presence or absence of rest or activity pain, and also night pain (see IDES documentation, Sect. 5.2).

It is helpful to record those activities the patient is unable to do as a result of his or her knee problem and the general activity level. In addition, the patients' goals and desires to perform activities as a result of surgery must be noted. Another important factor is past and current work requirements or occupational history, intake of oral analgesia or nonsteroidal anti-inflammatory drugs, frequency and response to intra-articular injections, physical therapy, bracing, and prior surgery. Finally, the patient's general health status must be recorded in depth because of anesthesia and postoperative treatment regimens.

Physical Examination

Initial observation of the patient's gait in terms of general strength, gait velocity, mobility, and apparent discomfort is important. The following should be documented accurately: ability to manage stairs, the type and degree of deformity, range of motion, other aspects of alignment, ligament balance, and conditions for skin incisions. A detailed examination of the lower extremity, including assessment of the hip joint and the ankle joint, general sensitivity, peripheral circulation, crepitation, and patellofemoral sensitivity, is important (Figs. 2.1–2.3). Standardized evaluation forms such as the HSS, the Knee Society Scoring system, or the IDES system (Sect. 5.2) are recommended and routinely utilized at our institution to measure outcomes.

Radiographic Examination

Evaluation for TKA includes routine anteroposterior and lateral weight-bearing radiographs, patellofemoral views, and longstanding weight-bearing views. Emphasis should be directed to general bone quality, varus/valgus alignment, genu flexum, joint space loss, appearance of osteophytes, evidence of effusion, size and position of the patella and other points

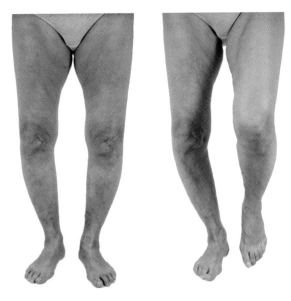

Fig. 2.1. Observation of the patient's gait in terms of gait velocity, mobility and apparent discomfort is important

(Fig. 2.4). General bone quality, such as osteoporosis, may indicate disease or inactivity atrophy and may suggest the impropriety of considering uncemented arthroplasty. Metaphyseal bone status is useful in evaluation of potential bone graft needs and ability to withstand loads. Flexion contracture is suggested if there is asymmetric enlargement of one knee on a bilateral anteroposterior view and on a weight-bearing

lateral view in maximal extension. The lateral view in flexion often shows an apparent narrowing of the medial or lateral joint space. Obtaining modified anteroposterior radiographs with the knee positioned in 30 degrees flexion can reveal loss of medial or lateral joint space (Fig. 2.5).

Medical history, physical examination, and radiographic studies should allow a basic assessment of the patient's knee problem. Preoperative questions should concentrate less on the severity of orthopedic pathologic factors, but rather on general medical and peripheral vascular status. Answers to these questions allow for better prediction regarding systemic risks, circulatory/vascular and healing problems. In the group of patients whose symptoms are out of proportion to objective findings, one must continue to search for other etiology, including hip and spine problems. Not infrequently, knee pain is referred from either hip arthritis or radicular spinal nerve entrapment due to lumbar spine degeneration. Other local etiologies include synovial disease, bony pathologic factors, tumors, fracture, menisci, cruciate ligaments, cartilage disease, tendinitis or bursitis, posttraumatic pain, unspecific reflex sympathetic dystrophy (or complex regional pain syndrome, CRPS), and pain of otherwise undetermined etiology. Bone scans, magnetic resonance imaging (MRI), computed tomography, or arthroscopy may be considered as additional and valuable investigations to determine the correct diagnosis.

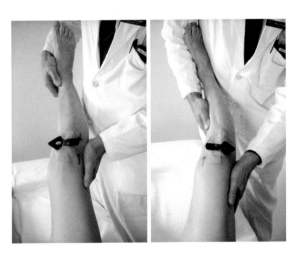

Fig. 2.2. In the physical examination, the type and degree of deformity, range of motion, other aspects of alignment and ligament balance are documented

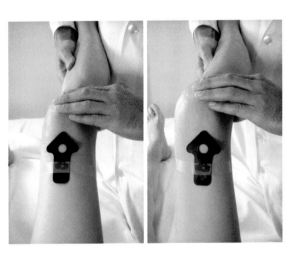

Fig. 2.3. Clinical data, such as patella tracking and crepitus, help form an opinion of the degree of wear of the joint. The tibiofemoral joint is examined in varus versus valgus stress

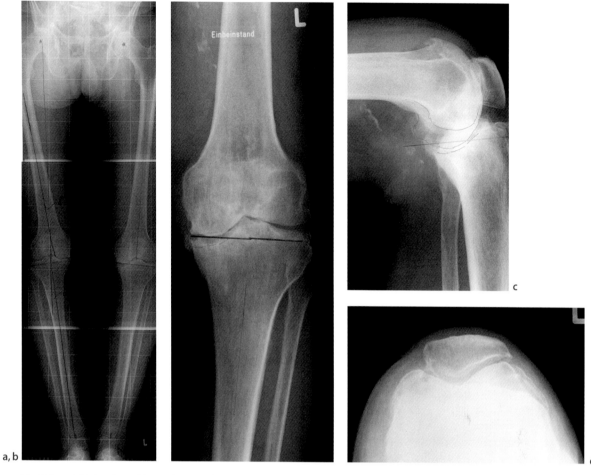

Fig. 2.4. a–d Evaluation of the patient requires routine anteroposterior and lateral x-ray films plus patellofemoral views, weight-bearing x-ray films, and long-standing x-ray views

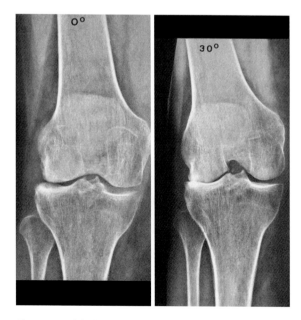

Fig. 2.5. Modified anteroposterior radiographs in 30° flexion can reveal loss of medial or lateral joint space

Treatment Options

Surgical options of joint surface degeneration include: arthroscopic wash-out and cartilage treatment, osteotomy, unicompartmental arthroplasty, patellofemoral arthroplasty, or TKA. Arthroscopic debridement in selected patients (locking, instability, elderly unable to tolerate TKA, etc.) may be of temporary benefit but does not treat the obvious problem.

Distal Femoral and Proximal Tibial Osteotomy

Proximal tibial osteotomy treatment can be considered in angular knee deformity, fixed deformity, and the presence of unicompartmental degeneration (Fig. 2.6). The patient should be negative for significant synovitis, meniscal pathology, or cruciate ligament tears. Arthroscopic partial medial or lateral meniscectomy should be performed in these cases. Preoperative MRI studies are recommended.

Other factors that may indicate osteotomy include:

1. Relatively long life expectancy. Patients in this category would typically be 65 years old or less with average health. Patients older than 65, with high physical activity, may also be considered for osteotomy.
2. Significant symptoms and moderate radiographic changes, together with high exercise tolerance.

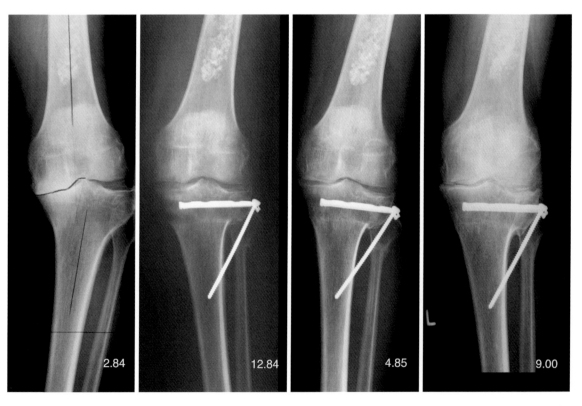

Fig. 2.6. 16-year result of a closing wedge tibial osteotomy in a highly active male patient who performs mountain hiking for 3 h five times a week

3. Fixed deformity in physiologically young patients or severe deformity for which satisfactory TKA outcomes would be less predictable. In these cases, osteotomy should be considered as a first-stage TKA, but often provides several years of satisfactory function and may be a permanent procedure.

Further factors that are not contraindications for tibial osteotomy are: (1) patellofemoral osteophytes, with clinical findings of patellofemoral sensitivity or pain; (2) presence of osteophytes and evidence of degenerative changes in the opposite compartment, or absence of clinical signs in the opposite compartment; (3) complete loss of articular cartilage in the concave side compartment (burned out). The patient with complete cartilage loss secondary to osteoarthritis frequently has smooth, polished joint surfaces and may do quite well with the diminution of compartment weight-bearing force consequent to osteotomy treatment.

Factors that are controversial or more variable regarding osteotomy treatment include:

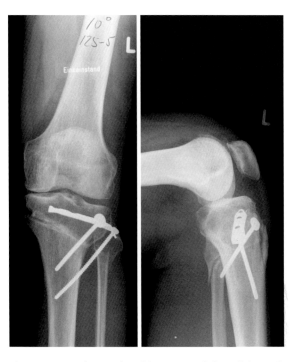

Fig. 2.7. One technique for addressing medial instability with medial osteoarthritis is a combined closing wedge on the lateral side with an opening wedge on the medial side

1. Presence of significant anterior instability causing pivot shift phenomenon. This can be managed by intra-articular or extra-articular anterior cruciate ligament reconstruction.
2. Medial instability partly secondary to attrition of medial compartment cartilage and bone, possibly in association with an old medial collateral ligament injury. This may be addressed by a combined closing wedge osteotomy on the lateral side with an opening wedge osteotomy on the medial side (Fig. 2.7) or an opening wedge on the medial side alone (Fig. 2.8).
3. Intra-articular pathology such as meniscal damage or condylar ridging in association with osteophytes and degeneration. Arthroscopic or even open treatment of these problems together with osteotomy can be very successful.

Factors that are clearly negative with respect to the osteotomy option include: (1) advanced age and decreased life expectancy; (2) patients with severely decreased range of motion, especially in conjunction with flexion contracture; and (3) significant synovitis. One must consider that osteotomy may be unsuccessful or of temporary benefit only. It is, therefore, important to consider the potential impact of osteotomy on future total knee replacement, and to obtain an informed consent from the patient if the option of osteotomy is offered.

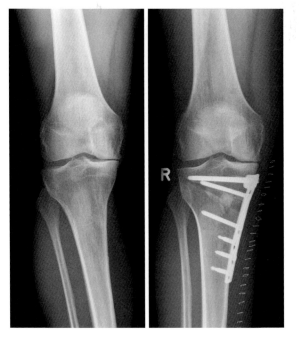

Fig. 2.8. The open wedge valgus osteotomy of the tibia is fixed with angle stable implants (Tomofix)

Unicompartmental Arthroplasty

Unicompartmental knee arthroplasty (UKA) is approached differently by individual surgeons. Whereas some have almost entirely abandoned osteotomy treatment in favor of UKA, others push the index osteotomy beyond the 65-year limit and elect UKA only in those patients who are "of arthroplasty age" with pure unicompartmental disease and intact cruciate ligaments (Fig. 2.9). Fixed deformity, not correctable with stress testing and/or flexion contracture, is considered to be a contraindication for UKA.

Laskin proposed four important questions that should be considered by the surgeon contemplating recommending UKA to a patient:

1. Does the patient have distinct unicompartmental disease?
2. Are clinical examinations sufficient?
3. Does patellofemoral pain exclude unicompartmental replacement?
4. Should arthroscopy be performed routinely prior to unicompartmental replacement?

Arthroscopy immediately followed by any arthroplasty may result in a higher rate of infection. For identifying articular surfaces, MRI is the investigation of choice. Technetium-99 bone scans usually show increased blood uptake in subchondral bone. If the scan indicates high uptake in both compartments or in the patellofemoral region, unicompartmental replacement should be contraindicated. The question that has to be answered is how much degeneration is acceptable for unicompartmental replacement.

Are there specific contraindications for unicompartmental replacement? Patients without an intact anterior cruciate ligament have abnormal knee kinematics with usually degenerative changes in the medial joint space. Based on Murray's experiences, absence of the anterior cruciate ligament should be a contraindication for unicompartmental replacement. The ideal patient for medial unicompartmental replacement should have symptoms and signs referable to the medial tibiofemoral joint space, minimal patellofemoral symptoms, less than a 10 degrees fixed flexion deformity, a flexion arc of at least 90 degrees, a body weight less than 80 kg, a low level of activity, no evidence of inflammatory arthropathy (including calcium pyrophosphate arthropathy), intact anterior cruciate ligament, and no fixed varus deformity.

What surgical technique is best for unicompartmental replacement? Many failures of unicompartmental replacement could be attributed to compo-

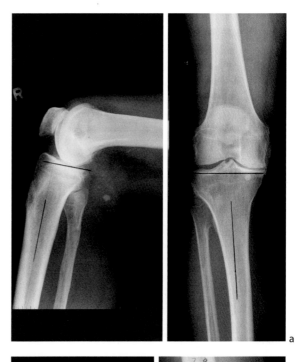
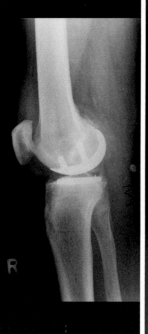
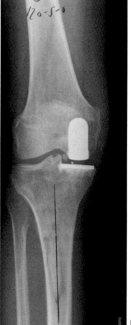

Fig. 2.9. Unicompartmental arthroplasty is considered in patients with unicompartmental disease and functioning cruciate ligaments. In case of failure, conversion to TKA is possible

nent malpositioning, often the result of poor instrumentation. Recent developments in instrumentation have increased the accuracy for implantation, which will increase the longevity of UKA.

What configuration of implant is optimal? The thickness of the polyethylene has been a major concern in UKA. The minimum thickness should be at least 6 mm, have a conforming design to the femoral component and may be mobile bearing. The advantages of UKA include a small incision and rapid recovery, making this procedure eligible for day-case surgery. There is less associated blood loss than in a total knee replacement, and if they fail, most are converted easily to a formal bi- or tricompartmental replacement.

Patellofemoral Arthroplasty

Isolated patellofemoral arthritis occurs in approximately 10% of patients with osteoarthritic knee symptoms. Conservative treatment can be rather frustrating, particularly in the early stages of osteoarthritis. Interestingly, pain may ease off when the patella and femoral groove articulate bone on bone, a phenomenon also found in rheumatoid arthritis (burn-out). Patients with patellofemoral osteoarthritis typically present with anterior knee pain, particularly on descending stairs or negotiating downslopes,

giving way, positive apprehension test, and aggravation on kneeling. In the 1960s and 1970s, patellectomy was a common treatment, a procedure often leading to significantly weakened knee joints and frequently reoccurrence of anterior knee pain. Literature reports cite successful outcomes in less than 50%. Patella-friendly anatomic femoral components have shown excellent long-term results, even when the patella is left unresurfaced (Sect. 3.2). Some surgeons favor TKA in isolated patellofemoral osteoarthritis without patella resurfacing with good outcomes (Sect. 3.4). Isolated patellofemoral arthroplasties have been available for some years but little attention has been paid to the patella treatment, patella tracking, and patellofemoral congruity (Fig. 2.10). Results from earlier designs do not reach those of modern TKA; however, more anatomical designs are available today (Sect. 2.5). Radiographical screening prior to operation identifies patients suitable for this procedure, but the final decision must be made at the time of arthrotomy. Minor degress of chondromalacia on the medial and lateral femoral condyles of the tibiofemoral joint are acceptable, but it is essential that the menisci and cruciates are intact and there is good range of movement of the joint. Like all arthroplasties, success depends on careful selection of appropriate cases, a technically competent procedure and carefully controlled rehabilitation.

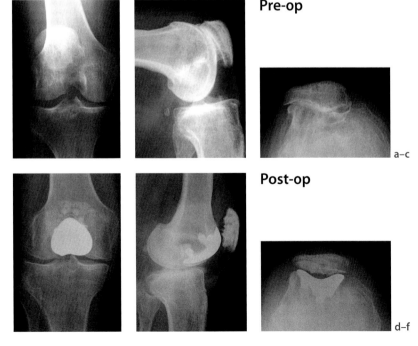

Fig. 2.10 a–f. Isolated patellofemoral arthroplasty for patellofemoral osteoarthritis. The congruity of the patellofemoral joint and the tracking of the patella are crucial

Pre-op

a–c

Post-op

d–f

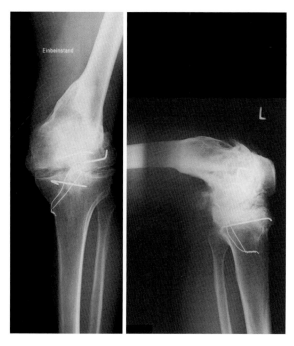

Fig. 2.11. The main indication for TKA in younger patients is post-traumatic injury that is severe enough to preclude osteotomy and other measures

Total Knee Arthroplasty

Total knee arthroplasty is indicated when all other options are unsuitable and should be seen as a last resort, with the exception of knee arthrodesis. This procedure should be offered cautiously to properly selected patients. Main symptoms for index TKA include pain caused by degeneration, appropriate radiographs, and unacceptable reduction of daily living activities. Deviation of mechanical axes must be appreciated in all cases prior to surgery (Figs. 2.11, 2.12). TKA may be suitable for patients in their 20s in cases of severe rheumatoid arthritis or arthritic knees post-trauma.

Bibliography

Krackow KA (1990) The Technique of Total Knee Arthroplasty. The C.V. Mosby Company

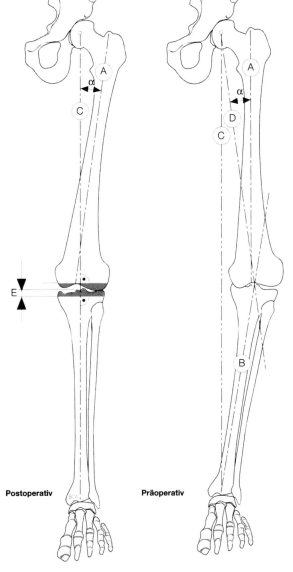

Fig. 2.12. Normal alignment involves restoration of the proper mechanical axis and joint line orientation, with the mechanical axis passing from the center of the femoral head through the center of the knee and on to the center of the ankle

2.2 Fixation: Cement, Hybrid or Cementless?
Peter A. Keblish, Jens G. Boldt

The issue of prosthetic fixation in total knee arthroplasty (TKA) is multifactorial and includes surgical options from cement to cementless to hybrid fixation (one component cemented, the other cementless). Preferences differ significantly and vary with respect to experience, training, interest and understanding of surgical technique, fixation, cost (if applicable to hospital), and other factors such as prosthetic design and its relation to interface fixation. Failures of the original fixed bearing TKA stimulated design changes to address issues of patella tracking, bearing overload, and fixation. Cementless fixation was introduced in the early 1980s to address cement-related failures in an attempt to allow for potential lifetime fixation. With improvements in design and technique, problems at the femoral and patella interface have been reduced to a point of minimal concern. However, design changes that increased constraint at the articulating interface also increased fixation stress and aseptic loosening, resulting in a decreased enthusiasm for cementless tibial fixation area. Tibial fixation problems in TKA are of primary concern, as the majority of failures (cemented and cementless) have been reported at the tibial side. Cement failures were usually related to undersizing (limited sizes), slight malposition and/or less than ideal surgical technique. Tibial fixation concerns without cement resulted in the addition of screws, fins, etc., to provide for initial stable fixation. Changes such as addition of tibial platform screws have led to other problems, including access of backside polyethylene wear and osteolysis. The addition of fins for early rotational stability has the relative disadvantage of obliterating radiographic visibility of the tibial interface, making interpretation more difficult.

Three basic options are available in TKA fixation: cemented TKA – all components, cementless TKA – all components, and cemented tibia (and patella) with cementless femur.

Cemented TKA – All Components

The surgeon performing standard fixed bearing TKA cements femur, tibia, and all polyethylene patella components. Reported results and findings support this approach (Whiteside 1995, Ranawat et al. 1986, Rand). Aseptic loosening and patella problems related to fixation, dislocation and/or maltracking remain an issue in metal-backed patellar components. Not resurfacing the patella is an option with proper design (such as the low contact stress, LCS) and is discussed in Sect. 3.1. Surgical patient selection varies with rationale related to age, bone quality, medicolegal issues, peer pressures, training, etc. Cement should be utilized if there is any question of stability/alignment at trial reduction. With proper sizing and surgical technique, cement fixation is reproducible at the 99% level in modern condylar components, which are well designed. Cement has disadvantages, which are well known, and failures remain.

Cementless TKA – All Components

There are many advantages to performing cementless arthroplasty, which include: (1) potential for lifetime fixation; (2) improved surgical technique; (3) shorter operating time; and (4) preservation of bone stock. The success of cementless TKA appears to be design dependent, therefore the surgeon must be knowledgeable of the prosthesis being used. Biological coatings such as hydroxyapatite may prove to be of value on porous-coated tibial surfaces.

Disadvantages include: (1) higher prosthetic costs depending on hospital contacts; (2) requirement of more precise surgical technique and prosthetic fit; (3) uncertainty of bone quality; (4) reports of increased (although low) primarily tibial failures secondary to tibial loosening; and (5) uncertainty in cases of unexplained periprosthetic pain, perhaps the most important clinical issue.

Cemented Tibia (and Patella) with Cementless Femur

This approach has evolved because of unpredictability of tibial fixation in some designs and predictability of femoral cementless fixation in most designs. Advantages include: (1) ease of surgery – especially in the obese and/or difficult primary TKA; (2) removing the primary source of potential problems such as unexplained pain and diagnostic dilemma presented with cementless tibial fixation; (3) technique – when resurfacing an all-polyethylene patella, the tibia and patella can be treated with a single batch of cement under direct vision. The femur is then press fit, which allows improved time considerations regarding exposure, cement setting time, and cement removal, therefore eliminating potential errors inherent in cementing all components at the same time.

Oligocement TKA – Tibial Component

The concept of cementing surfaces closest to the articulating areas (distal femur, proximal tibia) of short-stemmed components has been utilized and reported in primary TKA, based on success with use in long-stemmed revision components (Vince). This method has not been tested in most primary systems and is not recommended because of early failure rate. This concept is biomechanically unsound because upper tibial cancellous bone strength is less than optimum (Volz et al. 1988). Similarly, designs with cementless (porous-coated) undersurface and smooth non-porous-coated short stems have been unsuccessful. Weak central tibial metaphyseal bone is best treated with bone graft and/or cement or fully coated components. Stress shielding is not an issue when diaphyseal fixation is avoided, which is the case in most primary tibial designs.

Bone cement or polymethylmetracylate (PMMA) has stood the test of time in TKA. Some improvements have been made, but the basic polymer–monomer mixture as developed by John Charnley remains the standard in TKA, whereas it is being used less frequently in total hip arthroplasty (THA) worldwide because of improvement and proven results with cementless acetabular and femoral stem fixation. Femoral stem fixation has emerged as a more problematic area because higher rotational torque forces exist at the cement–prosthetic–bone interface. The well-documented fact that PMMA is weaker in stress (Collier, Fisher, Greenwald) and cement mantle continuity is less predictable remains of concern in femoral fixation. TKA cementation mixing techniques (centrifugation, vacuum, etc.) are also less critical since the technique is more of a "grouting" than in primary THA surfaces. In TKA, surfaces face more compressive loads throughout functional range of motion on the tibial side in well-designed components, especially mobile bearings. Therefore tibial fixation has been proven to be predictable.

Cementless fixation eliminates one of the variables (cement) and requires a biologic bonding at the prosthetic–bone interface. Variations in type of surface treatment (porous coating, grit blast, hydroxyapatite, fiber mesh, etc.), areas of surface treatment (partial, complete), and the time relationship after implantation must be understood to evaluate radiographs properly postoperatively. However, uncemented fixation remains a more controversial issue in TKA than in total hip replacements, especially at the tibial side (Schmalzried) (Figs. 2.13–2.15).

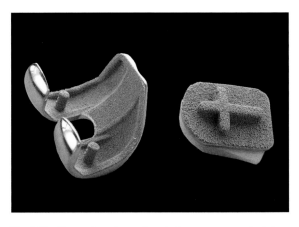

Fig. 2.13. Femoral and patellar design, porous-coated fixation surfaces

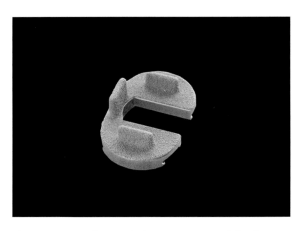

Fig. 2.14. Tapered cone design, porous-coated fixation surface of the tibial platform

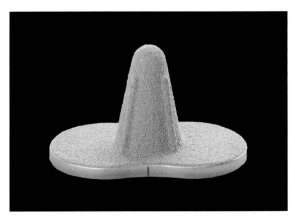

Fig. 2.15. Three-fin design, porous-coated fixation surface of tibial platform

The biology of the bone/implant fixation is multifactorial and has been widely studied and reported in the literature (Bloebaum et al. 1991, Gross, Barrack, Engh et al. 1988, 2002, Whiteside 1995, Ranawat et al. 1986, Ryd and Egund 1995). The interpretation of radiographic radiolucent lines (RLL) can be difficult and must be correlated to clinical findings. RLL at the interface in uncemented and cemented total joint arthroplasties and their interpretation have been of major interest since the beginning of total joint arthroplasty (Vyskocil et al. 1999, Whiteside 1994, Ecker et al. 1987, Matthews and Goldstein 1992). The appearance of RLL differs in cemented and uncemented TKA components. Fixation failures in cemented implants are frequently identified radiographically as extensive (global) lucent lines and zones at both the cement–prosthetic and cement–bone interface. Whereas cemented prostheses show fewer RLL early (first year of implantation) with a tendency to increase with time, uncemented prostheses have shown the opposite tendency. With uncemented implants, RLL are commonly seen within the first few months postoperatively and show radiographic improvement over time in successful cases (Kim 1990). These observations are generally accepted and have been shown in histological investigations of retrieved material by Engh et al. (1993), and classified as biological fibro-osseous integration. Histological investigations of retrievals of 1–2 mm RLL have shown a combination of both osseous and fibrous integration and represent biological remodeling (Cook et al. 1989, Engh et al. 1993). Occurrences of RLL in uncemented TKA are multifactorial and more critically dependent on the type of implant, the surgical technique, and the alignment of the components used.

Osseointegration is the goal of fixation at the interface of uncemented total joint components. Micromotion at the interface is a major contributing factor in the success or failure of osseointegration. Micromotion of up to 0.6 mm is considered acceptable and may positively influence fibrous–osseous integration (Ryd and Egund 1995), whereas micromotion of more than 1.9 mm has shown a higher incidence of RLL and clinical failure. When using cementless implants, osseointegration is required to eliminate the gasket effect (potential pumping of fluid and debris into the interface), that can lead to loosening and/or osteolysis. Occurrences of RLL in uncemented implants are highly dependent on the type of implant, the surgical technique, and the alignment of the components. Whiteside (1995) showed that circumferential porous coating was more resistant to the development of RLL at the tibial interface. Solid ingrowths of bone into porous-coated tibial implants was also studied by Ryd and Egund (1995) using roentgen stereophotogrammetric analysis, which demonstrated subsidence of 0.2–1.0 mm. These findings correspond with the theory of bone healing under limited micromotion (Farron et al. 1995).

Many mechanical factors influence fixation in uncemented TKA and include: (1) exacting interference fixation technique (Ranawat et al. 1986); (2) proper alignment of the knee joint; (3) prosthetic design, which allows for optimum surface area articulation (low contact stress) and low constraint (tension) forces at the bone–implant interface; and (4) adequate host bone quality to support the implant loads. Since mechanical fixation sets the stage for ultimate biologic osseointegration, cortical coverage and bone surface treatment are also important in achieving immediate mechanical fixation. Any deviation of technical accuracy can unfavorably influence outcomes. Bone surface treatment should include the generous use of morcelized cancellous autograft fill of the central tibia, cortico-cancellous strut grafts for slope-off deformities or soft zones (rheumatoid/osteopenic bone) of the distal femoral condyles or tibial plateaus, and bone paste for surface defects (Fig. 2.16). Bone graft material is readily available and can be harvested as needed. Bone paste is best collected from saw cuts and drillings. The use of autologous bone grafting has shown improvement in graft–host continuity. Bloebaum et al. (1992) demonstrated bony ingrowths of 8–22 % in retrieved tibial components 3–48 months after implantation. Cook et al. (1989) reported histological evidence of 50 % bone ingrowths into the porous coating in retrieved material, even in cases showing sclerotic lines close to the tibial component on radiographs.

Prosthetic design and component surface treatment are important considerations, especially in cementless TKA. Currently, the most common uncemented TKA designs are fixed bearings with various articulating geometries, often with screw fixation for "immediate fixation" on the tibial side (Whiteside 1994). Surface treatments of CoCr or treated titanium substrates, when used for cementless fixation, include porous coatings of various size and depths, fiber mesh, hydroxyapatite, or combinations. Partially or fully porous-coated prostheses have been used successfully in uncemented total joint arthroplasties. Size, shape, and bone ingrowths vary with different surface structures currently utilized for cementless implantation. Porous size, coating technique, and prosthetic interface design are very variable and most likely influence outcomes. Results must be

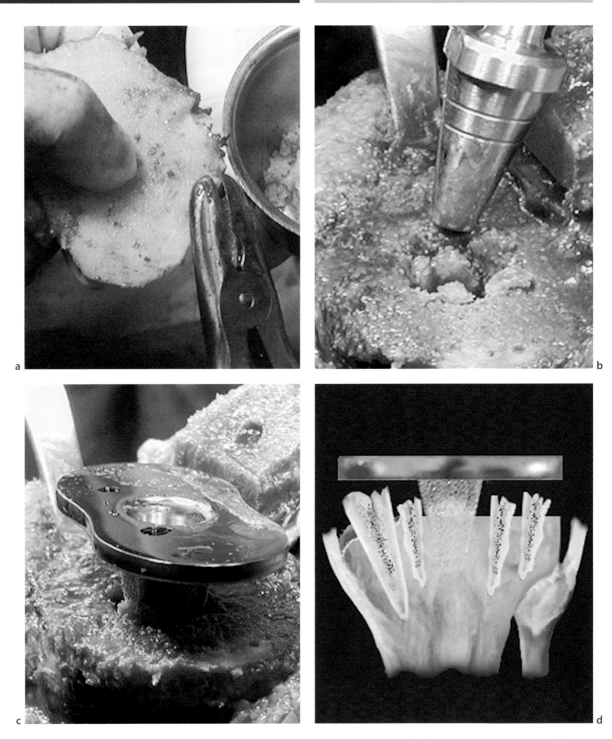

Fig. 2.16 a–d. Autologous bone graft technique. a Preparation of bone graft material; b impaction of morcellized bone chips into the instrumented tibial anchoring zone; c impaction of either morcellized graft, slurry, and/or bone paste on the tibial surface with the permanent component; d impaction of cortico-cancellous strut grafts in the softer central tibia metaphysis

measured for the specific prosthesis utilized. Therefore surgeons utilizing cementless implants must know the specifics and track record (results) of the prosthesis they are using.

Clinical Experience with Cementless LCS

We studied 709 consecutive primary cementless TKAs; 567 cases with complete radiographic and clinical review entered the study. All cases were performed by one senior author or under his direct supervision between May 1984 and December 1996. Mean follow-up was 5.7 years (2.0–14.9). There were 369 (65.1%) females and 198 (34.9%) males with a mean age of 68.6 years (32–94). The primary diagnosis was osteoarthritis (OA) in 502 (88.5%) cases, rheumatoid arthritis in 47 (8.3%) cases, and other non-inflammatory diagnoses in 18 cases (3.2%).

Prosthetic components utilized were the LCS anatomic femoral and metal-backed rotating patella designs (Fig. 2.13). Two different tibial designs were utilized. The tapered cone design (n=523) was utilized for both the posterior cruciate ligament (PCL) sacrificing rotating bearing (n=168) and the PCL retaining meniscal polyethylene bearing inserts (n=445). Both tapered cone designs are identical at the bone interface side (Fig. 2.14), but different on the bearing sub-surface side. The cruciate ligament sacrificing design is open centrally for accommodation of the rotating platform; the PCL retaining design has a posterior cut-out for the PCL retaining meniscal bearings with the same outer cone. The three-fin design (n=44) allows for the anterior cruciate ligament (ACL)/PCL meniscal bearing polyethylene inserts, which require retention of the cruciate bridge and, therefore, a different fixation interface surface (Fig. 2.15). The surface areas of the three-fin design, the tapered cone configuration, and the femoral and metal-backed patellar components are fully porous-coated with Porocoat (DePuy, Inc., Warsaw, Indiana, USA). The porous-coated implants described by Pilliar and Bratina consisted of a sintered porous bead coating with a volume porosity of 35–45% and an average pore size of 200–250 µm (Figs. 2.17–2.22).

Clinical results of all 567 cases were divided into non-inflammatory (OA) and inflammatory cases (rheumatoid arthritis). Of 520 OA cases, 493 (94.7%) had excellent or good results, 19 (3.7%) had fair results, and 8 (1.6%) had poor results. Mean preoperative score in the OA group was 54.7 points (27–85), and latest mean postoperative score was 87.3 points (51–99). Eleven patients had a decreased postoperative score at the latest evaluation, including those requiring revision surgery.

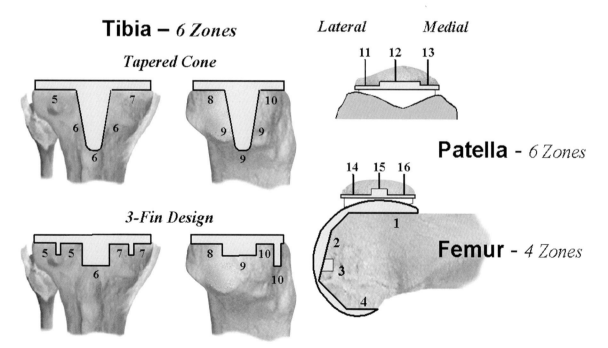

Fig. 2.17. Tibial interface zones of the tapered cone and three-fin design

Fig. 2.18. Femoral and patellar interface zones

Presence and Distribution of RLL in Femoral Zones 1 to 4.

Fig. 2.19. Presence and distribution of RLL in femoral zones 1–4

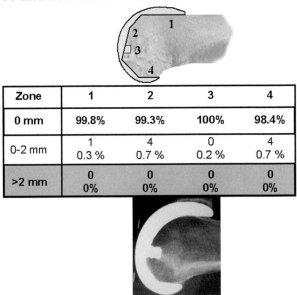

Zone	1	2	3	4
0 mm	99.8%	99.3%	100%	98.4%
0-2 mm	1 0.3 %	4 0.7 %	0 0.2 %	4 0.7 %
>2 mm	0 0%	0 0%	0 0%	0 0%

Presence and Distribution of RLL in Patella Zones 11-16

Fig. 2.20. Presence and distribution of RLL in patellar zones 11–16

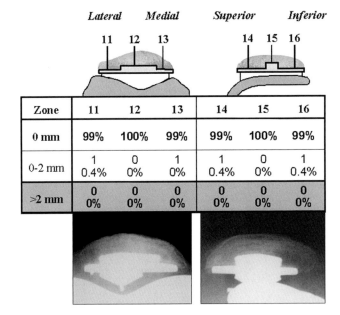

Zone	11	12	13	14	15	16
0 mm	99%	100%	99%	99%	100%	99%
0-2 mm	1 0.4%	0 0%	1 0%	1 0.4%	0 0%	1 0.4%
>2 mm	0 0%	0 0%	0 0%	0 0%	0 0%	0 0%

Complications

Thirty-two cases (5.6%) required revision surgery related to a combination of technical and/or polyethylene failures. Four cases (0.7%) were tibial fixation failures, as noted above; one (0.2%) septic loosening, and three (0.5%) aseptic loosenings. Three of the four aseptic loosening cases were bi-cruciate (ACL/PCL) retaining meniscal bearing devices with a three-fin design (Fig. 2.23), and one PCL-substituting rotating platform device (tapered cone) complicated by delayed sepsis. Three of the four cases that showed aseptic tibial loosening had a varus malposition of the tibial component of >6 degrees on immediate postoperative radiographs. One case of rheumatoid arthritis (0.3%) represented a late (metastatic) septic loosening of a tibial rotating platform device, which was superimposed on progressive varus subsidence

Fig. 2.21. Presence and distribution of RLL in tibial zones 5–7 evaluating tibial cone design

Presence and Distribution of RLL in Tibial Zones 5 to 10

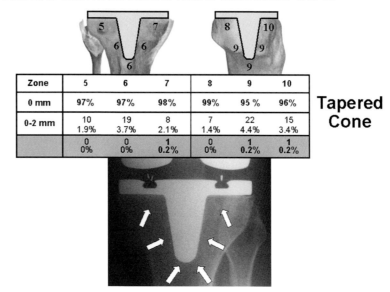

Zone	5	6	7	8	9	10	
0 mm	97%	97%	98%	99%	95 %	96%	**Tapered Cone**
0-2 mm	10 1.9%	19 3.7%	8 2.1%	7 1.4%	22 4.4%	15 3.4%	
	0 0%	0 0%	1 0.2%	0 0%	1 0.2%	1 0.2%	

Fig. 2.22. Presence and distribution of RLL in tibial zones 5–10 evaluating tibial three-fin design

Presence and Distribution of RLL in Tibial Zones 5 to 10.

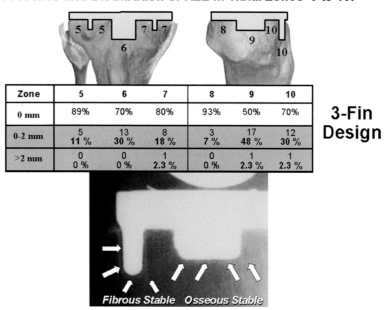

Zone	5	6	7	8	9	10	
0 mm	89%	70%	80%	93%	50%	70%	**3-Fin Design**
0-2 mm	5 11 %	13 30 %	8 18 %	3 7 %	17 48 %	12 30 %	
>2 mm	0 0 %	0 0 %	1 2.3 %	0 0 %	1 2.3 %	1 2.3 %	

Fibrous Stable   Osseous Stable

12 years after surgery. This case was considered to be a fixation failure prior to the infection. Tibial survivorships of 99 and 97 % were reported by Sorrells and Jordan et al. (1997) utilizing the LCS tapered cone meniscal and rotating platform designs. Personal results with LCS cementless knee implantation have been reported. However, neither of these studies addressed specific radiolucent zonal analysis, which this study evaluates in detail.

Fixation has evolved from a major to a relatively minor cause of poor outcomes and re-operation in TKA. The combination of better operating techniques, improved prosthetic design such as "stress relieving" mobile bearings, more sizes for optimum fit, improved bone cement, etc. have improved outcomes in cemented, cementless and hybrid fixation. Cement fixation remains the most predictable method in most designs with an expectation of 99 % success

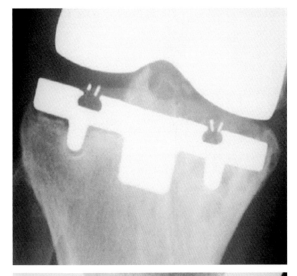

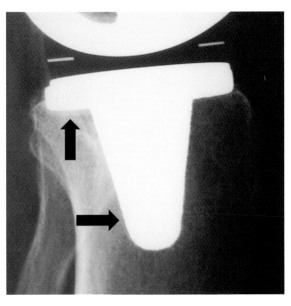

Fig. 2.24. Example of stable osseous and fibro-osseous fixation in tibial zones 8–10

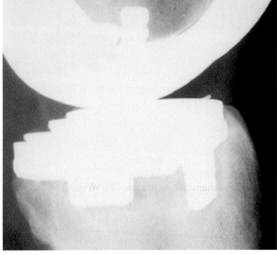

Fig. 2.23. Radiographs showing a fixation failure secondary to an aseptic loosening with subsidence and varus deformity

rates. Cementless fixation appears to be more design specific with results equal in systems such as the LCS mobile bearing. The current study reports a 99.3% overall success rate and a 99.8% success rate with a tapered cone design. Cementing all components or hybrid fixation should minimize or eliminate concerns of cementless failure (Figs. 2.24 and 2.25).

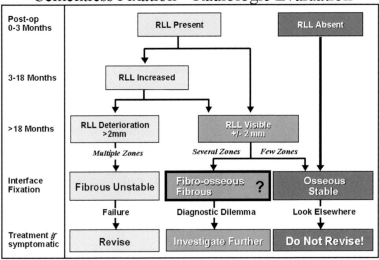

Fig. 2.25. Proposed algorithm for evaluation of treatment of cementless TKA utilizing RLL radiographic analysis

Bibliography

Aglietti P, Buzzi R (1988) Posterior stabilised total-condylar knee replacement. Three to eight years follow-up of 85 knees. J Bone Joint Surg [Br] 70B:211–216

Baldwin JL, El-Saied MR, Rubinstein RA Jr (1996) Uncemented total knee arthroplasty: report of 109 titanium knees with cancellous-structured porous coating. Orthopedics 19:123–130

Berger RA, Lyon JH, Jacobs JJ, Barden RM, Berkson EM, Sheinkop MB, Rosenberg AG, Galante JO (2001) Problems with cementless total knee arthroplasty at 11 years followup. Clin Orthop 392:196–207

Bizzini M, Boldt J, Munzinger U, Drobny T (2003) Rehabilitation guidelines after total knee arthroplasty. Orthopade 32(6):527–534

Bloebaum RD, Rhodes DM, Rubman MH, Hofmann AA (1991) Bilateral tibial components of different cementless designs and materials. Microradiographic, backscattered imaging, and histological analysis. Clin Orthop 268:179–187

Bloebaum RD, Rubman MH, Hofmann AA (1992) Bone ingrowth into porous-coated tibial components implanted with autograft bone chips. Analysis of ten consecutively retrieved implants. J Arthroplasty 7:483–493

Bloebaum RD, Bachus KN, Jensen JW, Hofmann AA (1997) Postmortem analysis of consecutively retrieved asymmetric porous-coated tibial components. J Arthroplasty 12:920–929

Boldt JG, Munzinger UK, Zanetti M, Hodler J (2004) Arthrofibrosis associated with total knee arthroplasty: gray-scale and power Doppler sonographic findings. AJR Am J Roentgenol 182(2):337–340

Boldt J, Munzinger U, Keblish P (2004) Comparison of isokinetic strength in resurfaced and retained patellae in bilateral TKA. J Arthroplasty 19(2):264

Buechel FF (1982) A simplified evaluation system for the rating of the knee function. Orthop Rev 11:9

Bugbee WD, Ammeen DJ, Engh GA (2001) Does implant selection affect outcome of revision knee arthroplasty? J Arthroplasty 16:581–585

Chockalingam S, Scott G (2000) The outcome of cemented vs. cementless fixation of a femoral component in total knee replacement (TKR) with the identification of radiological signs for the prediction of failure. Knee 7:233–238

Cook SD, Barrack RL, Thomas KA, Haddad RJ Jr (1989) Quantitative histological analysis of tissue growth into porous total knee components. J Arthroplasty 4 [Suppl]:S33–S43

Duffy GP, Berry DJ, Rand JA (1998) Cement versus cementless fixation in total knee arthroplasty. Clin Orthop 356:66–72

Ecker ML, Lotke PA, Windsor RE, Cella JP (1987) Long-term results after total condylar knee arthroplasty. Significance of radiolucent lines. Clin Orthop 216:151–158

Engh CA, Hopper RH Jr (2002) The odyssey of porous-coated fixation. J Arthroplasty 17 [Suppl 1]:102–107

Engh CA, Zettl-Schaffer KF, Kukita Y et al (1993) Histological and radiographic assessment of well functioning porous-coated acetabular components. A human postmortem retrieval study. J Bone Joint Surg Am 75A:814–824

Engh GA, Bobyn JD, Petersen TL (1988) Radiographic and histologic study of porous coated tibial component fixation in cementless total knee arthroplasty. Orthopedics 11:725–731

Ewald FC (1989) The Knee Society total knee arthroplasty roentgenographic evaluation and scoring system. Clin Orthop 248:9–12

Farron A, Rakotomanana RL, Zambelli PY, Leyvraz PF (1995) Total knee prosthesis. Clinical and numerical study of micromovements of the tibial implant. Rev Chir Orthop Reparatr Appar Mot 80:28–35

Fukuoka S, Yoshida K, Yamano Y (2000) Estimation of the migration of tibial components in total knee arthroplasty. A roentgen stereophotogrammetric analysis. J Bone Joint Surg Br 82B:222–227

Hartford JM, Banit D, Hall K, Kaufer H (2001) Radiographic analysis of low contact stress meniscal bearing total knee replacements. J Bone Joint Surg Am 83A:229–234

Jordan LR, Olivo JL, Voorhorst PE (1997) Survivorship analysis of cementless meniscal bearing total knee arthroplasty. Clin Orthop 338:119–123

Keblish PA. Schrei C, Ward M (1993) Evaluation of 275 low contact stress (LCS) total knee replacements with 2- to 8-year follow up. Orthop Int Edn 1:168–174

Khaw FM, Kirk LM, Gregg PJ (2001) Survival analysis of cemented Press-Fit Condylar total knee arthroplasty. J Arthroplasty 16:161–167

Kim YH (1990) Knee arthroplasty using a cementless PCA prosthesis with porous-coated central tibial stem. Clinical and radiographic review at five years. J Bone Joint Surg Br 72B:412–417

Konig A, Kirschner S, Walther M, Eisert M, Eulert J (1998) Hybrid total knee arthroplasty. Arch Orthop Trauma Surg 118:66–69

Matthews LS, Goldstein SA (1992) The prosthesis-bone interface in total knee arthroplasty. Clin Orthop 276:50–55

Matsuda S, Tanner MG, White SE, Whiteside LA (1999) Evaluation of tibial component fixation in specimens retrieved at autopsy. Clin Orthop 363:249–257

Parker DA, Rorabeck CH, Bourne RB (2001) Long-term followup of cementless versus hybrid fixation for total knee arthroplasty. Clin Orthop 388:68–76

Ranawat CS, Johanson NA, Rimnac CM, Wright TM, Schwartz RE (1986) Retrieval analysis of porous-coated components for total knee arthroplasty. A report of two cases. Clin Orthop 209:244–248

Rosenberg N, Henderson I (2001) Medium term outcome of the LCS cementless posterior cruciate retaining total knee replacements. Follow up and survivorship study of 35 operated knees. Knee 8:123–128

Rosenqvist R, Bylander B, Knutson K et al (1986) Loosening of the porous coating in patients with rheumatoid arthritis. J Bone Joint Surg Am 68A:538–542

Ryd L, Egund N (1995) Subsidence of tibial components in knee arthroplasty. A comparison between conventional radiography and roentgen stereophotogrammetry. Invest Radiol 30:396–400

Schroder HM, Berthelsen A, Hassani G, Hansen EB, Solgaard S (2001) Cementless porous-coated total knee arthroplasty: 10-year results in a consecutive series. J Arthroplasty 16: 559–567

Shaw JA (1995) Hybrid fixation modular tibial prosthesis. Early clinical and radiographic results and retrieval analysis. J Arthroplasty 10:438–447

Smith S, Naima VS, Freeman MA (1999) The natural history of tibial radiolucent lines in a proximally cemented stemmed total knee arthroplasty. J Arthroplasty 14:3–8

Stuchin SA, Ruoff M, Matarese W (1991) Cementless total knee arthroplasty in patients with inflammatory arthritis and compromised bone. Clin Orthop 273:42–51

Vigorita VJ, Minkowitz B, Dichiara JF, Higham PA (1993) A histomorphometric and histologic analysis of the implant interface in five successful, autopsy-retrieved, noncemented porous-coated knee arthroplasties. Clin Orthop 293:211–218

Volz RG, Nisbet JK, Lee RW, McMurtry MG (1988) The mechanical stability of various noncemented tibial components. Clin Orthop 226:38–42

Vyskocil P, Gerber C, Bamert P (1999) Radiolucent lines and component stability in knee arthroplasty. Standard versus fluoroscopically assisted radiographs. J Bone Joint Surg Br 81B:24–26

Whiteside LA (1995) Effect of porous-coating configuration on tibial osteolysis after total knee arthroplasty. Clin Orthop 321:92–97

Whiteside LA (1994) Four screws for fixation of the tibial component in cementless total knee arthroplasty. Clin Orthop 299:72–76

2.3 Patella and Extensor Mechanism

Peter A. Keblish, Jens G. Boldt

Patella management in total knee arthroplasty (TKA) remains controversial. Tri-compartmental TKA (with resurfacing of the patella) is performed most commonly, especially in the USA, primarily because of the potential for postoperative pain and early failure when the patella is left unresurfaced. However, since patellofemoral complications with resurfacing have resulted in major and, at times, catastrophic failures, the option of not resurfacing the patella has gained more popularity. If patella non-resurfacing (retention) is to be recommended, clinical outcomes must be equal or better than those of routine patella resurfacing in the specific prosthesis utilized. Different philosophies exist in different countries, regions, and centers regarding the treatment of the patella. Specific selection criteria for optimal treatment of the patella in TKA have not been clearly defined; therefore, options remain. The surgeon should understand patella biomechanics and the characteristics of the prosthesis being used.

The patella has been analyzed in many excellent studies, from normal to diseased states, as well as in TKA. The patella is an integral part of knee joint movements and plays a prominent role in total knee kinematics, whether retained or resurfaced. It acts as a guide for the quadriceps-patella-tendon (QPT) mechanism in centralizing the vector forces to the trochlear groove, protects the joint, and enhances the efficiency of the soft tissues of the extensor mechanism and the distal femur throughout the range of motion. Patella forces have been measured at up to seven times body weight (Reilly and Martens 1972), potentially increasing with TKA, whether resurfaced or retained. Control of these forces is influenced by many factors, including quadriceps–hamstring bal-

ance, the biomechanical axis (extremity), cruciate competence, bone quality, disease process, and others.

The patellofemoral joint is a highly complex articulation and requires equal attention in design at the femorotibial joint during total knee replacement surgery in terms of design, biomechanical, and physiological interaction. Patellar relationships (to the patellofemoral joint) change after TKA, even in an ideal situation. Component position placement (medial vs lateral, superior vs inferior), thickness, tilt, pre-existing "baja", design geometry, etc. can influence patella tracking, often in subtle ways. The success of patella retention is, therefore, multifactorial and dependent upon many factors, including: (1) "patella-friendly" femoral prosthetic design; (2) correct rotational positioning of the femoral component prosthetic design; (3) patella size and quality; (4) patella position (alta/baja); (5) soft tissue balancing; (6) surgical approach; and (7) patella bed management. Many TKA designs appear to treat the femoral–patellar relationship as a secondary thought, requiring patella resurfacing of various dimensions (usually dome-shaped) in order to adapt to different non-anatomical (patella-unfriendly) femoral designs.

Patella Resurfacing Options

Patella resurfacing in TKA was developed in the 1970s at the Hospital for Special Surgery because of a high rate of patella pain with early condylar designs (Insall et al. 1983, Aglietti et al. 1975). The cemented all-polyethylene dome-type patellae became the standard, but poor femoral trochlear designs led to other problems, primarily because of high contact stress and edge loading. The development of metal backing to dome patellae, to allow for cementless fixation (in the 1980s), led to an increasing number of wear failures. Many of these failures were catastrophic because of polyethylene "wear through" and metallosis. Failure rates of 5–15 % were often reported, usually with poor or "unfriendly patella" designs. Subsequently, many fixed bearing design changes were made to address the patella problem. A "second look" at patella retention was reported with many designs, but failure rates were often unacceptable. Femoral design and poor understanding of femoral rotation alignment were common factors in fixed bearing designs, with or without patella resurfacing. Incongruence and contact stress were looked at with renewed interest concerning design (Insall et al. 1983, Freeman et al. 1989). Therefore, most current designs are becoming more accommodating to the patella–femoral articulation.

Fig. 2.26. Comparisons of contact type with various fixed bearing patellofemoral articulations as compared to the LCS rotating design

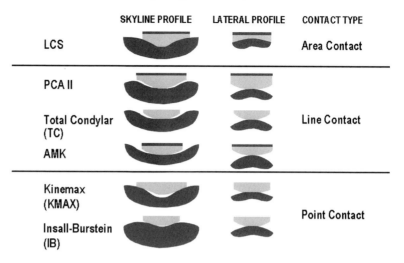

Fig. 2.27. Comparisons of patellofemoral contact stresses with various fixed bearing as compared to LCS mobile bearing prosthetic design

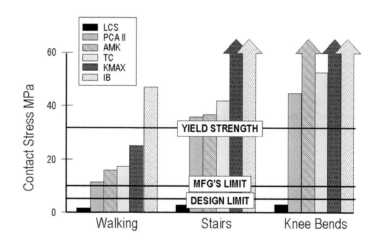

Patella Designs

The all-polyethylene cemented dome-shaped patella has remained the norm for most tri-compartmental knee systems. The surface geometries and contact stresses of the dome vary depending on the femoral trochlear anatomy, sizing, positioning, etc. The majority of designs produce line or point contact as shown in Fig. 2.26. Figure 2.27 shows computed contact stresses in various TKA designs that are frequently above the manufacturer's limit for ultra-high molecular weight polyethylene (Buechel et al. 1991, Pappas). These high-contact areas are accentuated with metal backing and less than ideal femoral rotation alignment, which is addressed in another chapter.

Dome patella results in most modern design TKAs have improved significantly with the improved understanding of soft tissue balancing, femoral–tibial positioning, flexion–extension gap balancing and more recently with mobile bearing TKA designs (other than the low contact stress, LCS). The dome patella has been used successfully with the LCS rotation platform by Johnston in an early experience (as a surgeon's choice) (Callaghan et al. 2000), before the all-polyethylene anatomic LCS design was available. Personal experience using a dome patella with the LCS meniscal and rotating platforms, for technical reasons (mainly spin-out with trial reduction), and in revision cases, supports the use of a dome-type patella with the LCS femoral flange, which was used prior to the development of the all-polyethylene anatomic patella. The compromise (less than perfect contact) appears to be tolerated because of the excellent patella tracking and deep sulcus of the LCS femoral flange, which will be discussed in the next section.

Low Contact Stress Patellofemoral Joint

The LCS patellofemoral and femorotibial articulations were designed by Pappas to accommodate interfaces that require absorption of high loads with angular torque forces. The patella articulates with an area of the femoral surface in deep flexion, which is the same surface the tibia "sees" in near full extension. To accommodate this articulation overlap, the LCS femoral component is designed as a common generating curve for the patella and tibial articulations and a common radius of curvature for most of the patellar articulation and part of the tibial articulation. The femoral component design, from its inception, was also felt to be most accommodating to an unresurfaced patella. The natural patella always articulates against the same surface shape (except near full extension) and therefore can more easily accommodate (with less remodeling) than most other designs that have non-anatomical, varying shapes. This femoral design concept has proven effective for patella function with the LCS moveable and fixed bearing patellar components as well as without resurfacing (Boldt et al. 2004, Keblish et al. 1994, Greenwald). Understanding these design principles is important and allows the operating surgeon patella options with the LCS system that are not available with any other design, namely: (1) metal-backed rotating; (2) all-polyethylene-modified anatomic; and (3) patelloplasty without resurfacing. As noted, the all-polyethylene dome-shaped patella resurfacing component appears to work equally well. These options will be discussed in more detail.

Low Contact Stress Metal-backed Rotating Patella

As noted in the chapter on the LCS design, the rotating patella has been part of the original system and has proven to be effective in multiple reported series (Hamelynk 1998, Keblish 1991, Greenwald, Sorrells 1996, Jordan et al. 1997). The unique design of a metal-backed rotating anatomic unit added a very different and controversial option in addressing the patellofemoral joint (Buechel et al. 1989), as noted in the

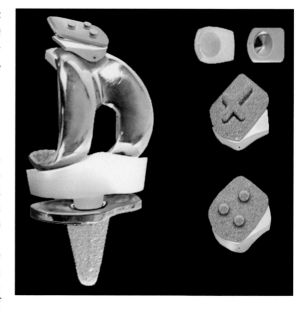

Fig. 2.28. Illustration of the LCS metal-backed rotating patella. Note the original cruciform and more current three-peg base plate, which is available for cement (matt finish) or cementless (porous coat) fixation. The trunnion type modular snap-on design allows for mobility and exchangeability

previous chapter on design. The coronal plane rotation allows for optimal congruent contact in keeping with the LCS principles. The base plate with the original cruciform and current three-peg configuration has been successful from a fixation and mobile articulation standpoint (Fig. 2.28). The trunnion bearing assembly allows for ease of exchange at the time of revision surgery, an option not available with other knee systems, and allows for upgrading with improved polyethylene at the time of revision for tibial or bearing problems, which are the most common indication for revision TKA (Fig. 2.29). The same polyethylene component replacement is available from the original design.

The design allows for options of cemented or cementless fixation, both of which have proven successful in long-term follow-up studies (Jordan et al. 1997, Sorrells 1996). Porous-coated backside (Porocoat, DePuy Orthopedics, Inc., Warsaw, IN, USA) has been modified from the original cruciform to a three-peg base plate for both cement and cementless fixation. The three-peg design allows for easier insertion and less bone removal. Both designs have proven successful. Cementless fixation has been extremely effective and failures are rare. Retrieval specimens have shown excellent osseous integration. Personal experience with fixation (cemented and cementless) over 20 years has shown no bone fixation failures with the

Fig. 2.29. Clinical example of revision surgery with simple trunnion polyethylene bearing exchange. Note excellent congruent tracking of new bearing in deep flexion

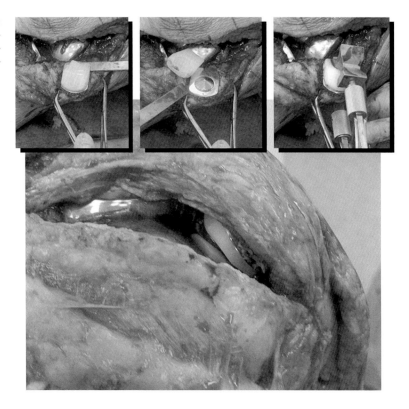

metal-backed components. Other studies have shown under 1% failure rates (Buechel et al. 1989, Pappas, Jordan et al. 1997, Sorrells 1996, Keblish 1991, Hamelynck 1998), most commonly related to patella maltracking. The LCS three-peg fixation system has been available for the past 5–6 years, without any reported changes in outcomes regarding fixation.

The downside of any metal-backed patella is the potential for wear secondary to abnormal tracking (under 1% problem). Rotation of the LCS design adds another potential complication, namely spin-out or edge-loading of the polyethylene insert. Therefore, polyethylene wear (due to a multitude of factors) can be addressed by replacement with superior materials and the same prosthetic design in revision TKA. Large series are not available since failure rates have been low for most LCS series, and patellofemoral complications under 1%.

The rotating patella complications have been low, but problems of spin-out and edge wear have a "potential complication" with a different dimension. Spin-out and/or metallic wear is a serious complication, which has been observed and reported (Hamelynck 1998, Keblish 1991, Jordan et al. 1997, Sorrells 1996). This complication can be avoided by careful trial testing of all component articulations prior to permanent implantation. If any question of edge loading is noted, an all-polyethylene patella should be used. High flexion requirements (eastern cultures) and significant patella baja (infera) are contraindications to use of rotating patella components. Recent reported and personally observed cases have shown an increased rate of polyethylene wear and fractures in this group.

Complications of the LCS rotating anatomic have been under 1% in previously cited series; it remains a treatment option in LCS tri-compartmental replacements. However, potential risks presented by any metal-backed patella, mal-tracking/wear issues and subsequent metal damage have not been totally eliminated. Many surgeons prefer the options of an all-polyethylene resurfacing or not resurfacing. As noted previously, personal experience with patellofemoral mal-tracking and a less than ideal patellofemoral articulation (at trial reduction) has led to the use of an all-polyethylene dome patella with the LCS system (Keblish 1991), with no known failures to date. The recent report by Callaghan et al. (2000) in primary LCS rotating platforms and success with well-fixed dome patellae in LCS revisions suggests that use of an all-polyethylene dome patella (although a minor compromise) is another option in both primary and revision TKA.

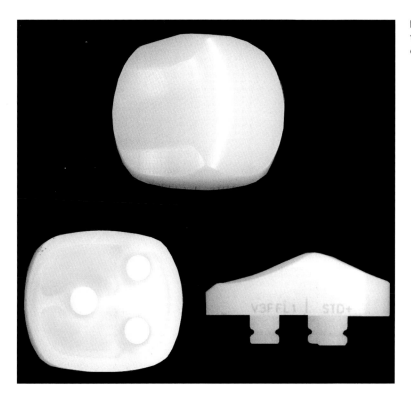

Fig. 2.30. Articulating, backside, and tangential projections of all-polyethylene LCS anatomic patella design

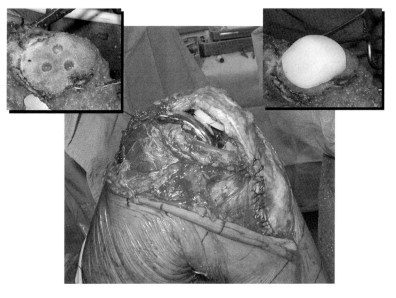

Fig. 2.31. Intraoperative views of preparation, fixation, insertion, and contact areas of the all-polyethylene anatomic design in deep flexion

Low Contact Stress Anatomic All-Polyethylene Patella

Because of the issues stated previously, a three-peg anatomic patella was designed by Pappas in the early 1990s and has had increasing use over the past 5 years. The design (Fig. 2.30) follows the principles of the LCS, namely optimizing area contact against the generating curve of the femoral sulcus (Fig. 2.31). The deep sulcus of the femoral component and soft tissue compliance allow for excellent/near congruent contact throughout the range of motion. Personal experience with the component in over 100 (unpublished) cases has been excellent, with no failures over a 6–7 year time period. This option is being selected as the preferred treatment by many surgeons who routinely resurface the patella and are fearful of metal backing for the reasons stated.

Patella Non-Resurfacing

The other option regarding patella management is retention or not resurfacing the patella bone. Key factors in patella outcomes include femoral component design and rotational positioning, femorotibial positioning and treatment of the extensor mechanism and patella (if left unresurfaced). Multiple designs exist, varying from extreme non-anatomic designs that are too flat to others that are too constrained and are not favorable for patella retention. The LCS femoral component was designed to the natural patella shape and contour with a common generating curve and deep trochlear groove, which best accommodates the unresurfaced patella. These design parameters contribute to patella tracking and stability, which allow for optimum contact with the retained patella or anatomic patella (rotating or non-rotating).

Biomechanical studies on cadaver knees published by Matsuda et al. (2000) demonstrated no change in contact stress independent of patella resurfacing. However, several biomechanical studies of the knee show significant alteration of forces following TKA, including the extensor mechanism and patella. Reuben et al. 1991 have shown that patella thickness reduced to less than 14 mm can decrease tensile strength by as much as 50%, which increases the likelihood of patella avulsions and fractures. Multiple problems of patella resurfacing such as fracture, QPT rupture, component loosening, dislocation, bearing edge wear, increased incidence of heterotopic ossification starting at the patella poles, etc. have been reported in 5–20% of metal-backed resurfaced patellae. Kinematic studies of the normal, anterior cruciate ligament-deficient, fixed bearing resurfaced and mobile bearing resurfaced and unresurfaced patellofemoral joint have shown that the unresurfaced patella with the LCS system best simulates normal (regarding patella tilt, tracking, and separation). The LCS metal-backed rotating patella was second best and fared better than all fixed bearings compared (Stiehl and Cherveny 1996).

Patelloplasty

When the patella is left unresurfaced, assessment of the size, shape, remodeling deformities, position and surface defects may be of importance. A method of treatment of the extensor mechanism including the patella bed has evolved (Boldt et al. 2001). It includes: (1) lateral rim release to include "filet" expansion of the vastus lateralis tendon; (2) circumferential rim cautery for partial denervation (Badalamente and Cherney 1989, Wojtys et al. 1990); (3) osteophyte removal; and (4) downsizing/contouring to original anatomy (Fig. 2.32). A formal lateral release (if required) can be made from outside-in (preferred) or inside-out, as advocated by other authors. The patelloplasty method/steps are modified when the direct lateral approach is utilized, since lateral releases and medial patella mobilization are performed with the arthrotomy (as noted in Sect. 4.12 on the valgus knee) (Buechel et al. 1991, Keblish 1991).

Recent publications have suggested that results of TKA without patella resurfacing can be equally satisfactory in many designs. Freeman et al. (1989) advocated the importance of improved patellofemoral design as early as 1973. Shoji et al. (1989) reported excellent to good results in patients with rheumatoid arthritis with and without resurfacing of the patella in the same patient and did not advocate routine resurfacing in these patients, since there were similar results in the contralateral knee. Keblish et al. (1994) and Boldt et al. (2004) found no significant difference between resurfaced and non-resurfaced patellae (same patient) in a prospective study of LCS knees. Isokinetic strength, however, was significantly greater with an unresurfaced patella when comparing bilateral TKA within the same patient, as reported by Boldt et al. (2004). Key advantages for clinical outcome of patellofemoral function, such as good tracking, improved range of motion, and higher level of activities, were described by those authors who did not find a benefit with patella resurfacing in their studies (Barrack et al. 1997, Shoji et al. 1989, Kajino et al. 1997, Keblish et al. 1994).

Indications and Contraindications for Patella Resurfacing

Setting absolute criteria for patella resurfacing vs non-resurfacing is difficult. In an attempt to establish some guidelines, strong and relative indications for patella resurfacing are suggested (Table 2.1). These criteria represent a combination of the subjective and objective. A near-normal appearance and contour of the patella theoretically favors patella non-resurfacing, and is the most commonly cited criteria advocating selective non-resurfacing. However, no published study has shown that a near-normal macroscopic appearance of the patella is related to better functional outcome. Dye has shown that the majority of patella pain is present primarily at the peripheral tendon insertions and fat pad, supporting the

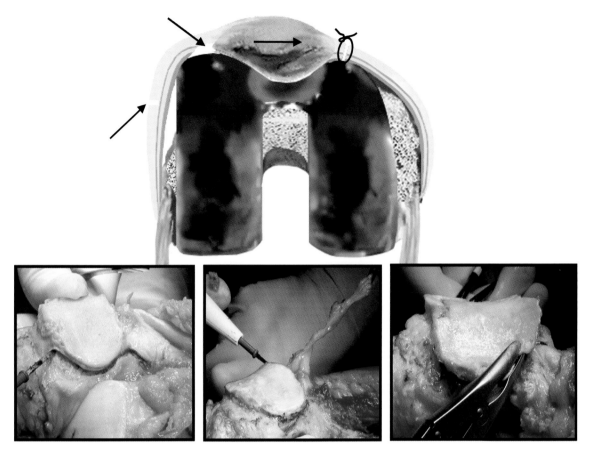

Fig. 2.32. Demonstration of patelloplasty procedure to include detilting with lateral rim release, circumferential cauterization, and osteophyte removal contouring, which allows for anatomic patella tracking. Formal lateral releases (seldom required) are performed preferably via the outside-in method as shown.

Table 2.1. Summary of indications for patella non-resurfacing vs resurfacing

	Patelloplasty (non-resurfaced)	Patella resurfacing
Strong	Small patellae	Wide and/or thick patellae
	Poor bone quality	Non-conforming patellae
	Vascular compromise, release	Severe preoperative patellar pain
	Complex QPT tracking	Multiply operated knee
	Minimal patellar pain	Complex knee pain (RSD)
	Patella baja	Poor patient compliance
Relative	Younger/higher demand patient	Overinformed patient
	Rheumatoid, poor bone stock	Rheumatoid, good bone stock
	Good patient compliance	Poor patient compliance

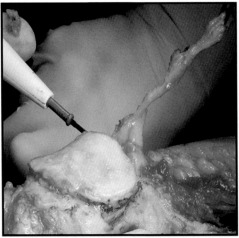

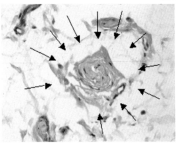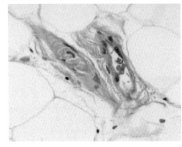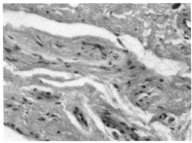

Fig. 2.33. Histologic appearance of extensive nerve supply with routine hematoxylin and eosin-stained patella rim tissue

concept of patelloplasty with appropriate prosthetic designs. Our personal histologic evaluation of patella rim tissue has confirmed a rich nerve supply in the peripheral patella rim tissue, which is also supporting evidence that the majority of patella pain emanates from soft tissue attachments (Fig. 2.33). Long-term evaluation of non-resurfaced patellae frequently demonstrates a neomeniscus-like fibrocartilage rim devoid of nerve supply (Fig. 2.34). If patella non-resurfacing is favored (or contemplated), patients should be advised of the advantages and potential risk factors (primarily anterior knee discomfort), which are slightly higher in non-resurfaced patellae. Therefore, potential informed consent/legal implications for patients with less than ideal outcomes are obviated.

Intraoperatively, patella options should be deferred until trial tibial and femoral reduction has been accomplished. Anatomic alignment and kinematic testing through the full flexion/extension arc will allow for more accurate evaluation of the patellofemoral articulation and influence the decision of whether or not to resurface. Patella options in revision TKA vary from leave alone, debridement when stable, re-resurfacing if the patella bed is sufficient, or reconstruction with autograft, allograft, or newer materials such as tantalum mesh attachments for a polyethylene patella resurfacing.

Surgeons should evaluate the pros and cons of patella management and options of non-resurfacing or resurfacing with various types of prosthetic designs. Key determinants of patellofemoral tracking and ultimate outcomes include attention to proper soft tissue balancing of the extensor mechanism and femoral rotational alignment (Stiehl et al. 2001), which is also addressed in another chapter. The surgeon's goal is to improve the risk/reward ratio and minimize potential complications that lead to less than optimum results and/or need for re-operation. Options presented in this chapter are generic to all TKAs, and also specific to the unique aspects of the LCS design that has proven favorable to long-term patella outcomes with and without resurfacing (Fig. 2.35). Knowledge of the prosthetic design and known results are important considerations in the surgeon's choice in the specific presenting clinical situation.

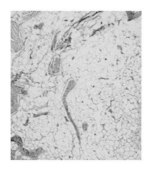

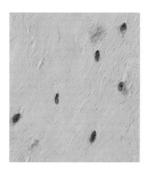

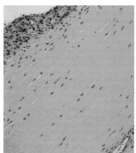

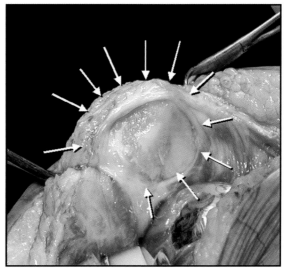

Fig. 2.34. Clinical example of non-resurfaced patella at 10-year follow-up for femorotibial bearing exchange. The patella was left unresurfaced. Histologic studies revealed absence of nerve tissue and highly organized fibrocartilage tissues similar to meniscus tissue

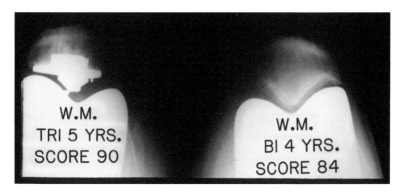

Fig. 2.35. X-ray examples of resurfaced and non-resurfaced patellae at long-term follow-up. Note the perfect contact and congruency

Bibliography

Aglietti P, Insall JN, Walker PS, Trent P (1975) A new patella prosthesis. Design and application. Clin Orthop 107:175–187

Badalamente MA, Cherney SB (1989) Periosteal and vascular innervation of the human patella in degenerative joint disease. Semin Arthritis Rheum 18:61–66

Barrack RL, Wolfe MW, Waldman DA, Milicic M, Bertot AJ, Myers L (1997) Resurfacing of the patella in total knee arthroplasty. A prospective, randomized, double-blind study. J Bone Joint Surg Am 79A:1121–1131

Bizzini M, Boldt J, Munzinger U, Drobny T (2003) Rehabilitation guidelines after total knee arthroplasty. Orthopade 32(6):527–534

Boldt J, Bezzini M, Drobny T, Munzinger U (2004) Comparison of isokinetic strength with/without patella resurfacing in bilateral TKA. AAOS 71st annual meeting, San Francisco, USA, Mar 2004

Boldt JG, Munzinger UK, Zanetti M, Hodler J (2004) Arthrofibrosis associated with total knee arthroplasty: gray-scale and power Doppler sonographic findings. AJR Am J Roentgenol 182(2):337–340

Boldt J, Keblish P, Drobny T, Munzinger U, Varma C (2001) Patella non-resurfacing in low-contact-stress (LCS) mobile-bearing total knee arthroplasty (TKA): results of 1777 TKAs with 2- to 15-year follow-up. Presented at AAOS 68th annual meeting, San Francisco, CA, 28 Febr – 4 March 2001

Boldt J, Munzinger U, Keblish P (2004) Comparison of isokinetic strength in resurfaced and retained patellae in bilateral TKA. J Arthroplasty 19(2):264

Buechel FF, Rosa RA, Pappas MJ (1989) A metal-backed, rotating-bearing patellar prosthesis to lower contact stress. An 11-year clinical study. Clin Orthop 248:34–49

Buechel FF, Pappas MJ, Makris G (1991) Evaluation of contact stress in metal-backed patellar replacement. A predictor of survivorship. Clin Orthop 273:190–197

Buechel FF Sr, Buechel FF Jr, Pappas MJ, D'Alessio J (2001) Twenty-year evaluation of meniscal bearing and rotating platform knee replacements. Clin Orthop 388:41–50

Buechel FF Sr, Buechel FF Jr, Pappas MJ, Dalessio J (2002) Twenty-year evaluation of the New Jersey LCS Rotating Platform Knee Replacement. J Knee Surg 15:84–89

Buechel FF Sr, Buechel FF Jr, Pappas MJ (2003) Ten-year evaluation of cementless Buechel-Pappas meniscal bearing total ankle replacement. Foot Ankle Int 24:462–472

Callaghan JJ, Squire MW, Goetz DD, Sullivan PM, Johnston RC (2000) Cemented rotating-platform total knee replacement. A nine- to twelve-year follow-up study. JBJS [Am] 82:705–711

Dye SF (1996) The knee as a biologic transmission with an envelope of load acceptance: a theory. Clin Orthop 325:10–18

Freeman MA, Samuelson KM, Elias SG, Mariorenzi LJ, Gokcay EI, Tuke M (1989) The patellofemoral joint in total knee prostheses. Design considerations. J Arthroplasty 4 [Suppl]:S69–S74

Hamelynck KJ (1998) The total knee prosthesis: indications and complications. Nederlands Tijdschr Geneeskd 142: 2030–2034

Hartford JM, Herfel C, Kaufer H (2002) Press-fit metal-backed rotating patella: seven- to 14-year followup. Clin Orthop 403:153–160

Insall JN, Aglietti P, Tria AJ Jr (1983) Patellar pain and incongruence. II. Clinical application. Clin Orthop 176:225–232

Jordan LR, Olivo JL, Voorhorst PE (1997) Survivorship analysis of cementless meniscal bearing total knee arthroplasty. Clin Orthop 338:119–123

Kajino A. Yoshino S. Kameyama S. Kohda M. Nagashima S (1997) Comparison of the results of bilateral total knee arthroplasty with and without patellar replacement for rheumatoid arthritis. A follow-up note. J Bone Joint Surg Am 79:570–574

Keblish P (1991) Results and complications of the LCS (Low Contact Stress) knee system. Orthop Belg 57 [Suppl 2]:124–127

Keblish PA (1991) The lateral approach to the valgus knee. Surgical technique and analysis of 53 cases with over two-year follow-up evaluation. Clin Orthop 271:52–62

Keblish PA Alternate surgical approaches in mobile-bearing total knee arthroplasty. Orthopedics (in press)

Keblish PA, Varma AK, Greenwald AS (1994) Patella resurfacing or retention in total knee arthroplasty: a prospective study of patients with bilateral replacements. J Bone Joint Surg [Br] 76:930–937

Kim BS, Reitman RD, Schai PA, Scott RD (1999) Selective patellar nonresurfacing in total knee arthroplasty. 10 year results. Clin Orthop 367:81–88

Matsuda S, Ishinishi T, Whiteside LA (2000) Contact stresses with an unresurfaced patella in total knee arthroplasty: the effect of femoral component design. Orthopedics 23:213–218

Munzinger UK, Petrich J, Boldt JG (2001) Patella resurfacing in total knee arthroplasty using metal-backed rotating bearing components: a 2- to 10-year follow-up evaluation. Knee Surg Sports Traumatol Arthrosc 9 [Suppl 1]:S34–S42

Rand JA, Trousdale RT, Ilstrup DM, Harmsen WS (2003) Factors affecting the durability of primary total knee prostheses. J Bone Joint Surg Am 85A:259–265

Reilly DT, Martens M (1972) Experimental analysis of the quadriceps muscle force and patello-femoral joint reaction force for various activities. Acta Orthop Scand 43:126–137

Reuben JD, McDonald CL, Woodward PL, Hennington LJ (1991) Effect of patella thickness on patella strain following total knee arthroplasty. J Arthroplasty 6:251–258

Shoji H, Yoshino S, Kajino A (1989) Patellar replacement in bilateral total knee arthroplasty. A study of patients who had rheumatoid arthritis and no gross deformity of the patella. J Bone Joint Surg Am 71A:853–856

Sorrells RB (1996) The rotating platform mobile bearing TKA. Orthopedics 19:793–796

Stiehl JB, Cherveny PM (1996) Femoral rotational alignment using the tibial shaft axis in total knee arthroplasty. Clin Orthop 331:47–55

Stiehl JB, Komistek RD, Dennis DA, Keblish PA (2001) Kinematics of the patellofemoral joint in total knee arthroplasty. J Arthroplasty 16:706–715

Wasielewski RC (2002) The causes of insert backside wear in total knee arthroplasty. Clin Orthop 404:232–246

Wojtys EM, Beaman DN, Glover RA, Janda D (1990) Innervation of the human knee joint by substance-P fibers. Arthroscopy 6:254–263

2.4 Unicondylar Knee Arthroplasty

Peter A. Keblish

Historical Background

The concept of unicondylar resurfacing was developed by McKeever and Elliot in the 1950s and utilized through the 1960s (McKeever and Elliot 1960). Cemented hemiarthroplasty (femoral and tibial surfaces) was first reported in the early 1970s in North America by Gunston and Marmor, utilizing the fixed bearing knee with different geometry (Fig. 2.36). The Gunston failed early because of the straight tracks, which failed to allow rotation. During this development period (late 1970s), a few negative reports on unicompartmental knee arthroplasty (UKA) appeared and proved to be damaging to the concept. Most centers abandoned UKA (and its teaching) as a viable treatment option. Therefore, many "trained orthopedists", especially in the USA, have little or no exposure to the procedure. Surgeons from many centers around the world, especially Scandinavia, continued to have a satisfactory experience with hemiarthroplasty. They, and others, have continued to teach and recommend the procedure as an excellent treatment option in angular knee deformity. Moveable bearing arthroplasty was introduced by Goodfellow and O'Connor (Oxford knee) in 1975 (Goodfellow and O'Connor 1982) and subsequently enhanced by Buechel and others (New Jersey LCS; Buechel and Pappas 1989) to improve contact stress kinematics and wear (Fig. 2.37).

Why the difference in approach? Is there a variable population base? Are expectations different? These questions and others are of interest since results and opinions regarding successful UKA vary from surgeon to surgeon, center to center, and country to country. There has been renewed interest in UKA with "minimally invasive" techniques and newer instrumentation, which is reviewed in another chapter.

We have always favored a minimally invasive technique (mid- or subvastus), but one adequate to perform the procedure accurately. Surgeons should be cautioned not to jump on the "minimally invasive" approach for the wrong reasons. UKA is a technically demanding procedure and patient selection is critical. Small incisions, poor patient selection with "oversell", and small technical errors can lead to less than ideal results. Early to intermediate results are now being reported for the "minimally invasive" approach (Repicci). However, the procedure is being hyped by

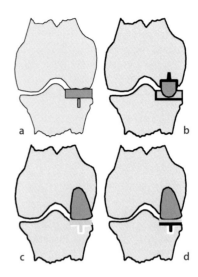

Fig. 2.36 a–d. Fixed bearing UKA designs. **a** McIntosh partial hemicondylar replacement, **b** Gunston straight track (cemented), highly constrained, **c** Marmor type cemented non-metal backed, constrained, **d** metal backed tibial – flat to slightly dished with different models

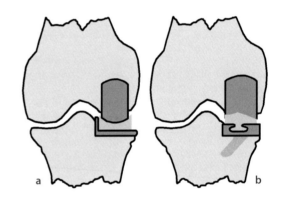

Fig. 2.37 a, b. Mobile bearing UKA. **a** Oxford design fully congruent without track. **b** Design with dovetail radial track and cementless option

many centers previously not familiar with UKA, and caution remains. Is a smaller incision better if it compromises any aspect of the procedure?

Introduction: Surgical Options for Angular Knee Deformity

When angular knee deformity with unicompartment involvement is present, surgical options include total knee arthroplasty (TKA), osteotomy, and UKA. Indications for TKA are well established. High tibial osteotomy (HTO) for genu varum deformity has proven to be effective and remains a well-accepted proce-

Table 2.2. Patient selection factors for angular knee deformity

Factors	Osteotomy	UKA
Deformity	Fixed	Correctable (without releases)
Range of motion	Near normal; age and diagnosis dependent	Normal
Disease process	Osteoarthritis, post-traumatic arthritis, selective inflammatory arthritis (juvenile rheumatoid arthritis, hemophilia)	Osteoarthritis
		Post-traumatic arthritis
		Osteonecrosis
Opposite compartment	Variable near normal; age dependent	Peripheral osteophytes acceptable; normal/near normal
Patellofemoral compartment		
ACL/PCL	Variable; age dependent	Normal; intact and functional
Weight	No limit	Reasonable height/weight ratio
Activity level	No limit	Active with reasonable limits

dure. Supracondylar varus osteotomy for genu valgum is performed less commonly, but is also effective, especially in the young obese female. Literature reviews report satisfactory results of HTO, ranging from 28% (Matthews et al. 1988) to 77% (Coventry 1987), with a general consensus that the procedure is 60–70% successful. Technical problems, need for immobilization, longer rehabilitation, and other factors have dampened the enthusiasm for the procedure (if other options are available) and emphasized the stricter criteria (Table 2.2) required in selecting the best procedure for a given patient.

Unicompartmental arthroplasty provides an alternative to HTO and TKA for angular knee deformity. Criteria and selection factors in the literature to date have been conservative. The procedure is usually recommended for relatively inactive, elderly patients. An increasing number of patients, however, are more youthful, more active, will live longer, and desire to maintain an active lifestyle, including recreational athletics such as tennis, skiing, etc. These patients may be too young for TKA and may not meet the treatment criteria for HTO or newer approaches such as autologous cartilage autotransplantation and allograft (bone-cartilage-meniscal) transplantation, which remain experimental for the intermediate term regarding durability. Improvements in prosthetic design, materials, instrumentation, and surgical technique have renewed interest in UKA for this patient group.

The philosophy of UKA is to realign minimal, correctable angular deformity while preserving normal kinematics. The procedure entails a resurfacing to re-establish the normal ligament environment (cruciates, collaterals) and the mechanical axis to the premorbid alignment, which is dictated by collateral ligament tension. Flexion–extension balancing must be accomplished without lengthening releases, subtle elevation of the joint line, overloading the opposite compartment, overcorrection, or creating patellofemoral impingement.

The advantages of UKA include preservation of: (1) bone stock, (2) normal articulating surfaces of the uninvolved compartments, (3) near-normal kinematics, and (4) normal or near-normal range of motion. In addition, surgical trauma is minimal, blood replacement is not required, rehabilitation is rapid, hospitalization is shorter, and the procedure is cost-effective.

Factors Influencing UKA Outcomes

Patient selection is perhaps the most important factor, followed by prosthetic design and surgical technique if consistent results are to be achieved. All authors have stressed that UKA patient selection is most important, including proper diagnosis, age, activity level, weight, and at times appropriate imaging studies (magnetic resonance imaging, computed tomography) to confirm non-inflammatory single compartment disease. The patient should be well motivated with a good understanding of the philosophy of the procedure. Many patients have had previous arthroscopic surgery with well-documented compartment pathology and overall joint assessment.

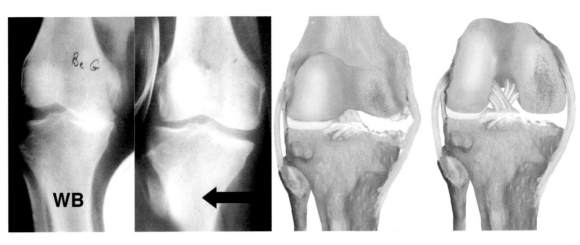

Fig. 2.38. Ideal patient for UKA. Note correctable varus instability with stress x-rays. Ideal anatomic candidate for UKA with isolated compartment disease, a correctable deformity and intact ligaments

Patient permission for conversion to TKA at surgery, if believed to be indicated, should be agreed upon, as more extensive disease may be present than had been anticipated.

Selection Factors for UKA

Based on 30 years of personal experience and supporting literature, the most important criteria for selecting UKA are: (1) a correctable deformity with minimal to no ligament releases, (2) an intact anterior cruciate ligament (ACL), (3) avoiding over-correction and subsequent overload of the opposite compartment, and (4) the surgeon's experience (Fig. 2.38). The operating surgeon must be a "believer" in UKA and be familiar with the technique and system being utilized. He or she must communicate the controversial but conservative nature of the procedure to the patient and family if UKA is not commonly performed in the community. Patients must be well informed and give preoperative consent in all cases to allow conversion to TKA at the time of surgery if the factors listed above prove to be less than ideal, except perhaps in younger patients who understand the risk and are willing to accept discomfort with increased activity.

Prosthetic Design

Prosthetic design is another key factor in achieving successful UKA and must allow for unconstrained motion without mechanical (translational or rotational) blocks. Designs that have attempted to intro-

duce increased stability without allowing for mobility have resulted in premature mechanical failures, while designs with high contact stress have led to failures secondary to polyethylene wear. Two basic designs have stood the test of time: round-on-flat or slightly dished fixed bearing and meniscal bearing with more congruent geometry. Fixed bearing designs include all-polyethylene tibial components (Marmor prototype) and metallic-backed polyethylene tibial components (Brigham prototype), which have been modified to allow for cementless fixation and modularity. Fixed bearing devices that have attempted to add increased congruity may lead to increased torque and tensile forces, high contact stresses with potential loosening and/or subluxation. Meniscal bearing designs include the Oxford (Goodfellow and O'Connor 1982) cemented straight track constant radius and the low contact stress (LCS; DePuy, Leeds, UK) radial track with decreasing radius of curvature.

Mobile Bearing Rationale

Consequences of polyethylene wear have been the primary initiating cause of TKA and UKA failures. Mobile bearing UKA addresses problems of wear with improved congruent mobility, kinematics, stability and potentially normal range of motion. The LCS provides the option of cementless fixation. The biomechanics of the original and second-generation modifications, which have a 25-year follow-up (with no change in articulating geometry), are shown in Figs. 2.39 and 2.40. The ability to exchange polyethylene bearings (Fig. 2.41) is a major advantage, and

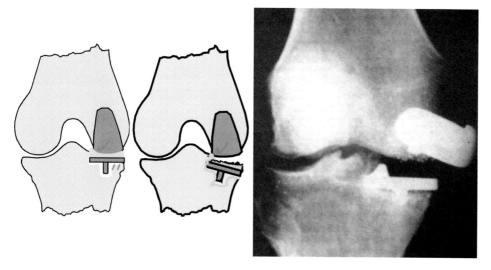

Fig. 2.39. Fixed bearing UKA with built-in constraint on left. Rotational forces can lead to failures in the femoral and/or tibial side

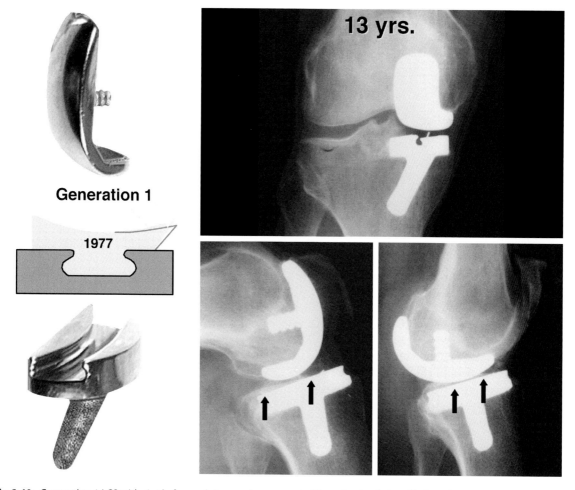

Fig. 2.40. Generation 1 LCS with single femoral stem and unsupported lateral polyethylene lip. Note long-term follow-up with bearing movement posterior in flexion and anterior in extension. There is natural kinematic rollback of the femur

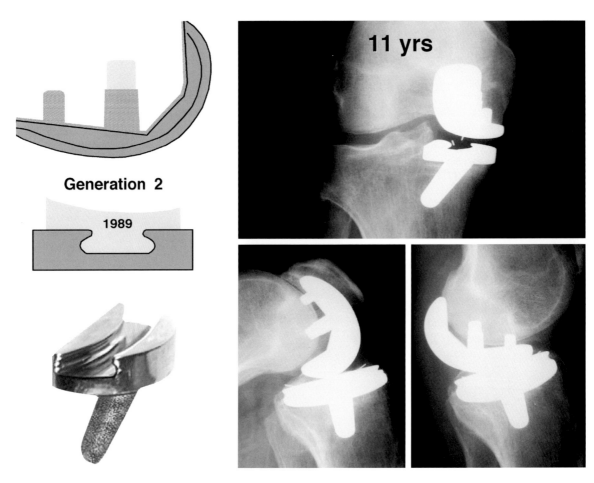

Fig. 2.41. Generation 2 LCS with additional femoral peg and supportive polyethylene edges. Eleven-year cementless follow-up showing no polyethylene wear/osteolysis and normal kinematics in flexion and extension

allows the active young patient an option for longer-term success with minimal operative downtime. Conversion to TKA has not been a problem and is less challenging than HTO conversion in this author's opinion.

Fixed and meniscal bearing knees have been used successfully for over 25 years and provide options for the orthopedic surgeon who believes in the concept of UKA. Both fixed and meniscal bearing knees present the surgeon with the challenge of proper implantation. (More precise instrumentation and improved prosthetic design have enhanced the surgeon's ability to achieve a better outcome.)

Surgical Approach

Surgical technique and principles of accurate surgical alignment in UKA are important factors that are basic to satisfactory outcomes. The technique of UKA is more challenging, and experience with operative techniques is frequently limited in residencies and/or fellowships. Basic surgical principles apply to all design systems and will be addressed with the LCS system (Fig. 2.42).

Medial UKA

A midline anterior skin incision is preferred. The incision is angled distally to the medial side of the tibial tubercle. Minimal undermining is required. The arthrotomy incision can be performed via the standard parapatellar, subvastus or a short midvastus variation, which is the current approach of choice. The midvastus approach, popularized by Engh et al. (1997), splits the medial quadriceps and capsule from the anteromedial attachment of the patella proximally along a natural cleavage plane. A limited medial sleeve release of the upper tibia enhances the expo-

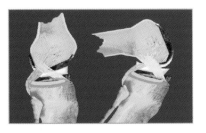
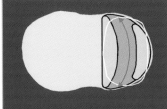
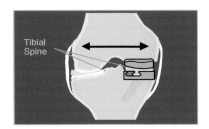
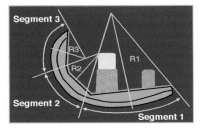
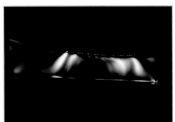
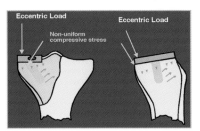

Fig. 2.42. Summary of design and biomechanical rationale of kinematics, movement, geometry, contact stress, and fixation of the LCS unicompartment arthroplasty

sure. The status of the lateral and patellar femoral compartments can be assessed without everting the patella. Patella eversion and extensive exposure are not required in UKA. However, if the surgeon is more comfortable with a more extensive exposure, it is easily accomplished with the midvastus approach. The advantages of patella translocation (rather than eversion) include minimizing the external tibial rotation, which improves rotational positioning, and protecting the normal articular cartilage. Maintaining the bulk of the medial quadriceps to the central tendon allows for better patella control intraoperatively, less postoperative pain, and more rapid rehabilitation.

Lateral UKA

Lateral compartment replacement for valgus instability is best performed via a modified direct lateral approach, which accomplishes the lateral release with the exposure. The skin incision is proximal midline ending distally at a point between Gerdy's tubercle and the tibial tubercle. The arthrotomy incision splits the retinaculum (superficial layer) at the medial border of Gerdy's tubercle and extends proximally, 1–2 cm lateral to the patella. The deep capsular layer is released from the patellar rim. The proximal arthrotomy can be completed by splitting the vastus lateralis, subvastus, or a limited lateral parapatellar incision made obliquely through the central tendon.

The direct lateral approach allows for direct soft tissue release, adequate exposure without everting the patella, improved patellofemoral tracking, minimal soft tissue trauma, and rapid rehabilitation. The approach can be extended if TKA is required, as described in the chapter on the lateral approach and previously by Keblish (2002) and Insall et al. (1994).

Technique Principles

The technical principles of UKA are similar to but subtly different from those of TKA. Re-establishing the joint line of the diseased compartment and restoring the altered anterior cruciate ligament, posterior cruciate ligament, and collateral (medial and lateral) kinematics are key goals of implantation. When proper indications exist, normal knee function is possible. Instrumentation systems plus surgical expertise must provide for accurate compartment resurfacing of the femoral condyle and tibial plateau. Technical errors of malposition (rotational, varus–valgus, flexion–extension) and gap imbalance (depth of resection) will negatively affect stability, mobility, wear, and fixation, with less than satisfactory clinical outcomes (Fig. 2.43). Since few UKAs are performed, even by so-called experts, more attention to detail is required. Excellent long-term results can be appreciated when patient selection, prosthetic design, and surgical technique are optimal. This section addresses the key technical aspects of UKA that will affect clinical results (Keblish 2002).

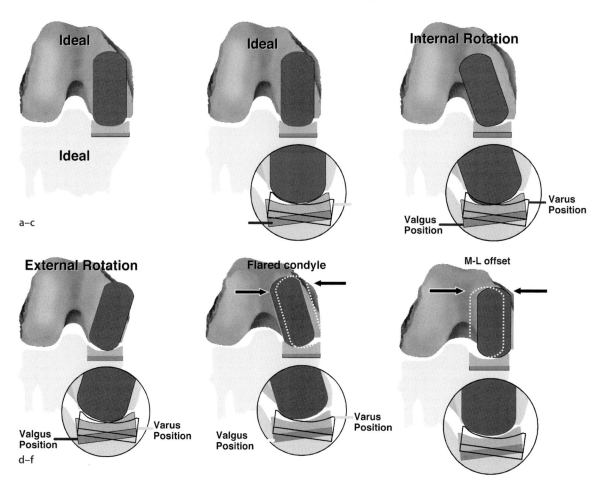

Fig. 2.43. Bone resection (prosthetic position) variables from ideal femoral and tibial placement (in flexion), to malresection potentials. Malresection is compounded if (1) femoral geo- metry is atypical, (2) gaps are unequal, and become less than ideal as the knee ranges from flexion to extension

Bone Resections

Position and Orientation Variables

Effective instrumentation should reliably establish the correct size, position, and orientation of the femoral and tibial components. The variables of axial rotation, varus-valgus tilt, flexion-extension orientation, anteroposterior (A-P) position, and joint line level must be correctly defined by the surgeon using instruments designed for these purposes. Proper flexion-extension gap balancing should allow for unimpeded motion with normal kinematic control. Bone resections are the key element in preparing implantation surfaces and dictate final positioning. The potential for malresection exists on both femoral and tibial sides (Fig. 2.40) and will be described in more detail. Errors are compounded if instrument malposition (malresection) is made on both sides and are more common with anatomic variations such as flared femoral condyles, which may be a contraindication to UKA.

Tibial first or femoral first approaches can be utilized, depending on the UKA system (Stulberg 1990, Cartier et al. 1997, Laskin 1976) and instrumentation philosophy/rationale. Most implantation systems, however, have similar guidelines, which include: (1) referencing off the subchondral bone, which is more consistent, or a fixed point such as the ACL insertion, maintaining the proper joint line; (2) correct tibial rotation to reproduce a perpendicular mediolateral plane with a 5–7 degrees posterior slope; (3) extramedullary instrumentation for the tibial resection; and (4) mating the femoral resection to the tibial resection plane via appropriate resection blocks. Femoral orientation can employ either extramedullary or intramedullary instrumentation. An intramedullary system requires a more extensive

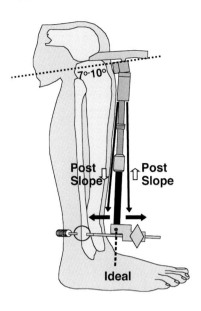

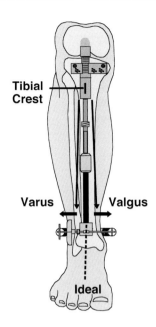

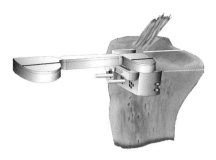

Fig. 2.44. Tibial resection guide emphasizing the proper anteroposterior and lateral positions. *Central illustration* shows the proper depth, plane and rotation of the L-resection, which re-establishes the normal joint line (at the ACL insertion) to allow an 8 mm polyethylene bearing

approach and violation of the femoral canal, both potential disadvantages.

Exposure of the tibial plateau is enhanced by a sleeve elevation that is adequate enough to allow for exposure and removal of peripheral osteophytes to normal anatomy. Preservation of the outer meniscal rim is recommended to maintain the integrity of the medial sleeve, preserve optimal stability, and avoid geniculate vessels.

Tibial and femoral osteophytes are best removed with a reciprocating saw and/or rongeurs to re-establish pre-morbid anatomy. External tibial rotation will improve access to the posterior corner. Loose bodies or remaining posterior osteophytes are removed. Anatomic variants, pathological erosions, the tibial slope, and bone quality are assessed. Articular (cartilage and bone) high points or irregularities should be removed to subchondral bone, since referencing is more accurate and the bone surfaces are more accessible for instrumentation.

The Tibial "L" Resection

Accuracy of the tibial resection is critical and will be determined by proper instrument positioning for variables of rotation (coronal plane), varus–valgus tilt, flexion–extension (A-P slope), horizontal limit (sizing), and depth of resection (Fig. 2.44). Rotational orientation influences varus–valgus and the A-P positions (posterior slope) and, therefore, should be

established first. Malposition of the rotational setting can lead to subtle or obvious changes in the varus–valgus and A-P slope cuts, which may lead to less than ideal resections. Malresections will result in higher contact stress at the articulating surface and increased torque forces at the bone (cement)–prosthetic interface, especially in fixed bearings with round-on-flat or dished geometries.

Tibial Resection Guide Positioning

Extramedullary guide systems are the norm. Lower profile UKA tibial resection guides, as utilized in the LCS system, allow for instrumentation with more limited compartment exposure as recommended. The resection guide should allow for small adjustments of the alignment rod to fine-tune rotation, varus–valgus, and A-P positions. The guide should allow for an adjustable resection block to accommodate the depth of resection changes (Fig. 2.42).

Rotation Alignment

The sagittal plane of the "L" resection dictates the rotational orientation of the tibial component; therefore, this setting is critical. Internal or external positioning will result in rotational malalignment that will be accentuated with the knee in extension.

Varus–Valgus Alignment

The mediolateral resection should be made perpendicular to the anatomic (mechanical) axis of the tibia. The alignment rod is best referenced distally (ankle level) to the tibialis anterior tendon. The lateral border of the tibialis anterior tendon is easily palpable and centers over the midpoint of the talus. This point is slightly medial to the midpoint of the malleus and centers over the second metatarsal when the foot is normal. Medial rod placement will result in a valgus position, and lateral rod placement, which is more common, will result in a varus position. An ideal (perpendicular) resection is critical; therefore, the alignment rod should be rechecked prior to final resection.

Flexion–Extension (A-P) Alignment

Reproducing the patient's normal posterior slope (5–10 degrees) is the goal and is important for restoration of normal kinematics of the ACL/PCL and the so-called four-bar linkage. Alignment systems should allow for A-P adjustment. The LCS resection block is set for a 7 degrees posterior resection when the alignment rod is parallel to the tibial crest and/or fibular shaft as viewed from the lateral side. Anterior placement of the rod will increase the posterior slope while posterior rod alignment will decrease the posterior slope. Some "eye-balling" may be required if external landmarks are obscured. Remember that a neutral or decreased posterior slope will limit roll back and flexion, increase contact stress on the posterior bearing surface, increase polyethylene wear, and increase the potential for prosthetic lift off and prosthetic fixation failure.

The depth of resection is best determined after having confirmed the other variables. The goal is to resect enough bone to allow space for the "total tibial prosthetic thickness" without elevating the joint line (femoral–tibial articulating surface). The most consistent landmarks for establishing the proper depth of resection are the ACL insertion and the upper slope of the tibial spine. The final joint line (articulating interface) should be located at this level to allow for optimal kinematics. The space is more finite in UKA (ACL–PCL controlled) and relates most critically to the normal opposite compartment. Final selection of the tibial component size is determined following completion of the "L" resection. Optimal peripheral bony rim contact should be obtained with abutment of the sagittal tibial surface against the vertical arm of the "L" resection (Fig. 2.44). The ACL insertion must be preserved and the final tibial articulating surface adjusted to the original tibial plateau

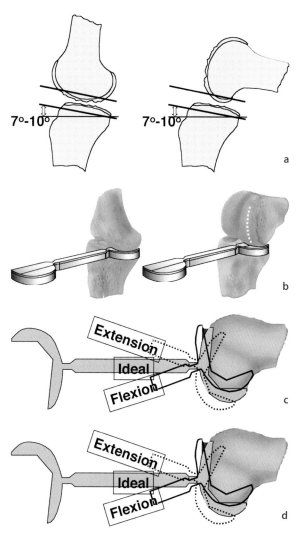

Fig. 2.45. Spacer block placement following tibial resection. Mapping the tibial from flexion to extension confirms the rotational position and flexion/extension gaps

surface. The spacer block of appropriate size and depth is inserted to check all tibial resection variables. A drop rod attached to the guide rechecks the varus–valgus and the A-P slope (Fig. 2.45). Ranging the knee from 90 degrees to full extension rechecks the level and orientation of the tibial resection and maps the rotational tracking to the femoral surface before instrumentation of the femoral side. The tibial resection should be rechecked when the femoral resections are referenced from the tibia, and vice versa if a femoral first approach is used.

Fig. 2.46. The femoral shell/drilling guide is set and the cutting gig is impacted to the subchondral surface to establish the proper depth and plane of the distal campher and posterior cuts (*top* and *bottom left*). Drilling templates are secured and rotation and flexion/extension gap stability is rechecked. Anchoring holes are made for trial and final prosthetic insertion (*top* and *bottom right*).

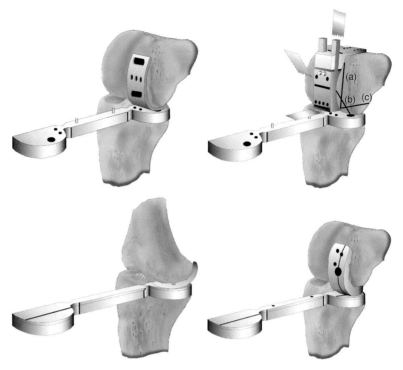

Femoral Preparation and Size Selection

The femoral condyle is frequently irregular, with bony and/or articular cartilage high spots. Referencing from the subchondral bone is more consistent and is recommended with use of most instrument systems, whether a femoral first or tibial first approach is utilized. Removal of irregular high spots from the femoral condyle surfaces is accomplished utilizing an oscillating saw (Fig. 2.46). Smoothing of the subchondral surface allows for better seating of alignment shells or cutting jigs.

Femoral size selection that best approximates the existing bony geometry is initially estimated by use of an A-P template and mediolateral sizing shells (Fig. 2.47). It is important to keep in mind that it is the shape of the subchondral bone and not the articular cartilage that is to be re-established. Rotational (coronal and sagittal) planes are checked. Care must be taken to avoid over-correction and over-sizing, which increases the risk of soft tissue and/or patella impingement. The medial and lateral prosthetic borders should lie flat or just within the femoral condyles. The most superior medial edge is often flush with the condyle in the typical medial UKA. Overhang must be avoided. Flared condyles may present a problem.

Flexion–Extension Gap Balancing

The A-P femoral position (resection) dictates the flexion gap, and the distal position dictates the extension gap. Condylar resections (thickness) must accommodate the prosthetic mass. Checking the flexion and extension gap with a shell positioner assures that the proper amount of bone is resected. If the flexion gap is tight, the sizing template can be moved anteriorly to, but not beyond, the limiting point previously described. Downsizing the femoral component may be required if the flexion gap is too tight or there is impingement anteriorly. It is important to recognize this potential error prior to femoral resection, although it can be corrected following trial component placement. Reattachment of the resection block, however, may be less exact, recuts less precise, and the final fit compromised if previous fixation holes need to be redone.

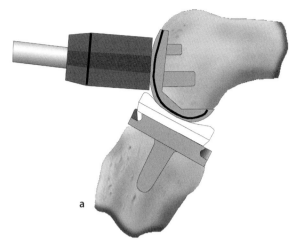

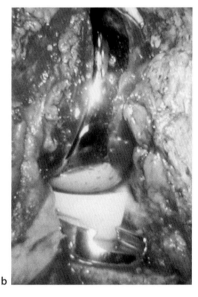

Fig. 2.47 a, b. a The permanent components are driven to the bone surfaces with or without cement. b Final clinical result in deep flexion; excellent contact with posterior bearing movement allows for ideal kinematics.

Femoral Rotation Considerations

The femoral component can be placed correctly, too far medially or laterally, internally or externally rotated (coronal plane), and flexed or extended in the sagittal plane (Fig. 2.43). Malrotation will be exacerbated if these resections are additive and/or combined with tibial malpositioning. As noted above, recognition of these potential errors, by mapping the rotation plane from 90 to 0 degrees, will avoid the initial malresections, as previously illustrated. Internal malrotation of the femoral component will result in: (1) high contact stress on the more central articulation; (2) increased

torque on the prosthetic component; (3) flexion gap instability; and (4) rotational incongruence in extension. External malrotation will result in: (1) high contact stress on the peripheral articulating surface; (2) increased torque; (3) flexion gap instability; and (4) increased potential for soft tissue impingement due to proximal overhang of the prosthesis. Flexion positioning of the femoral component will result in bearing impingement anteriorly in extension. Conversely, extension positioning of the femoral component will result in bearing impingement posteriorly in flexion. Lateral (central) positioning will result in impingement on the tibial spine, whereas medial (peripheral) component positioning will result in medial tibial component overload. Both will increase the potential for patella and/or medial soft tissue impingement. These malrotations (malresections) may lead to increased wear and loosening, the primary cause of failure in UKA.

Femoral Resection

Coronal plane orientation (axial positioning) of the femoral component must align to the tibial component in flexion and extension. Resection blocks should be oriented to the femoral axis and allow for proper flexion–extension position (referencing parallel to the anterior femoral cortex). Take care to set the resection block flush to the subchondral bone. If the block is proud (setting on high points), the distal resection will be inadequate and/or rotationally malaligned. These malpositions will result in a tight extension gap with overcorrection and overload of the opposite compartment and/or an abnormal articulation at the prosthetic interface. Femoral referencing is accomplished with the LCS resection block as an extramedullary approach. Systems using an intramedullary approach are also referencing the anatomic femoral axis and the anterior femoral cortex. Both systems work. Understanding the principles is most important because anatomical variances may require fine adjustments, which are more technically subtle with UKA than TKA.

Final Positioning and Trial Reduction

The trial tibial component should be inserted first, followed by the bearing and the femoral component (Fig. 2.45). Final impaction will position the tibial component against the sagittal resection. A stemmed unit, such as the LCS, may require rotational maneuvering. External rotation of the tibia will aid in exposure and insertion of the tibial component. The bearing is inserted by placing a valgus stress from flexion to extension and back to extension in order to clear the femoral condyle. The femoral component is then impacted, beginning at 100 degrees and completed with the knee at 60–70 degrees. The patella is then reduced and the knee ranged from extension to maximum flexion. Normal, natural range of motion with meniscal bearing movement, anterior in extension and posterior in flexion, confirms normal kinematic control. There should be no patella impingement and no component lift off from either tibial or femoral sides with extremes of motion. The most common cause of lift off or a tight flexion block is failure to slope the A-P resection 7–10 degrees as recommended. Fine-tuning of any resection variables should be completed before permanent prosthetic placement.

Clinical Results of UKA

Surgical outcomes of UKA have varied from the dismal failure rate reported by Insall and Walker (1976), Insall and Aglietti (1980), Swank et al. (1993), and Laskin (1976), to the more optimistic reports of Lewold et al. (1993), Marmor (1988), Kozinn et al. (1989), Scott et al. (1991), Buechel and Pappas (1989), Goodfellow and O'Connor (1982), and others. Why are reported results so variable? Critiques of the negative papers highlight patient selection, surgical technique, and prosthetic design as major causes of failure. The Insall and Walker (1976) report of 24 UKAs is faulted for having a poor design (blunted anterior flange causing patellar abutment), producing overcorrection with thick tibial components and having 15 patellectomies in their series. The Insall and Aglietti (1980) report of 32 knees included the original 24 patients with ten lost to follow-up. The Laskin (1976) report of 37 knees included 35 obese patients with a high incidence of subsidence and failure of the opposite compartment (probable overcorrection and overload). Swank et al. (1993) reported poor results (cementless design) with failure due to dissociation, fixation and medial subluxation. The issue of prosthetic design and ACL competence must be raised in these series.

The positive UKA experience in the literature addresses the factors summarized above and reports satisfactory (good/excellent) results of between 85 and 90%. Perhaps these results can be improved with more strict selection criteria, surgical technique, and improved prosthetic design.

Personal experience with cemented Marmor modular UKA (1972–1980) and the LCS meniscal bearing UKA (1980 to present) at the Lehigh Valley Hospital has been very positive. Prospective evaluation of 109 LCS UKAs followed for a mean of 5.2 years has shown 93% good/excellent results. Ninety-six medial and 13 lateral replacements were performed with cemented (49) and cementless (65) fixation. A longer-term study, being prepared for publication, suggests that cementless and cemented LCS meniscal bearing UKA in a more active population is equal to or better than previous UKA reports and comparable to current TKA results (Sisto et al. 1993). Prosthetic design, fixation, and future improvements in materials are also factors that may improve outcome.

Discussion/Conclusion

Unicompartmental knee arthroplasty remains controversial and its application varies from country to country, region to region, and within orthopedic training centers. Literature reports have been variable, ranging from the negative studies of Insall et al. (1976, 1980), Laskin (1976), and Swank et al. (1993) to multiple positive studies. Advocates of UKA site the multiple advantages, which include: (1) restoration of normal kinematics; (2) preservation of normal structures; (3) avoidance of major problems reported with TKA; (4) maintaining and/or improving functional range of motion, which is frequently decreased following TKA; (5) lower morbidity with no need for blood transfusions, less soft tissue damage, etc.; and (6) lower prosthetic costs and shorter hospitalization. Non-advocates of UKA cite higher failure rates, problems of selection and technique, and difficulty in revision to TKA. Conversion of UKA, however, is reported to be less difficult than revision TKA (Levine et al. (1996), Otte et al. 1997), which has also been this author's personal experience.

All authors agree that patient selection and prosthetic design can influence outcomes. Grelsamer and Cartier (1992) stressed that UKA is not "half a total knee", with major differences mostly related to technical factors, which have been discussed and illustrated. The Swedish knee study (Lindstrand et al. 2000, Lewold et al. 1993) reported improved results of a large series (1,969 cemented Marmor fixed bearing) of UKAs relative to the time of implant. Five-year cumulative revision rates were reduced from 11% (1975–1983 cases) to 5% (1983–1989 cases), suggesting that experience, patient selection, and surgical techniques are major determinants of clinical results.

Materials, improved fixation, and design improvements such as meniscal bearings, which combine controlled motion with matching spherical geometry (Fig. 2.47) and are illustrated in this section, provide potential for improved results (Cohen et al. 1991, Keblish 1994) and early bearing exchange without component removal in the extremely active, younger patient population. Results of the Oxford and LCS UKA compare with or exceed best results reported in the literature. Improvements in technique and experience should further improve outcomes as UKA becomes a more accepted alternative in correctable angular knee deformity. The surgical technique of UKA is more demanding but should not be a deterrent to learning and offering this conservative option to patients who meet the selection criteria.

A philosophy of the UKA concept, good judgment, and understanding of the surgical principles and instrumentation systems of a proven prosthetic design, along with exacting surgical technique, should decrease failures in UKA that are due to surgeon-dependent technical factors. However, slightly higher failure rates must be anticipated if the procedure is extended to the younger, more active patient. The LCS, with potential for bearing exchange, offers an excellent option in this difficult patient group.

Bibliography

Berger RA, Nedeff DD, Barden RM, Sheinkop MM, Jacobs JJ, Rosenberg AG, Galante JO (1999) Unicompartmental knee arthroplasty. Clinical experience at 6- to 10-year followup. Clin Orthop 367:50–60

Beverland D (2002) Advanced mobile-bearing surgical technique. Orthopedics 25 [Suppl 2]:s265–s271

Bohm I, Landsiedl F (2000) Revision surgery failed unicompartmental knee arthroplasty: a study of 35 cases. J Arthroplasty 15:982–989

Bowman P, Coventry MB (1978) Upper tibial osteotomy: long-term results in the non-rheumatoid knee. J Bone Joint Surg Br 60B:437

Buechel FF, Pappas MJ (1989) New Jersey low contact stress knee replacement system. Ten-year evaluation of meniscal bearings. Orthop Clin North Am 20:147–177

Cartier P, Sanouiller JL, Grelsamer RP (1996) Unicompartmental knee arthroplasty surgery. 10-year minimum follow-up period. J Arthroplasty 11:782–788

Cartier P, Epinette JA, Deschamps G et al (eds) (1997) Unicompartmental knee arthroplasty. Expansion Scientifique Francaise, Paris

Cohen M, Buechel F, Pappas MJ (1991) Meniscal-bearing unicompartmental knee arthroplasty. An 11-year clinical study. Orthop Rev 20:443–448

Coventry MB (1987) Proximal tibial varus osteotomy for osteoarthritis of the lateral compartment of the knee. J Bone Joint Surg Am 69A:32–38

Dorr LD (2002) Contrary view: wear is not an issue. Clin Orthop 404:96–99

Engh GA, Holt BT, Parks ML (1997) A midvastus muscle-splitting approach for total knee arthroplasty. J Arthroplasty 12:322–331

Goodfellow JW, O'Connor JJ (1982) The Oxford knee: a clinical trial. J Bone Joint Surg Br 64B:620

Grelsamer RP, Cartier P (1992) A unicompartmental knee replacement is not "half a total knee": five major differences. Orthop Rev 21:1350–1356

Heck DA, Marmor L, Gibson A et al (1993) Unicompartmental knee arthroplasty. A multicenter investigation with long-term follow-up evaluation. Clin Orthop 286:154–159

Heck DA, Marmor L, Gibson A, Rougraff BT (1993) Unicompartmental knee arthroplasty. A multicenter investigation with long-term follow-up evaluation. Clin Orthop 286:154–159

Hodge WA, Chandler HP (1992) Unicompartmental knee replacement: a comparison of constrained and unconstrained designs. JBJS [Am] 74:877–883

Insall J, Aglietti P (1980) A five to seven-year follow-up of unicondylar arthroplasty. J Bone Joint Surg Am 62A:1329–1337

Insall J, Walker P (1976) Unicondylar knee replacement. Clin Orthop 120:83–85

Insall JN, Joseph DM, Msika C (1984) High tibial osteotomy for varus gonarthrosis. J Bone Joint Surg Am 66A:1040–1048

Insall JN, Scott WN, Keblish PA et al (1994) Total knee arthroplasty exposures and soft tissue balancing. In: Insall JN, Scott WN (eds) VideoBook of knee surgery. Lippincott, Philadelphia

Keblish PA (1991) The lateral approach to the valgus knee. Surgical technique and analysis of 53 cases with over two-year follow-up evaluation. Clin Orthop 271:52–62

Keblish PA (1994) The case for unicompartmental knee arthroplasty. Orthopedics 17:853–855

Keblish PA (2002) Surgical approaches: lateral approach. In: Scuderi GR, Tria JA (eds) Surgical techniques in total knee arthroplasty. Springer, Berlin Heidelber New York

Kisslinger E, Justen HP, Wessinghage D (2001) Better than their reputation? 5 to 20 years outcome with single compartment knee joint endoprostheses in medial osteoarthritis of the knee. Z Orthop Ihre Grenzgeb 139:97–101

Knight JL, Atwater RD, Guo J (1997) Early failure of the porous coated anatomic cemented unicompartmental knee arthroplasty. Aids to diagnosis and revision. J Arthoplasty 12:11–20

Kozinn SC, Marx C, Scott RD (1989) Unicompartmental knee arthroplasty: a 4.5-6-year follow-up study with a metal-backed tibial component. J Arthroplasty 4 [Suppl]:S1–S10

Laskin RS (1976) Modular total knee-replacement arthroplasty. J Bone Joint Surg Am 58A:766–773

Levine WN, Ozuna RM, Scott RD et al (1996) Conversion of failed modern unicompartmental arthroplasty to total knee arthroplasty. J Arthroplasty 11:797–801

Lewold S, Knutson K, Lidgren L (1993) Reduced failure rate in knee prosthetic surgery with improved implantation technique. Clin Orthop 287:94–97

Lewold S, Knutson K, Lidgren L (1993) Reduced failure rate in knee prosthetic surgery with improved implantation technique. Clin Orthop 287:94–97

Lindstrand A, Stenstrom A (1992) Polyethylene wear of the PCA unicompartmental knee. Prospective 5 (4–8) year study of 120 arthrosis knees. Acta Orthop Scand 63:260–262

Lindstrand A, Stenstrom A, Lewold S (1992) Multicenter study of unicompartment knee revision. PCA, Marmor, and St. Georg compared in 3,777 cases of arthrosis. Acta Orthop Scand 63:256–259

Lindstrand A, Stenstrom A, Ryd L, Toksvig-Larsen S (2000) The introduction period of unicompartmental knee arthroplasty is critical: a clinical multicentered and radiostereometric study of 251 Duracon unicompartmental knee arthroplasties. J Arthroplasty 15:608–616

Marmor L (1979) Marmor modular knee in unicompartmental disease. Minimum four-year follow-up. JBJS [Am] 61:347–353

Marmor L (1988) Unicompartment arthroplasty of the knee with a minimum ten-year follow-up period. Clin Orthop 228:171–177

Marmor L (1990) Patient selection for osteotomy, unicompartmental replacement, and total knee replacement. Am J Knee Surg 3:206–213

Matthews LS, Goldstein SA, Malvitz TA, Katz BP, Kaufer H (1988) Proximal tibial osteotomy. Factors that influence the duration of satisfactory function. Clin Orthop 229:193–200

McKeever DC, Elliot RB (1960) Tibial plateau prosthesis. Clin Orthop 18:86–95

Ohdera T, Tokunaga J, Kobayashi A (2001) Unicompartmental knee arthroplasty for lateral gonarthrosis: midterm results. J Arthroplasty 16:196–200

Otte KS, Larsen H, Jensen TT et al (1997) Cementless AGC revision of unicompartmental knee arthroplasty. J Arthroplasty 12:55–59

Perkins TR, Gunckle W (2002) Unicompartmental knee arthroplasty: 3- to 10-year results in a community hospital setting. J Arthroplasty 17:293–297

Psychoyios V, Crawford RW, O'Connor JJ, Murray DW (1998) Wear of congruent meniscal bearings in unicompartmental knee arthroplasty: a retrieval study of 16 specimens. JBJS [Br] 80:976–982

Robertsson O, Borgquist L, Knutson K, Lewold S, Lidgren L (1999) Use of unicompartmental instead of tricompartmental prostheses for unicompartmental arthrosis in the knee is a cost-effective alternative. 15,437 primary tricompartmental prostheses were compared with 10,624 primary medial or lateral unicompartmental prostheses. Acta Orthop Scand 70:170–175

Robertsson O, Dunbar M, Pehrsson T, Knutson K, Lidgren L (2000) Patient satisfaction after knee arthroplasty: a report on 27,372 knees operated on between 1981 and 1995 in Sweden. Acta Orthop Scand 71:262–267

Robertsson O, Knutson K, Lewold S, Lidgren L (2001) The routine of surgical management reduces failure after unicompartmental knee arthroplasty. JBJS [Br] 83:45–49

Scott RD, Cobb AG, McQueary FG, Thornhill TS (1991) Unicompartmental knee arthroplasty. Eight- to 12-year follow-up evaluation with survivorship analysis. Clin Orthop 271:96–100

Sisto DJ, Blazina ME, Heskiaoff F et al (1993) Unicompartment arthroplasty for osteoarthritis of the knee. Clin Orthop 286:149–153

Sorrells RB (2002) The clinical history and development of the low contact stress total knee arthroplasty. Orthopedics 25 [Suppl 2]:s207–s212

Stern SH, Becker MW, Insall JN (1993) Unicondylar knee arthroplasty: an evaluation of selection criteria. Clin Orthop 286:143–148

Stulberg SD (1990) Unicompartmental knee replacement. Techn Orthop 5:1–74

Svard UC, Price AJ (2001) Oxford medial unicompartmental knee arthroplasty. A survival analysis of an independent series. JBJS [Br] 83:191–194

Swank M, Stulberg SD, Jiganti J et al (1993) The natural history of unicompartmental arthroplasty. An eight-year follow-up study with survivorship analysis. Clin Orthop 286:130–142

Swank M, Stulberg SD, Jiganti J, Machairas S (1993) The natural history of unicompartmental arthroplasty. An eight-year follow-up study with survivorship analysis. Clin Orthop 286:130–142

Tabor OB Jr, Tabor OB (1998) Unicompartmental arthroplasty: a long-term follow-up study. J Arthroplasty 13:373–379

Thornhill TS, Scott RD (1989) Unicompartmental total knee arthroplasty. Orthop Clin North Am 20:245–256

Van Dalen J, Krause BL (1991) Medial unicompartment knee replacement. Minimum five year follow-up. Aust NZJ Surg 61:497–500

Weale AE, Murray DW, Baines J, Newman JH (2000) Radiological changes five years after unicompartmental knee replacement. JBJS [Br] 82:996–1000

Weale AE, Murray DW, Crawford R, Psychoyios V, Bonomo A, Howell G, O'Connor J, Goodfellow JW (1999) Does arthritis progress in the retained compartments after 'Oxford' medial unicompartmental arthroplasty? A clinical and radiological study with a minimum ten-year follow-up. JBJS [Br] 81:783–789

Weale AE, Murray DW, Newman JH, Ackroyd CE (1999) The length of the patellar tendon after unicompartmental and total knee replacement. JBJS [Br] 81:790–795

2.5 Patella Femoral Arthroplasty

Alan C. Merchant

A new modular prosthesis has been designed to treat severely disabled patients who have isolated end-stage arthrosis or failed surgeries of the patellofemoral joint. The younger patients of this group are not good candidates for total knee arthroplasty (TKA), and the older patients will benefit from replacement of only those joint surfaces that are damaged. Because this new prosthesis was designed to be modular with the low contact stress (LCS) total knee system, it has an important advantage. Some patients who have had successful operations using this modular design will require revision to a TKA in the future because of deterioration of the femorotibial compartments. At that revision surgery, only the trochlear component will need to be removed and replaced by an LCS femoral component. The patellar component can be left intact because it has been designed to articulate exactly with the new femoral component, thus eliminating the high risks and complications associated with patellar component revision.

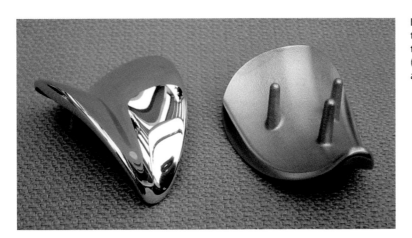

Fig. 2.48. Trochlear components of the modular LCS patellofemoral prosthesis showing the articular surface (left) and the reverse with the three fixation pins (right)

Eight patients who have had total patellofemoral arthroplasty using this new design have been followed for more than 2 years (24–45 months). Seven patients (88%) had excellent or good results, and one was fair. Based on the success of this small initial sample, and the fact that any one surgeon does not perform total patellofemoral arthroplasty frequently, the current author has started a prospective multicenter outcome study. This prospective protocol will use data gathered in a similar manner, the same outcome instrument to measure knee function, and a common database.

Design Considerations

During the past two decades, various authors (Blazina et al. 1979, Lubinus 1979, Arciero and Toomey 1988, Cartier et al. 1990, Argenson et al. 1995, Kracja-Radcliffe and Coker 1996, and Tauro et al. 2001) have reported on three different designs of patellofemoral prostheses. The good or excellent results ranged from a low of 45% (Tauro et al. 2001) to a high of 96% (Kracja-Radcliffe and Coker 1996). A careful review of these studies showed that implant design and patient selection are the two most important factors for success. None of these earlier patellofemoral prostheses have been designed to be modular with a total knee replacement system in order to take advantage of safer and easier revision surgery should it be needed in the future.

Patients disabled by isolated patellofemoral arthritis and failed patellofemoral surgeries tend to be much younger than those considered to be good candidates for TKA. Their relative youth demands a prosthetic design that will provide maximum longevity and survivorship. The LCS rotating patella (Buechel et al. 1989) has the best long-term survivorship,

greater than 99% at 12-year follow-up, as well as the lowest reported complication rate, 0.9% (Jordan et al. 2000). The current author modified the polyethylene bearing for use as a patellofemoral implant. Then a trochlear component (Fig. 2.48) was designed to articulate exactly with that patellar component. This new combination for total patellofemoral arthroplasty (TPFA) takes advantage of the design features that have led to such excellent survivorship and freedom from complications. These design features are: (1) an anatomic trochlear groove that is deeper than most other implants, reducing the risk of patellar dislocation; (2) components with broad and congruent area contact loading, as opposed to point or line contact loading, reducing the wear rate; and (3) the self-aligning feature of the rotating patellar bearing that reduces stress on the bone–implant interface, reducing the risk of loosening.

However, the most important feature of this new prosthesis is the modularity designed into the trochlear component. If a patient with this prosthesis should require revision to a TKA in the future because of deterioration of the femorotibial compartments, the trochlear component can be removed and the femoral component of the LCS knee system implanted, leaving the patellar component intact (Fig. 2.49). This is not just a theoretical advantage. Berry and Rand (1993) have shown that patellar revision has an unacceptably high complication rate of 33%. The new modular knee replacement system avoids this source of complications. Furthermore, the rotating polyethylene bearing can be snapped off from its base plate and exchanged for a new one if wear is found. If a size change is planned, a custom bearing can be ordered.

The trochlear component is inlaid flush with the remaining normal joint surfaces after preparing the osseous bed with small osteotomes and a motorized

Fig. 2.49. An LCS femoral component (left) and the modular LCS patellofemoral joint prosthesis (right) demonstrating the modularity of all the components

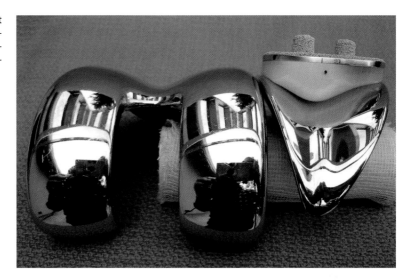

Fig. 2.50. The modified LSC rotating patella bearing (left) compared to the standard LCS patella (right). Both shown in a side view from the medial aspect

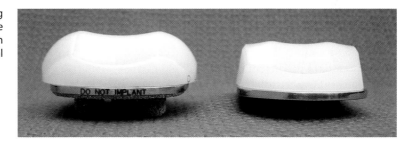

burr. It is impacted into position secured by its three small fixation pins and bone cement. Because very little bone is removed for implantation, conversion to a total knee femoral component, if necessary at a later date, will be straightforward.

The patella is implanted in the usual manner using a porous coated, press-fit technique or cement at the surgeon's preference. Because the polyethylene patellar bearing slides off the metallic trochlear component to articulate with the remaining normal femoral cartilage during full flexion, the author has redesigned the shape and contour of this bearing. The superior–inferior dimension of the rotating bearing has been increased somewhat so that the bearing will remain in contact with the metal trochlear implant a little longer during acute knee flexion. The sharp, angular superior and inferior edges of the standard LCS rotating bearing have been rounded off or contoured to avoid gouging the femoral articular cartilage during acute flexion (Fig. 2.50). Because the polyethylene patellar bearing articulates with normal cartilage in full flexion, all patients are warned repeatedly to avoid weight bearing when the knee is flexed more than 90 degrees, that is, avoid full squatting. Half squats are acceptable.

Indications

Patellofemoral replacement is a salvage procedure, and patient selection is the single most important factor determining a successful result. There are four major indications for TPFA and all four must be present to qualify a patient for this operation.

The surgeon must prove that the source of pain is from patellofemoral arthrosis or chondrosis. All other causes for anterior knee pain, such as tendinitis, neuromata, reflex sympathetic dystrophy, etc., must be ruled out or treated first. The patellar and trochlear damage must be severe, grade III or IV chondromalacia, or true osteoarthrosis. Objective evidence from arthroscopic observation or radiographic joint narrowing, sclerosis, and perhaps osteophytes, must be present. The amount of pain must limit the patient's ability to perform the activities of daily living. The goal of TPFA is to return the patient to normal daily activities, not competitive sports. The candidate must agree to low demand activities after surgery. Frequently, these patients are relatively young and they tend to overutilize the knee once it is pain free. They must understand the dangers of running, jumping, and squatting. Mild to moderate recreation is allowed, such as hiking, golf, moderate cycling with the seat adjusted to avoid flexion beyond 90 degrees, and perhaps doubles tennis without tournaments. All alternative treatments must either have been tried and failed or are contraindicated. For instance, a relatively simple lateral release can give significant and long-lasting relief if the patient has a tight lateral retinaculum along with the isolated patellofemoral arthrosis. On the other hand, if the surgeon is considering anterior or anteromedial tibial tubercle transfer, Pidoriano et al. (1997) have shown that the presence of proximal patellar articular lesions is a contraindication to these procedures. In the young patient with patellofemoral plus medial or lateral arthrosis, patellofemoral replacement can be combined with a tibial osteotomy.

Contraindications

The usual contraindications for joint replacement also apply to total patellofemoral arthroplasty: infection, reflex sympathetic dystrophy, and psychogenic pain. Patella infera is a relative contraindication. It must be corrected to normal before the total patellofemoral arthroplasty, or correction can be achieved at the same surgery and the postoperative rehabilitation modified to protect the repair until it has healed. Patients with rheumatoid or inflammatory arthritis should be considered carefully and individually. Usually it is a mistake to leave any articular cartilage to act as a stimulus for further synovial reaction. However, if the inflammatory process is well controlled or "burned out" and the other criteria have been met, this modular total patellofemoral arthroplasty may be appropriate. Certainly the patient's age and general health play important roles in this complex decision.

Results

Eight patients of those selected for this new arthroplasty have been followed for a minimum of 2 years (24–45 months). All were female. The average age at surgery was 51 years (range 26–81 years). During hospitalization the patients followed a standard TKA protocol with full weight bearing as tolerated. After discharge, the patients were given a home exercise program to regain knee flexion and quadriceps strength. Understandably, they recovered more rapidly than TKA patients. Because this modular TPFA is a salvage procedure, a simple outcome assessment was used.

- Excellent: Able to perform activities of daily living and light recreation using no medication.
- Good: Able to perform activities of daily living and light recreation using over-the-counter medications.
- Fair: Improved, but still requiring non-narcotic prescription medication for activities of daily living.
- Poor: No better, or worse than before surgery.

At the latest follow-up, seven (88%) patients rated excellent (6) or good (1), and all were very happy with their result. One patient required a prepatellar bursectomy and removal of foreign body suture material under local anesthesia 10 months postoperatively. She continues to have unexplained anterior pain and has a fair result. One patient (Case 1 below) required a patellar tendon lengthening 23 months after her index arthroplasty, changing her good result to excellent. There have been no major complications from the procedure itself, and there have been no implant failures.

Illustrative Case Reports

Case 1

A 26-year-old woman had a 6-year history of chronic left anterior knee pain aggravated by an injury 4 years previously. Arthroscopic surgery shortly after that injury revealed a grade IV lesion of the femoral trochlear cartilage. During the next 4 years, she had a total of five more unsuccessful surgeries including two anteromedializations of the tibial tubercle to treat this severely painful patellofemoral chondrosis. She improved significantly after her modular LCS patellofemoral replacement. Because the severity of a patella infera had not been recognized at the time of her arthroplasty, she required a 1.0 cm Z-plastic patellar tendon lengthening 23 months later, changing her result from good to excellent. At 2.5 years follow-up she is even enjoying mild recreational activities (golf, bicycling, hiking, etc.), without signs of implant loosening or wear.

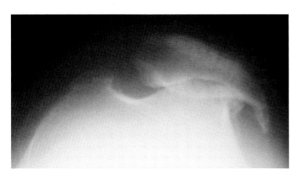

Fig. 2.51. The preoperative axial view radiograph of the right knee of Case 2. Diagnosis: chronic subluxation of the patella with secondary patellofemoral osteoarthrosis

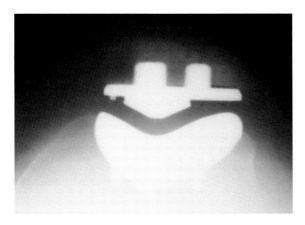

Fig. 2.52. The post-operative axial view radiograph of the right knee of Case 2

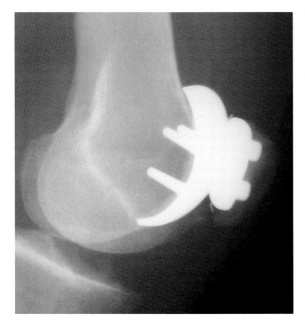

Fig. 2.53. The post-operative lateral view radiograph of the right knee of Case 2

Case 2

A 41-year-old woman had been involved in sports since childhood and always remembered having had anterior knee pain. She had a solitary dislocation of the right patella at age 14. At age 30 she had a lateral release and patellar exostectomy on the left knee. The diagnosis was bilateral chronic patellar subluxation with secondary patellofemoral arthrosis. A modular LCS patellofemoral replacement on the left produced an excellent result. She has since had the same arthroplasty on the right knee (Figs. 2.51, 2.52, and 2.53).

Conclusions

The modular LCS patellofemoral arthroplasty offers a more conservative alternative compared with TKA, both for the younger patient for whom TKA is inappropriate and for the older patient who has no disease in the medial or lateral compartments. Laskin and van Steijn (1999) and others (Oberlander et al. 1998, Mont et al. 2000) have advocated TKA for older patients who have only isolated patellofemoral arthritis. It makes no sense to perform a more major operation to remove normal medial and lateral compartments if a less destructive operation, such as TPFA, will provide equally good results.

Based on these encouraging initial results, a prospective multicenter protocol study has been started. Because no one surgeon will perform patellofemoral joint replacement frequently, meaningful numbers of patients cannot be accumulated over a reasonable time without pooled data. All surgeons interested in using this new modular design are being asked to join this prospective study. The data gathering has been simplified to a one-page outcome form. The outcome assessment instrument is a patient-reported Activities of Daily Living (ADL) Scale created by Irrgang et al. (1998). These authors have validated their ADL scale against the Lysholm Knee Scale and the International Knee Documentation Committee guidelines for global function. Others (Marx et al. 2001) have confirmed its reliability, validity, and responsiveness compared with three other commonly used knee outcome scales. The ADL Scale expresses the function of the tested knee as a percentage of normal. Pooling this outcome data in a common database will allow a reliable assessment of this new modular LCS patellofemoral joint prosthesis in the future.

Bibliography

Arciero R, Toomey H (1988) Patellofemoral arthroplasty; a three to nine year follow-up study. Clin Orthop 236:60–71

Argenson J-NA, Guillaume J-M, Aubaniac J-M (1995) Is there a place for patellofemoral arthroplasty? Clin Orthop 321:162–167

Berry DJ, Rand JA (1993) Isolated patellar component revision of total knee arthroplasty. Clin Orthop 286:110–115

Blazina ME, Fox JM, Del Pizzo W, Broukhim B, Ivey FM (1979) Patellofemoral replacement. Clin Orthop 144:98–102

Buechel FF, Rosa RA, Pappas MJ (1989) A metal-backed, rotating-bearing patellar prosthesis to lower contact stress, an 11-year clinical study. Clin Orthop 248:34–49

Cartier P, Sonouiller JL, Grelsamer R (1990) Patellofemoral arthroplasty. J Arthroplasty 5:49–55

Irrgang JJ, Snyder-Mackler L, Wainner RS, Fu FH, Harner CD (1998) Development of a patient-reported measure of function of the knee. J Bone Joint Surg 80A:1132–1145

Jordan LR, Olivo JL, Voorhorst PE (2000) Survivorship analysis of a metal-backed rotating anatomic patella in total knee arthroplasty: a 14-year follow-up. Paper no 183, Am Acad Orth Surg, 67th annual meeting, Orlando, FL

Krajca-Radcliffe JB, Coker TP (1996) Patellofemoral arthroplasty; a two to eighteen year follow-up study. Clin Orthop 330:143–151

Laskin RS, van Steijn M (1999) Total knee replacement for patients with patellofemoral arthritis. Clin Orthop 367:89–95

Lubinus HH (1979) Patella glide bearing replacement. Orthopedics 2:119–127

Marx RG, Jones EC, Allen AA, Altchek DW, O'Brien SJ, Rodeo SA, Williams RJ, Warren RF, Wickiewicz TL (2001) Reliability, validity, and responsiveness of four knee outcome scales for athletic patients. J Bone Joint Surg 83A:1459–1469

Mont MA, Haas S, Mullick T, Hungerford DS, Krackow K (2000) Total knee arthroplasty for patellofemoral arthritis. Paper no 288. Am Acad Orth Surg, 67th annual meeting, Orlando, FL

Oberlander MA, Baker CL, Morgan BE (1998) Patellofemoral arthrosis: the treatment options. Am J Orthop 27:263–270

Pidoriano AJ, Weinstein RN, Buuck DA, Fulkerson JP (1997) Correlation of patellar articular lesions with results from anteromedial tibial tubercle transfer. Am J Sports Med 25:533–537

Tauro B, Ackroyd CE, Newman JH, Shah NA (2001) The Lubinus patellofemoral arthroplasty, a five- to ten-year prospective study. J Bone Joint Surg 83B:696–701

2.6 Patella Graft Options in Patellectomized Knees

Jens G. Boldt, Urs K. Munzinger

Patellectomized knees perform poorly with respect to extensor mechanism function. Reconstruction options and literature reports are limited. The purpose of this study was to describe and review bone graft patella reconstruction in total knee arthroplasty (TKA). Since 1990, nine previously patellectomized patients underwent cementless low contact stress (LCS) TKA with autologous patella reconstruction. One patient died 5 years post-surgery. Mean follow-up was 8.0 years (6–12). Autologous bone graft was taken in five cases from the iliac crest, in two cases from the posterior femoral condyle and in two cases from the opposite patella at the time of simultaneous bilateral TKA. Postoperative evaluation included clinical and radiographic analysis and bilateral comparative isokinetic strength measurement at 60 degrees per second (Biodex). Clinical scores had a mean of 27 points (max. 30) and mean isokinetic extension strength of 71 Newtonmeter (Nm) (81%) compared with the opposite healthy patella site. One patient with bilateral patellectomy and unilateral patella reconstruction showed a 50% increase of strength on the grafted side. Radiographs showed minor signs of neopatella bone resorption, but a maintained lever arm. Reconstruction of a neopatella in TKA with autograft provides marked improvement of isokinetic extensor strength, little evidence of autograft resorption, excellent or good clinical outcome and high patient satisfaction after a mean of 8 years. The results of this study indicate encouraging data for reconstructing a new patella and lever arm in patellectomized knees during primary or revision TKA. Cosmetic improvement in females is another subjective advantage.

From 1990 to 1995, ten patients (eight females, two males; mean age 56.8 ± 11.3 years) with a previous patellectomy required TKA for tibiofemoral arthritis (LCS, DePuy, Warsaw, IN, USA). The reason for patellectomy was severe patellofemoral chondromalacia in six patients, patellofemoral osteoarthritis after patella dislocation in two cases, and multipart patellar fracture in a further two patients. The interval between patellectomy and TKA averaged 16 years (± 8.5). The mean number of knee operations before TKA was 4.2. Mean age at index surgery was 55 years (38–68), which was relatively younger than the general patient profile in this center. Mean body mass index was 29 (22–47), which was comparable with the

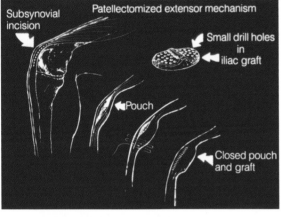

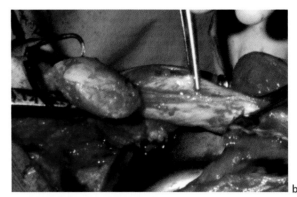

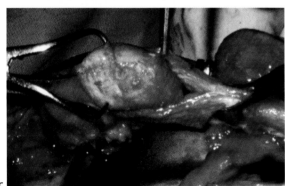

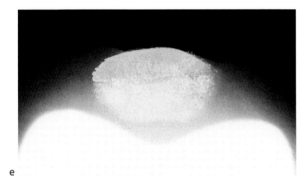

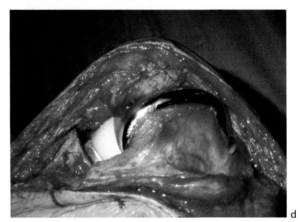

Fig. 2.54 a–e. Surgical technique of patella bone autografting in patellectomized knees during TKA. Insertion and suture of bone autografts into a subsynovial pouch at the previous anatomical position of the patella. TKA is performed with the neopatella articulating in the anatomical groove of the femoral knee implant. The autograft may be harvested from the iliac crest, the posterior femoral resections, or the opposite patella resection in a bilateral simultaneous TKA procedure

overall patient profile. None of the patients had rheumatoid arthritis, but osteoarthritis was an indication for TKA. All femoral components were implanted without cement and had an identical anatomic patellar groove design. Three TKAs had rotating platforms inserted and seven received meniscal bearings. In all cases, a new patella (neopatella) was reconstructed utilizing the patient's own bone graft. The autograft was taken in five cases from the iliac crest (corticocancellous bone block), in three cases from the posterior femoral condyle (sandwich technique), and in two cases from the opposite patella when both knees had a TKA at the same time with resurfacing of the existing patella. The bone shell had the shape of a

normal patella and was inserted into a subsynovial pouch underneath the patella tendon. After a mean of 16 years between patellectomy and TKA surgery, there was a thick synovial layer and scar tissue covering the patella tendon. The bone graft itself was not fixed within the pouch, but was secured with tight closure of the pouch with vicryl sutures (Figs. 2.54–2.56).

One patient died at study date cut off, leaving eight patients who had a clinical and radiological examination after a mean follow-up of 8.0 years (6–12). For each patient a modified Hospital for Special Surgery (HSS) knee arthroplasty rating scale was evaluated (30 points for pain, 25 points for function, 15 points

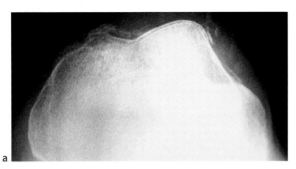

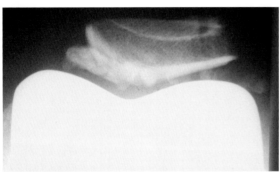

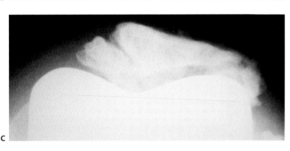

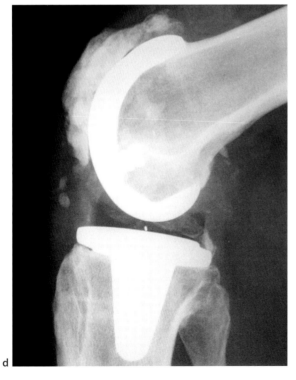

a

b

c

d

Fig. 2.55 a–d. Clinical example of a previously (18 years) patellectomized knee, in which autologous bone grafting from the iliac crest was performed during TKA procedure (**a, b**). Same patient 11 years after patella grafting, showing remarkable preservation and survival of the autologous patella bone in both size and shape (**c, d**)

for range of motion, 12 points for deformity, 10 points for stability, 8 points for strength). The clinical result was graded as excellent (85–100 points), good (70–84 points), fair (60–69 points), or poor (less than 60 points) (Buechel 1982).

Radiological data were analyzed according to the radiographic evaluation system of the Knee Society. In-depth analysis of lateral and axial patella radiographs preoperatively, immediate postoperatively and at latest follow-up included patella graft shape, size, structure, fragmentation, sclerosis, bone density, evidence of retrabeculation or avascular necrosis taking individual x-ray magnification factors into account. In addition, the strength of the quadriceps and hamstrings was measured on both knees using the Cybex II isokinetic dynamometer at 60 degrees per second. Peak torque forces were evaluated in both flexion and extension in Nm. An independent statistician analyzed all the data. All the metric data in each group showed a normal distribution (one-sample Kolmogorov-Smirnov test). As such, parametric statistical analysis was employed. Differences between groups for metric parameters such as maximal torque in extension and flexion were examined using the unpaired Student's t-test. Significance was accepted at the 5% level. All eight patients in the group attended investigations, except one, who died 5 years postoperatively.

None of the eight patients required any further knee surgery. Two knees required a manipulation under anesthesia for releasing adhesions and improving the postoperative range of motion. The mean preoperative modified HSS score (max. 100 points) improved significantly ($p<0.001$) from 47.8 to 92.4 points at a mean of 8 years follow-up with six excellent and two good clinical results; the specific patella score (max. 30 points) also improved highly significantly ($p<0.001$) from 10.8 points preoperatively to 27.1 points at latest follow-up (all excellent). A subjective questionnaire demonstrated that all patients were satisfied with the clinical outcome and all patients would undergo the same surgery again. Five of six women specifically appreciated the improved cosmesis of the knee joint and leg.

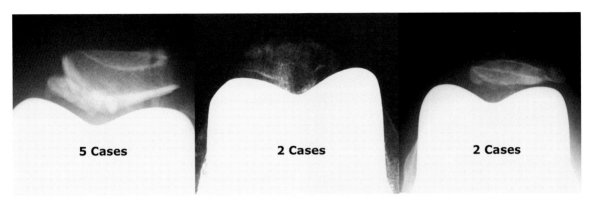

5 Cases | **2 Cases** | **2 Cases**

Fig. 2.56. All autologous neopatellae were inserted into a pouch of the horizontally split extensor mechanism retinaculum. Three different methods were used for reconstructing a new (neo) patella. In five cases a corticocancellous block was taken from the iliac crest of the same patient. In two cases the new bone was taken from the opposite patella during total knee arthroplasty with patella resurfacing. In another two cases the bone was taken from both posterior femoral condyle resections, creating a "sandwich"

All patella bone grafts showed radiological changes with time. Sclerosis had increased in six neopatellae, loss of thickness (axial views) averaging 4.6 mm. In three cases there was a slight fragmentation of the neopatella; however, those knees did not indicate a reduction during the isokinetic strength testing over time. One case presented considerable radiographic fragmentation, although a respectable patella thickness was maintained. In this patient we measured the lowest peak torque in extension (14 Nm). The average extension peak torque at the final follow-up was compared with the opposite knee of the same patient, which in all but one case had a normal patella without knee arthroplasty. On average peak extension, the strength of the neopatella TKA was 70.9 Nm compared with 88 Nm on the opposite side, counting for 85% of the normal strength (or only 15% weaker). Flexion strength was increased to compensate and was 14% stronger on the neopatella side. Studies performed at the Schulthess Clinic showed that peak torque extension strength in patellectomized knees was up to 65% weaker when compared with the healthy knee in the same patient. Our data indicate that reconstruction of a new patella during TKA helped in near normalizing the significant 50% loss of extension strength (Figs. 2.57–2.59).

Other centers have confirmed that patients perform poorly after patellectomy with respect to knee joint function, stability, and pain (Hungerford 1994, Leopold et al. 1999). Patellectomized knees demonstrate inferior kinematics mainly because of a considerably reduced lever arm for extension forces, leading to increased patellofemoral (tendon) compressive forces, increased pain and instability. Fur-

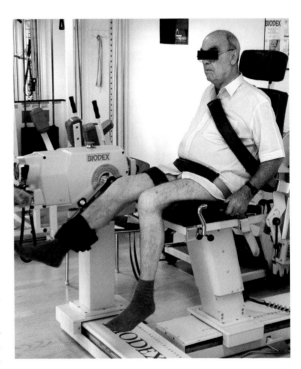

Fig. 2.57. Each patient had to warm up for 10 minutes on a stationary bike. Isokinetic strength of knee extension and flexion was measured using the BIODEX machine run by one independent observer, who was not aware which knee was the one with the neopatella (single blind)

thermore, increased patella tendon compression in the femoral groove leads to increased synovial response, scarring and discomfort. Vice versa, an increase of the quadriceps lever arm reduces quadriceps forces and can facilitate activities of daily living

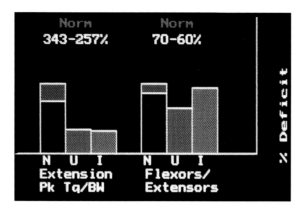

Fig. 2.58. Bar diagrams showing peak torque, overall power and total work in comparison with the opposite knee. Data were similar in both knees. Knees with neopatellae were significantly stronger than patellectomized knees

(D'Lima et al. 2001). Particularly in TKA, the patella lever arm should be maintained in order to warrant best clinical outcomes (Hsu et al. 1996, Jiang et al. 1993).

There is general agreement that clinical outcomes of TKA in patellectomized knees are significantly inferior to those in normal knees, independent of whether the patella is resurfaced or retained (Lennox et al. 1987, Larson et al. 1991). Further kinematic problems in patellectomized TKA include difficulties in climbing stairs, rising from chairs, deep bends, full active extension of the knee joint, increased discomfort (pain), and cosmesis (Martin et al. 1995, Insall, Keblish). Kang et al. (1993) noted that significantly reduced peak extension forces reflected the patient's difficulty in managing stairs and Huang et al. (1996) reported that the hamstring to quadriceps ratios in patellectomized TKA were not the same as those of the healthy group, even after long-term (6–13 years) functional adaptation. Joshi et al. (1994) compared the outcome of TKA in 19 patients who had had previous patellectomy with a matched healthy group and found poor outcomes in five cases, instability in three and persistent pain in four. Three supracondylar fractures occurred in his group, with an overall complication rate of 36%. Larson et al. (1991) concluded that TKA in patellectomized knees is justified; however, patients without patellae may be at a higher risk for failure of the prosthesis, as seen in his study.

There appears to be consensus in favoring posterior stabilized knee components in patellectomized patients and less predictable results when utilizing bicruciate sacrificing components (Paletta and Laskin 1995, Insall). When a patellar component could

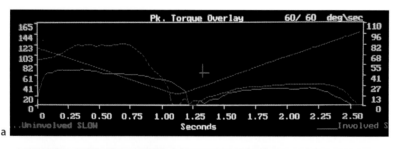

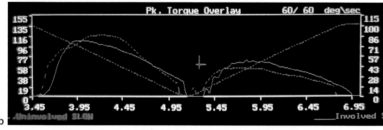

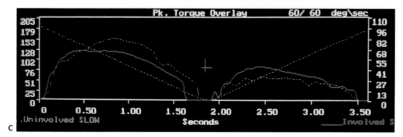

Fig. 2.59 a–c. Peak torque at 60 degrees/s under isokinetic strength exercise, demonstrating less than 50% strength in patellectomized knees (a), and close to normal strength of the neopatella TKA knee, with an average of 84% power in extension compared with the opposite knee (b, c). There was compensatory increased flexion in the neopatella knee

not be implanted in revision total knee arthroplasty, a lower quality result was observed (Barrack et al. 1998). Another observation made by Paletta noted better results after TKA when the patellectomy resulted from trauma rather than osteoarthritis. However, increased pain, flexion contracture, lack of extension, increased revision rate, and significantly worse clinical results were observed in TKA after patellectomy. Larson et al. (1991) and Lennox et al. (1987) also recommended braces or arthrodesis in patellectomized knees rather than performing TKA.

When the lever arm in patellectomized knees is increased during TKA, resulting reduced quadriceps forces lead to reduced patellofemoral forces, which can have a beneficial effect on anterior knee pain, patellar component wear, and loosening, as well as postoperative rehabilitation (D'Lima et al. 2001).

Surgical techniques of patella reconstruction during TKA were first published by Buechel (1991), who suggested the insertion and suture of bone autografts into a subsynovial pouch at the previous anatomical position of the patella. TKA is then performed without patella resurfacing, with the graft articulating in the anatomical groove of the LCS knee prosthesis. The autograft may be harvested from the iliac crest, the posterior femoral resections, or the opposite patella resection in bilateral simultaneous TKA procedure. A French group recommends a technique consisting of an iliac crest bone graft screwed into the remaining patella shell (if existent) followed by cementation of a polyethylene dome-shaped patella button (Tabutin 1998). Other patella bone grafting procedures have been reported recently by Hanssen (2001), who describes impaction allografting of patella cysts in revision TKA surgery.

In summary, patellar tendon bone grafting improves quadriceps leverage in previously patellectomized knees and is useful in significantly improving extensor function, clinical overall outcomes, patient satisfaction, postoperative rehabilitation and knee joint cosmesis. Because to date there is no downside to this procedure, we routinely recommend patella reconstruction in patellectomized patients in both primary and revision cases.

Acknowledgements. I thank U. Munzinger MD and T. Drobny MD for clinical data and support, and M. Bizzini PT, MA for physiotherapeutic advice.

Bibliography

Barrack RL, Matzkin E, Ingraham R, Engh G, Rorabeck C (1998) Revision knee arthroplasty with patella replacement versus bony shell. Clin Orthop 356:139–143

Berman AT, Bosacco SJ, Israelite C (1991) Evaluation of total knee arthroplasty using isokinetic testing. Clin Orthop 271:106

Berry DJ, Rand JA (1993) Isolated patellar component revision of total knee arthroplasty. Clin Orthop 286:110–115

Bizzini M, Boldt J, Munzinger U, Drobny T (2003) Rehabilitation guidelines after total knee arthroplasty. Orthopade 32(6):527–534

Björkström S, Goldie IF (1980) A study of the arterial supply of the patella in the normal state, in chondromalacia patellae and in osteoarthrosis. Acta Orthop Scand 51:63–70

Boldt JG, Bezzini M, Keblish PA, Munzinger UK (2004) Isokinetic strength in resurfaced and retained TKA. Scientific exhibition, AAOS annual meeting, San Francisco, USA, Mar 2004

Boldt JG, Keblish PA, Munzinger UK (2003) Patella bone graft reconstruction in patellectomized knees undergoing primary TKA. Scientific poster, AAOS annual meeting, New Orleans, Feb 2003, USA

Boldt JG, Munzinger UK, Zanetti M, Hodler J (2004) Arthrofibrosis associated with total knee arthroplasty: gray-scale and power Doppler sonographic findings. AJR Am J Roentgenol 182(2):337-40

Boldt J, Munzinger U, Keblish P (2004) Comparison of isokinetic strength in resurfaced and retained patellae in bilateral TKA. J Arthroplasty 19(2):264

Buechel FF (1982) A simplified evaluation system for the rating of knee function. Orthop Rev 11:9

Buechel FF (1991) Patellar tendon bone grafting for patellectomized patients having total knee arthroplasty. Clin Orthop 271:72–78

Buechel FF Sr, Buechel FF Jr, Pappas MJ, D'Alessio J (2001) Twenty-year evaluation of meniscal bearing and rotating platform knee replacements. Clin Orthop 388:41–50

Buechel FF Sr, Buechel FF Jr, Pappas MJ, Dalessio J (2002) Twenty-year evaluation of the New Jersey LCS rotating platform knee replacement. J Knee Surg 15:84–89

D'Lima DD, Poole C, Chadha H, Hermida JC, Mahar A, Colwell CW Jr (2001) Quadriceps moment arm and quadriceps forces after total knee arthroplasty. Clin Orthop 392:213–220

Elia EA, Lotke PA (1991) Results of revision total knee arthroplasty associated with significant bone loss. Clin Orthop 271:114–121

Ewald FC (1989) The Knee Society total knee arthroplasty roentgenographic evaluation and scoring system. Clin Orthop 248:9

Hanssen AD (2001) Bone-grafting for severe patellar bone loss during revision knee arthroplasty. J Bone Joint Surg Am 83A:171–176

Hirano A, Fukubayashi T, Ishii T, Ochiai N (2001) Relationship between the patellar height and the disorder of the knee extensor mechanism in immature athletes. J Pediatr Orthop 21:541–544

Huang CH, Cheng CK, Lee YT, Lee KS (1996) Muscle strength after successful total knee replacement: a 6- to 13-year followup. Clin Orthop 328:147–154

Hungerford DS (1994) Management of extensor mechanism complications in total knee arthroplasty. Orthopedics 17:843–844

Hsu HC, Luo ZP, Rand JA, An KN (1996) Influence of patellar thickness on patellar tracking and patellofemoral contact characteristics after total knee arthroplasty. J Arthroplasty 11:69–80

Jiang CC, Chen CH, Huang LT, Liu YJ, Chang SL, Wen CY, Liu TK (1993) Effect of patellar thickness on kinematics of the knee joint. J Formos Med Assoc 92:373–378

Joshi AB, Lee CM, Markovic L, Murphy JC, Hardinge K (1994) Total knee arthroplasty after patellectomy. J Bone Joint Surg Br 76:926–929

Kang JD, Papas SN, Rubash HE, McClain EJ Jr (1993) Total knee arthroplasty in patellectomized patients. J Arthroplasty 8:489–501

Kim BS, Reitman RD, Schai PA, Scott RD (1999) Selective patellar nonresurfacing in total knee arthroplasty. 10 year results. Clin Orthop 367:81–88

Larson KR, Cracchiolo A 3rd, Dorey FJ, Finerman GA (1991) Total knee arthroplasty in patients after patellectomy. Clin Orthop 264:243–254

Lennox DW, Hungerford DS, Krackow KA (1987) Total knee arthroplasty following patellectomy. Clin Orthop 223:220–224

Leopold SS, Greidanus N, Paprosky WG, Berger RA, Rosenberg AG (1999) High rate of failure of allograft reconstruction of the extensor mechanism after total knee arthroplasty. J Bone Joint Surg Am 81:1574–1579

Marmor L (1987) Unicompartmental knee arthroplasty following patellectomy. Clin Orthop 218:164

Martin SD, Haas SB, Insall JN (1995) Primary total knee arthroplasty after patellectomy. J Bone Joint Surg Am 77:1323–1330

Munzinger UK, Petrich J, Boldt JG (2001) Patella resurfacing in total knee arthroplasty using metal-backed rotating bearing components: a 2- to 10-year follow-up evaluation. Knee Surg Sports Traumatol Arthrosc 9 [Suppl 1]:S34–S42

Paletta GA Jr, Laskin RS (1995) Total knee arthroplasty after a previous patellectomy. J Bone Joint Surg Am 77:1708–1712

Parvizi J, Seel MJ, Hanssen AD, Berry DJ, Morrey BF (2002) Patellar component resection arthroplasty for the severely compromised patella. Clin Orthop 397:356–361

Rand JA, Trousdale RT, Ilstrup DM, Harmsen WS (2003) Factors affecting the durability of primary total knee prostheses. J Bone Joint Surg Am 85A:259–265

Railton GT, Levack B, Freeman MA (1990) Unconstrained knee arthroplasty after patellectomy. J Arthroplasty 5:255–257

Ritter MA, Keating EM, Faris PM (1989) Clinical, roentgenographic, and scintigraphic results after interruption of the superior lateral genicular artery during total knee arthroplasty. Clin Orthop 248:145

Ritter MA, Herbst SA, Keating EM, Faris PM, Meding JB (1996) Patellofemoral complications following total knee arthroplasty. Effect of a lateral release and sacrifice of the superior lateral geniculate artery. J Arthroplasty 11:368–372

Stiehl JB, Komistek RD, Dennis DA, Keblish PA (2001) Kinematics of the patellofemoral joint in total knee arthroplasty. J Arthroplasty 16:706–714

Tabutin J (1998) Osseous reconstruction of the patella with screwed autologous graft in the course of repeat prosthesis of the knee. Rev Chir Orthop Reparatr Appar Mot 84:363–367

Walker PS, Haider H (2003) Characterizing the motion of total knee replacements in laboratory tests. Clin Orthop 410:54–68

Watkins MP, Harris BA, Wender S, Zarins B, Rowe CR (1983) Effect of patellectomy on the function of the quadriceps and hamstrings. J Bone Joint Surg 65A:390–395

Wendt PP, Johnson RP (1985) A study of quadriceps excursion, torque, and the effect of patellectomy on cadaver knee. J Bone Joint Surg 67A:726–732

CHAPTER 3

Clinical Outcomes

Jens G. Boldt · Jeannette Petrich-Munzinger
Peter A. Keblish · Mario Bizzini · Urs K. Munzinger
N.W. Thompson · A.L. Ruiz · E. Breslin
D.E. Beverland · Yaw Jakobi · Thomas Guggi

3.1 Patella Resurfacing Utilizing LCS Prostheses

Jens G. Boldt, Jeannette Petrich-Munzinger

Routine patella resurfacing in total knee arthroplasty (TKA) has been the standard management in TKA and is considered the gold standard in most centers worldwide. However, studies have reported comparable long-term results in TKA without resurfacing the patella. When resurfaced, the patella component consists of either full polyethylene (PE) with a button or a more anatomical shape, or is metal backed with or without mobile PE bearings. Despite hypothetical advantages, mobile bearing metal-backed components have yet to prove acceptable outcomes, since considerable problems have been reported, such as increased PE wear, metallosis, fracture, or dissociation (spinout) requiring revision surgery.

A congruent fixed PE patella bearing provides low contact stress and therefore less PE wear. However, constraint forces on the prosthesis are greater, with potential development of increased radiolucent lines at the implant–bone interface, which ultimately increases the risk of component loosening. A less congruent fixed bearing (button shape, femoral component with box design) has higher PE contact stress, leading to increased PE wear. Constraint forces are less, and component loosening is less likely to occur. A congruent mobile patellar bearing provides low contact stress with reduced PE destruction and less constraint forces at the implant–bone interface, providing improved long-term fixation [5, 9]. The mobile bearing LCS patella component consists of a polished metal base plate with an interchangeable moveable PE bearing device, which permits rotational adaptation of the bearing into the femoral trochlear groove during full range of knee joint motion. The metal-backed plate can be implanted more independently and "anatomically fitting" into the patellar bone regarding alignment due to rotational adaptation of the bearing. The major goal is a reduction in component loosening caused by both PE wear parti-

cles and constraint forces at the implant-bone interface.

Patellar failures remain a challenge in TKA regardless of whether resurfaced or not. The outcome of resurfaced patellae should be compared with that without resurfacing of the patella, which shows similar or better results in the recent literature. Indications for resurfacing the patella are varied and include: (1) the presence of specific anterior knee pain, (2) workmen's compensation type patients, (3) medicolegal concerns, (4) patient's specific choice to resurface, (5) evaluation of LCS moveable bearing patella, (6) malfunctioning of patella at trial reduction (e.g., height, width, severe deformity), and (7) evaluation of resurfacing vs non-resurfacing of the patella. Fewer than 10 % of patellae have been resurfaced at this center since 1989. The present study investigated 105 cases of LCS TKA with metal-backed rotating bearing patella components.

At the Schulthess Clinic in Zurich, Switzerland, a total of 2,293 cases of TKA have been performed since 1988 using LCS (DePuy, Leeds, UK). Of these, 235 (10.2 %) involved patella resurfacing with a metal-backed rotating bearing component. The criteria for resurfacing the patella were independent of diagnosis, age, activity, and body mass index and included patients with preoperative anterior knee pain, evaluation of the same patient with and without patella resurfacing, and the patient's specific desire for resurfacing of the patella. In 40 % of the cases there had been previous knee joint surgery, including arthroscopic intervention with or without arthrotomy, cruciate ligament reconstructions, high tibial osteotomies, and surgery for trauma. We analyzed clinical and radiographic results in the 105 patients whose follow-up was longer than 2 years (73 % women, 27 % men; mean age 68.1 years, range 32–87). The diagnosis was primary osteoarthritis or other non-inflammatory disease in 97 patients (92.3 %) and rheumatoid arthritis in eight (7.6 %). A modified 100-point Hospital for Special Surgery knee scoring system was used (total knee score 100; pain 30, function 25, motion 15, deformity 12, stability 10, and strength 8 points); excellent scores were those of 85–100 points, good 70–84, fair 60–69, and poor less than 60 points.

Pre- and postoperative clinical evaluations were performed by a physician. Patients with complications were evaluated in depth. Radiographic evaluation of all cases was performed retrospectively to examine the appearance and outcome of the resurfaced patella. The method assessed lateral, anteroposterior, and skyline views of the patella, with measurement of congruency, tilt, tracking (patella crown to femoral sulcus of 0–2 mm was considered as perfect), patella height, length, and symmetry of the patellar bone cut.

Surgical Technique

The LCS moveable bearing system, either cemented or uncemented, was used in all cases. The patella was partially denervated via circumferential rim cautery, detilted with lateral release maneuvers where necessary, and downsized. The management of the extensor mechanism varied according to the alignment and knee joint pathology. In valgus deformity and in cases with subluxation or lateral maltracking of the patella (27%), a lateral retinacular approach as described by Keblish (1991) was used. In all other cases (63%), a medial retinacular approach was carried out. The posterior cruciate was retained in 36% and sacrificed in 64%. The vast majority (95%) of patellae were fully porous coated with either a three-peg or a cross-bar design; 5% of patellae were fixed with cement.

Of the 105 cases, there were 98 (93.3%) with excellent or good results, four (3.8%) with fair results, and three (2.9%) with poor results. The mean preoperative LCS score was 53.0 points (range 21–78), and the latest mean postoperative score was 84.3 points (range 45–99). Seven patients had a decreased postoperative score at the latest evaluation. Mean preoperative pain improved from 13 to 28 points postoperatively, function improved from 13 to 20 points, mobility improved from 103 to 110 degrees motion, deformity improved from 9 to 11 points, strength improved from 5 to 6 points, and stability improved from 8 to 9 points.

Radiographic analysis focused on patella tracking, congruency, and patella tilt on comparable pre- and postoperative skyline radiographs (Knutsson technique). Congruency of patella tracking was studied via a method of radiographic skyline-view analysis [6, 10]. Radiographic assessment revealed congruent tracking in more than 90% of cases, considering less than 2 mm lateral subluxation, less than 3 degrees of

lateral tilt, and more than 95% patellofemoral contact area on axial views as the limits. Tracking improvement, according to the alignment of the femoral trochlear sulcus and the tip of the patella, was measured in millimeters of lateral subluxation on comparable pre- and postoperative skyline views. Of the patellae, 26.4% had a lateral subluxation of more than 2 mm, compared with a mean of 13 mm preoperatively, which improved to 11% postoperatively that showed less than 6 mm subluxation. All of the nine (8.6%) dislocated patellae were relocated postoperatively.

Complications

Revision surgery related to patella complications was required in seven of 235 (3%) cases, including two of PE bearing spinout and one each of infection, patella necrosis, PE breakage, patella maltracking, and traumatic patella component loosening. Four (1.7%) patella complications were related to patellofemoral maltracking, excluding the infected, traumatic, and patella necrosis cases (Figs. 3.1–3.4). Prosthesis-related complications were noted in 10% of the 235 cases, including hematoma in 8% and delayed wound healing in 2%. Mobilization under anesthesia was required in 17% of TKA cases within the first postoperative year. One patient required a closed relocation of the patella after traumatic dislocation. Complications that were not prosthesis-related, such as medical impairments and thromboembolic events, were encountered in 17 of 235 cases (7.2%).

Management of the patella in TKA has become an important issue. The longevity of tibiofemoral prosthetic components has improved over the past three decades. However, patella-related complications remain a major concern and are frequently the reason for secondary intervention, whether resurfaced or not. When resurfaced, the options of patella resurfacing include cemented full PE components such as the button type and more anatomical designs, and cemented or uncemented metal-backed PE components with fixed or mobile bearings (Fig. 3.5). Common modes of failure include increased PE bearing edge wear, PE fractures, component dissociation (loosening or PE spinout), increased heterotopic ossification at the patella poles, and patella fractures. Early TKA designs were bicompartmental duocondylar excluding the patellofemoral joint. Complication rates have been high for various reasons, leading to the development of tricompartmental (total condylar) TKA with patella components in the mid-

Fig.3.1. a Traumatic patella fracture treated with open reduction and internal fixation. b Figure-of-eight tension band wiring

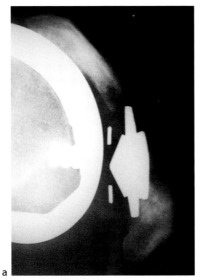
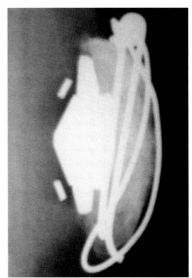

a

b

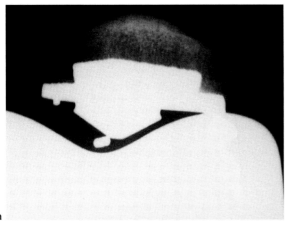

a

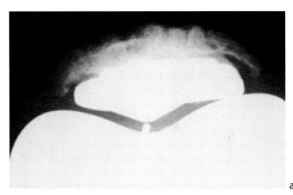

a

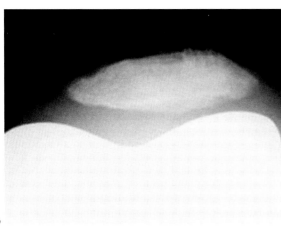

b

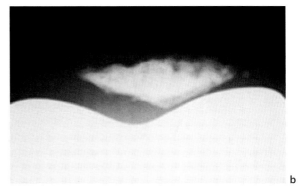

b

Fig.3.2. a Patella baja with lateral subluxation and aseptic loosening of patella component, b treated with removal of patella implant and shaving of patella

Fig.3.3. a Postoperative avascular necrosis of patella with loosening of patella component. b Subsequent removal of patella implant and contouring of remaining patella bone. Excellent clinical outcome after patella contouring and non-resurfacing

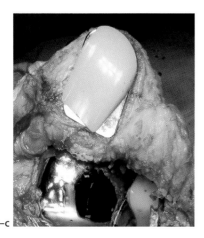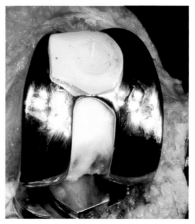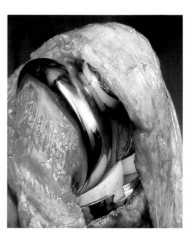

a–c

Fig. 3.4. a Edge wear of rotating patella bearing after 10 years without causing osteolysis. **b** Removal of worn bearings. **c** Demonstration of patellofemoral contact. Exchange of bearing with compression clamp

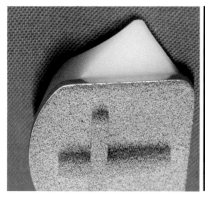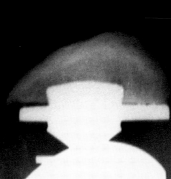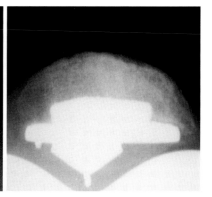

Fig. 3.5. Well fixed and aligned mobile bearing insert patella component with cementless fixation on lateral and axial views

1970s. This reduced the patella-related complication rate from an estimated mean of 25% to one of 6%. Tricompartmental TKAs are currently the most commonly performed, particularly in osteopenic or rheumatoid patients. However, patella retention has recently become more popular because of complications related to the resurfaced patella, including PE bearing failures (excessive wear, fracture, spinout), component loosening, and patellar bone fracture. Most of these complications may cause clinical symptoms and are either of concern and/or require surgical intervention.

The frequency of problems at the patellofemoral joint in TKA has decreased over the past 20 years as a result of improvements such as more conforming prosthetic designs (both femoral groove and patellar bearing), more durable materials, and understanding of femoral component rotation in relation to patellar articulation. The patella orientation changes during flexion and extension of the knee joint in all planes including coronal rotation. If the patella is resurfaced with a fixed dome-shaped bearing, implantation in an "intermediate" position is required to allow tracking close to optimum, as the patella rotates over the full range of motion. A button-type design may adapt more easily to rotation of the patella but is usually less comforting. A fixed, more congruent designed PE bearing would provide decreased contact stress but increased constraint forces at the bone-implant interface (in contrast to a button-type design). The philosophy of a rotating bearing patella component is to take advantage of both worlds: increased congruency of the patellofemoral articulation and decreased constraint forces at the bone-implant interface, particularly when stressed with coronal patella rotation during knee joint motion. Disadvantages of moveable PE bearings, which can lead to further surgical intervention, include fracture of the PE, spinout of PE, and increased wear particles due to two PE contact surfaces.

Mechanical Studies

The patella articulates as a sesamoid in the femoral trochlear groove and centralizes vector forces of the quadriceps-patella-tendon extensor mechanism. In active knee flexion and extension, both compressive and tensile forces act on the patellar bone, with a resulting tendency of lateral subluxation. Compression forces have been measured up to seven times body weight, whether resurfaced or not. The mechanical situation may be further compromised in pathological changes, including extensor–flexor muscle group imbalances, non-physiological biomechanical axes, cruciate ligament and/or capsulo-ligamentous insufficiencies, and arthritic diseases. A laboratory simulation performed at the Mt Sinai Medical Center investigated the normal lateral stability of the rotating patella and found that the rotating patella design offers sufficient resistance to lateral subluxation in the normal knee.

Acceptable contact stress levels for PE bearings in the patellofemoral articulation should not exceed 5 MPa to avoid the risk of PE failure. Forces less than 5 MPa have been measured only in the congruent patella and femoral designs. PE-related complications are increased contact stress including PE yielding, wear, fracture, and disintegration from the metal-backed bed or cement. Constraint forces at the bone–implant interface may cause fixation-related complications and ultimate loosening. Fractures of patellae appear to occur more frequently when resurfaced because the biomechanical features of the natural patella are distorted in both thickness and absence of one cortex. Rubens et al. (1991) reported increased tensile strength of up to 50% if the patella thickness is less than 14 mm, thus increasing the likelihood of patella fracture. Computed mathematical contact stress analyses performed at the New Jersey Institute of Technology have revealed lower contact stresses using a rotating patella than with dome-shaped patella designs. Contact stress was further increased in cases with non-ideal patellofemoral tracking.

In summary, the metal-backed rotating patella component with anatomical PE design provides increased congruent load distribution and decreased constraint forces at the bone–implant interface. In comparison to full PE (non-metal-backed) patellae, some fixed and all rotating bearings may be exchanged without interference of the patella bone–implant fixation, thus preserving patellar bone stock. However, in our group of patients and other published reports, this metal-backed patella component led to a number of complications that were not encountered when the full PE patella component was utilized or when the patella was treated with the patelloplasty procedure. Therefore, patella non-resurfacing or cemented full PE patella components are preferred by the author.

Acknowledgements. We thank U. Munzinger MD, and T. Drobny, Schulthess Clinic, Zurich, Switzerland for clinical data and support.

Bibliography

Aglietti P, Baldini A, Buzzi R, Indelli PF (2001) Patella resurfacing in total knee replacement: functional evaluation and complications. Knee Surg Sports Traumatol Arthrosc 9 [Suppl 1]:S27–S33

Barrack RL, Bertot AJ, Wolfe MW, Waldman DA, Milicic M, Myers L (2001) Patellar resurfacing in total knee arthroplasty. A prospective, randomized, double-blind study with five to seven years of follow-up. J Bone Joint Surg Am 83A:1376–1381

Bayley JC, Scott RD (1988) Further observations on metal-backed patellar component failure. Clin Orthop 236:82–87

Berend ME, Ritter MA, Keating EM, Faris PM, Crites BM (2001) The failure of all-polyethylene patellar components in total knee replacement. Clin Orthop 388:105–111

Bizzini M, Boldt J, Munzinger U, Drobny T (2003) Rehabilitation guidelines after total knee arthroplasty. Orthopade 32(6):527–534

Boldt JG, Bizzini M, Keblish PA, Munzinger UK (2004) Isokinetic strength with or without patella resurfacing in the same patient. AAOS Scientific exhibition SE43, San Francisco, USA, Mar 2004

Boldt JG, Munzinger UK (2003) Patella resurfacing in LCS mobile bearing TKA. A 2 to 12 year evaluation. EFORT, Helsinki, Finland

Boldt JG, Keblish PA, Drobny T, Munzinger UK Patella non-resurfacing in LCS mobile bearing TKA. Evaluation of 1777 cases with 2 to 15 year follow-up

Boldt JG, Keblish PA, Munzinger UK (2003) Bone graft options during TKA in patellectomized knees. ISTA, San Francisco, USA

Boldt J, Munzinger U, Keblish P (2004) Comparison of isokinetic strength in resurfaced and retained patellae in bilateral TKA. J Arthroplasty 19(2):264

Boldt JG, Munzinger UK, Zanetti M, Hodler J (2004) Arthrofibrosis associated with total knee arthroplasty: gray-scale and power Doppler sonographic findings. AJR Am J Roentgenol 182(2):337–340

Boyd AD Jr, Ewald FC, Thomas WH, Poss R, Sledge CB (1993) Long-term complications after total knee arthroplasty with or without resurfacing of the patella. J Bone Joint Surg Am 75:674

Bristol-Myers-Squibb/Zimmer Orthopedic Symposium Series, Lippencott-Raven Philadelphia, pp 47–63

Buechel FF (1982) A simplified evaluation system for the rating of the knee function. Orthop Rev 11:9

Buechel FF, Pappas MJ, Makris G (1991) Evaluation of contact stress in metal-backed patellar replacements. A predictor of survivorship. Clin Orthop 273:190–197

Crites BM, Berend ME (2001) Metal-backed patellar components: a brief report on 10-year survival. Clin Orthop 388: 103–104

Ewald FC (1989) The Knee Society total knee arthroplasty roentgenographic evaluation and scoring system. Clin Orthop 248:934

Hirano A, Fukubayashi T, Ishii T, Ochiai N (2001) Relationship between the patellar height and the disorder of the knee extensor mechanism in immature athletes. J Pediatr Orthop 21:541–544

Keblish PA (1991) The lateral approach to the valgus knee. Surgical technique and analysis of 53 cases with over two-year follow-up evaluation. Clin Orthop 271:52

Keblish PA, Greenwald AS (1990) Patella retention versus patella resurfacing in total knee arthroplasty. AAOS Scientific Exhibit, New Orleans, Febr 1990

Kelly MA (2001) Patellofemoral complications following TKA. Instr Course Lect 50:403–407

Kulkarni SK, Freeman MA, Poal-Manresa JC, Asencio JI, Rodriguez JJ (2000) The patellofemoral joint in total knee arthroplasty: is the design of the trochlea the critical factor? J Arthroplasty 15:424–429

Kulkarni SK, Freeman MA, Poal-Manresa JC, Asencio JI, Rodriguez JJ (2001) The patello-femoral joint in total knee arthroplasty: is the design of the trochlea the critical factor? Knee Surg Sports Traumatol Arthrosc 9 [Suppl 1]:S8–S12

Larson CM, Lachiewicz PF (1999) Patellofemoral complications with the Insall-Burstein II posterior-stabilized total knee arthroplasty. J Arthroplasty 14:288–292

Laskin RS (2001) Lateral release rates after total knee arthroplasty. Clin Orthop 392:88–93

McNamara JL, Collier JP, Mayor MB, Jensen RE (1994) A comparison of contact pressure in tibial and patellar total knee components before and after service in vivo. Clin Orthop 299:104–113

Merchant AC, Mercer RL, Jacobsen RH, Cool CR (1974) Roentgenographic analysis of patellofemoral congruence. J Bone Joint Surg Am 56:1391

Muller W, Wirz D (2001) The patella in total knee replacement: does it matter? 750 LCS total knee replacements without resurfacing of the patella. Knee Surg Sports Traumatol Arthrosc 9 [Suppl 1]:S24–S26

Munzinger UK, Petrich J, Boldt JG (2001) Patella resurfacing in total knee arthroplasty using metal-backed rotating bearing components: a 2- to 10-year follow-up evaluation. Knee Surg Sports Traumatol Arthrosc 9 [Suppl 1]:S34–S42

Rosenberg AG, Andriacchi TP, Barden R, Galante JO (1988) Patellar component failure in cementless total knee arthroplasty. Clin Orthop 236:106–114

Rubens JD, McDonald CL, Woodard PL, Hennington LJ (1991) Effect of patella thickness on patella strain following total knee arthroplasty. J Arthroplasty 6:251

Scuderi GR, Insall JN, Scott WN (1994) Patellofemoral pain after total knee arthroplasty. J Am Acad Orthop Surg 2:239–246

Shoji H, Yoshino S, Kajino A (1989) Patellar replacement in bilateral TKA. A study of patients who had rheumatoid arthritis and no gross deformity of the patella. J Bone Joint Surg Am 71:853

Steubben CM, Postak PD, Greenwald AS (1993) Mechanical characteristics of patello-femoral replacements. Orthopedic Research Laboratories, Mt Sinai Medical Center, Cleveland

Stiehl JB, Komistek RD, Dennis DA, Keblish PA (2001) Kinematics of the patellofemoral joint in total knee arthroplasty. J Arthroplasty 16:706–714

Stulberg SD, Stulberg BN, Hamati Y, Tsao A (1988) Failure mechanisms of metal-backed patellar components. Clin Orthop 236:88–105

Tanzer M, McLean CA, Laxer E, Casey J, Ahmed AM (2001) Effect of femoral component designs on the contact and tracking characteristics of the unresurfaced patella in total knee arthroplasty. Can J Surg 44:127–133

Theiss SM, Kitziger KJ, Lotke PS, Lotke PA (1996) Component design affecting patellofemoral complications after total knee arthroplasty. Clin Orthop (326):183–187

Thompson NW, Ruiz AL, Breslin E, Beverland DE (2001) Total knee arthroplasty without patellar resurfacing in isolated patellofemoral osteoarthritis. J Arthroplasty 16:607–612

3.2 Patella Non-resurfacing Utilizing Mobile Bearing Prostheses

Jens G. Boldt, Peter A. Keblish, Urs K. Munzinger

Patella management in total knee arthroplasty (TKA) is of concern when resurfaced (multiple problems) or when non-resurfaced (pain). Tricompartmental TKA with resurfacing of the patella is performed most commonly, especially in the USA, primarily because of the unpredictability of postoperative pain and fear of early failure. Studies with various TKA component designs continue to favour patella resurfacing, particularly in the rheumatoid patient. However, patellofemoral complications with resurfacing have resulted in major and at times catastrophic failures in TKA. Different philosophies exist regarding selection criteria and specifics of patella treatment in TKA. Since patellofemoral problems remain a major concern, patella non-resurfacing has been gaining popularity and reported as an option in TKA. If patella non-resurfacing (retention) is to be recommended, clinical outcomes must be equal to or better than those of routine patella resurfacing.

The patellofemoral joint is a highly complex articulation and requires equal attention to the femorotibial joint during total knee replacement surgery in terms of design, biomechanical, and physiological interaction. The patellar relationship changes after TKA, even in an ideal situation. Component position placement (medial versus lateral, superior versus inferior), thickness, tilt, pre-existing "baja", design geometry, etc. can influence patella tracking, often in subtle ways. The success of patella retention is multifactorial and is dependent on many factors, including: (1) prosthetic design; (2) rotational positioning of the femoral component; (3) patella size, quality, and position (alta/baja); (4) soft tissue balancing; (5) surgical approach; and (6) patella bed management (Fig. 3.6). Many TKA designs require patella resurfacing of various dimensions (usually dome shaped) in

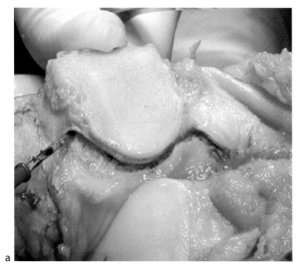

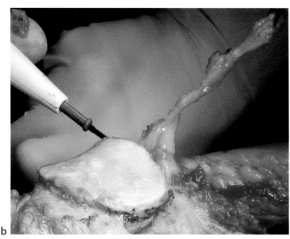

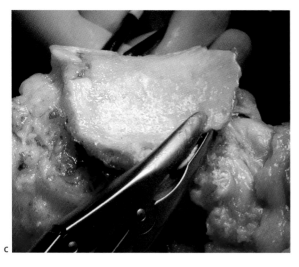

Fig. 3.6 a–c. Patelloplasty procedure utilized with medial approach. a Detilting manoeuvre extended into vastus lateralis as needed. b Denervation (partial) of patellar rim with cautery or scalpel. c Cheilectomy and downsizing to premorbid anatomy or contouring of oversized/severely deformed patella to accommodate femoral groove

order to adapt to different non-anatomical femoral designs.

Acceptable patella outcomes in TKA include: (1) good patella congruence, both clinically and radiologically; (2) minimal patellofemoral symptoms; (3) minimal patella-related complications (patella fractures, rupture of patella/quadriceps tendons, bone resorption, bearing edge wear, component dissociation/loosening); (4) minimal reoperation rate; (5) unimpaired functional activities, such as stair climbing; and (6) good patient acceptance. When the patella is not resurfaced, the main outcome factor is the reoperation rate for patella pain attributable to the non-resurfaced patella. Prosthetic design, femoral component positioning, surgical approach and management of the extensor mechanism represent important factors in successful patella outcome in TKA. Most publications continue to suggest that patella resurfacing is superior to non-resurfacing. However, the prostheses studied are frequently patella unfriendly and factors of femoral positioning and patella bed management are seldom addressed. This study evaluates the results of patella non-resurfacing in TKA using the same anatomic femoral design, technique, and similar selection criteria.

We reviewed 1,777 TKAs without resurfacing of the patella using the low contact stress (LCS) mobile bearing knee system (DePuy, Warsaw, IN, USA) in two large total joint centres. Criteria for non-resurfacing the patella varied somewhat. In centre A, criteria for patella non-resurfacing varied because of: (1) evaluation of the LCS moveable bearing concept, which included the rotating patella bearing in an early Food and Drug Administration (FDA) trial; (2) evaluation of the same patient with and without resurfacing in a reported study independent of diagnosis; (3) more recent evaluation and use of a cemented three-peg all-polyethylene anatomic patella; (4) patient selection with criteria to include the over-informed patient; and (5) intraoperative factors such as the extremely wide and/or thick patella and the distorted patella with good bone. In centre A, 68% were treated without patella resurfacing. Criteria for non-resurfacing the patella in centre B were independent of primary diagnosis, intraoperative appearance, age, activity, and body mass index. TKA without resurfacing of the patella was used, except in those cases where there was: (1) significant preoperative anterior knee pain; (2) evaluation study of the same patient with and without patella resurfacing; and (3) patient request for resurfacing the patella. In centre B, 91% of all TKAs were treated without patella resurfacing.

Combined Data from Both Centres

Of 3,621 TKAs without resurfacing of the patella in both centres, 1,777 had a follow-up of 2.0–15.3 years (mean 3.7). There were 70.3% females and 29.7% males. Diagnosis was primary osteoarthritis (OA) in 1568 cases (88.2%), rheumatoid arthritis (RA) in 144 cases (8.1%), and secondary OA due to trauma, crystalloid diseases, or other factors in 65 cases (3.7%). The mean age was 68 years (19–87). Fifteen cases (of 19 failures) with reoperations less than 2 years post-index procedure were included.

Prosthetic Components and Surgical Technique

The LCS moveable bearing system, both cemented and uncemented, was utilised in all cases (rotating bearing for posterior cruciate ligament (PCL)-compromised and meniscal bearing for PCL-competent knees). The non-resurfaced group was treated with a method of patelloplasty (Fig. 3.6) that included detilting (lateral rim release), partial denervation via circumferential rim cautery, selected multiple drilling in sclerotic bone, downsizing to normal contour (osteophytes removed), and/or contouring (to adapt to the femoral sulcus). The management of the extensor mechanism varied according to the alignment and knee joint pathology. In varus or neutral knees, a medial retinacular approach with patelloplasty was performed. In fixed valgus deformity or in cases with subluxation or lateral maltracking of the patella, a lateral retinacular approach was used in centre A. Centre B surgeons used the direct lateral approach with a lateral to medial tubercle osteotomy in the valgus knee.

Clinical and Radiographic Evaluation

Patients were followed clinically using a modified Hospital for Special Surgery (HSS; 100 points) knee scoring system initially designed for the FDA protocol, with evaluation factors of pain 30, function 25, motion 15, deformity 12, stability 10, and strength 8 points. Excellent scores rated from 100 to 85, good from 84 to 70, fair from 69 to 60, and poor results 59 or fewer points. All surgery in centre A was performed by one author or residents under his direct supervision. In centre B, all surgery was performed by two authors or fellows under their direct supervision. Similar indications and surgical techniques were used with minor variations as previously noted. Pre- and postoperative clinical evaluations were performed by physician assistants or physical therapists at centre A and by a physician at centre B. Specific radiographic analysis for all cases with patella complications and in 200 cases with the longest follow-up (100 from each centre) was carried out by the first author.

Results from Both Centres

Of the 1,628 OA cases, 1,540 (94.6%) had excellent or good results, 60 (3.7%) fair, and 28 (1.7%) poor results. The mean LCS scores improved from 60.6 (21–91) points preoperatively to 86.6 (43–100) points at the latest evaluation. Twenty patients had a decreased postoperative score at the latest evaluation. Mean preoperative pain score improved from 13.7 to 28.1 points, function from 13.2 to 20.0, deformity from 9.1 to 10.9, strength from 4.5 to 6.6, stability from 8.4 to 9.6, and mobility from 100 to 111 degrees.

Of the 149 RA cases, 134 (89.9%) had excellent or good results, 14 (9.4%) fair, and one (0.7%) had a poor result. Mean LCS scores improved from 56.3 (23–89) points preoperatively to 87.4 (43–100) points. No patient had a decreased postoperative score at the latest evaluation. Mean preoperative pain in this RA group improved from 15.2 to 28.0 points, function from 12.1 to 16.7, deformity from 9.4 to 11.2, strength from 4.5 to 5.7, stability from 7.6 to 8.9, and mobility from 96 to 108 degrees. Overall, RA patients had higher scores postoperatively compared with the OA group.

Complications: Centre A

Complications were evaluated as general, prosthetic non-patella-related and patella-related. Non-patella-related complications counted for 27 (4.6%), and included 13 problems related to bearing failure or a combination of progressive ligament instability/bearing wear or malpositioning, three failures were related to tibial problems (primarily aseptic loosening and/or subsidence), seven wound problems without deep infection, and four cases with arthrofibrosis. Of these 27 re-interventions, nine (1.5% of 591 cases) patellae were resurfaced incidental to revisions for other reasons, all after 2 years. These cases are not considered as failures attributed to the non-resurfaced patella, but included in worst-case scenario results regarding secondary patella resurfacing for any reason.

There were six (1.0%) patella failures requiring patella resurfacing due to severe anterior knee pain. Five of these six failures underwent secondary resurfacing within 2 years after surgery. These cases are considered to be failures of the non-resurfaced patella. Of the six (1.0%) cases requiring resurfacing, five were in the OA non-inflammatory group. Four patients improved their symptoms and are considered successes, confirming the patella as the cause of the failure. Two of the six patients had minimal/no improvement after surgery and may represent those cases for which a definitive diagnosis is ill-defined. The specifics of each failure are summarised as follows: one patella failure represented a highly active 48-year-old obese male heavy vehicle driver with post-traumatic arthritis and previous anterior cruciate ligament (ACL) autograft reconstruction, who developed anterior knee pain 1–2 years after ACL/PCL retaining TKA. X-ray changes of the lateral aspect of the patella revealed reduced patella height and increased sclerosis. His symptoms improved after patella resurfacing. Two female OA patients had postoperative anterior knee pain and reduced mobility secondary to synovitis/chondrolysis. Both showed clinical improvement after patella resurfacing. One male OA patient developed considerable cardiac impairment postoperatively, which limited early rehabilitation and resulted in arthrofibrosis and anterior knee pain. He underwent arthrotomy and removal of adhesions and fibrotic scar tissues with patella resurfacing, but did not improve postoperatively. Another male OA patient with diabetic neuropathy presented with severe anterior knee pain, persistent effusion without response to conservative management. His symptoms remained unchanged despite debridement and patella resurfacing. One RA female patient had a generalised rheumatoid flare-up within 6–12 months postoperatively. She had a fair to good response after revision surgery with synovectomy, meniscal bearing exchange, and patella resurfacing. The non-resurfaced patella was attributed as the cause for her revision, but the situation was not clear-cut, as there was also synovitis in the non-replaced joints (hands, opposite knee).

Complications: Centre B

Non-patella-related complications counted for 36 cases (3%) and included eight patients with progressive ligamentous insufficiency (PLI), eight wound-healing problems, two early infections, 14 patients with arthrofibrosis, and four patients with aseptic loosening or bearing failure of the tibial component. These complications were considered to be unrelated to the non-resurfaced patella. Of these 36 cases, 11 patellae were resurfaced incidental to tibiofemoral revisions for mechanical or instability failures after 2 years. These cases are not considered as failures attributed to the non-resurfaced patella, but are included in worst-case scenario results regarding secondary patella resurfacing for any reason.

True patella failures requiring reoperation in this group numbered 13 (1.1%). Secondary resurfacing was required in nine cases. Thirteen failures occurred within 2 years and four failures occurred more than 3 years after surgery. These cases are considered to be failures of the non-resurfaced patella. All of the 13 (1.1%) cases were in the OA non-inflammatory group. Specifics of the failures are summarised. Nine (69%) patients improved their symptoms and are considered successes, confirming the patella as the cause of the failure. Four (31%) of the 13 patients had no improvement after surgery (Fig. 3.7). Two cases had specific findings of anterior fat pad impingement, but have been included as true patella failures in our study. The two patients who did not improve included one with non-specific anterior knee pain and no specific intraoperative findings. The second patient had an extremely large patella, which was felt to be the problem. Revision surgery at 17 months included patella downsizing and contouring without resurfacing. Resurfacing at 21 months after index TKA (4 months after revision surgery) failed to improve the anterior knee pain at latest follow-up (18 months).

Of the four cases requiring resurfacing after 2 years, two were true isolated patella failures. Two patients had increased laxity secondary to PLI after 3 and 5 years. It is felt that the PLI was secondary to a combination of ligament stretch-out and/or bearing wear, which increased forces on the patellofemoral joint, with subsequent pain, synovitis, and mild maltracking. Both cases improved with tibial bearing exchange of an increased height and patella resurfacing. These cases are included as true patella failures in this study, but are not clear-cut, isolated patella failures.

Complications: Both Centres

Reoperation (secondary resurfacing) for anterior knee pain in TKA was noted in 19 (1.1%) of 1,777 cases, only 13 (0.7%) of which reported unequivocal clinical improvement postoperatively. Six (32%) of 19

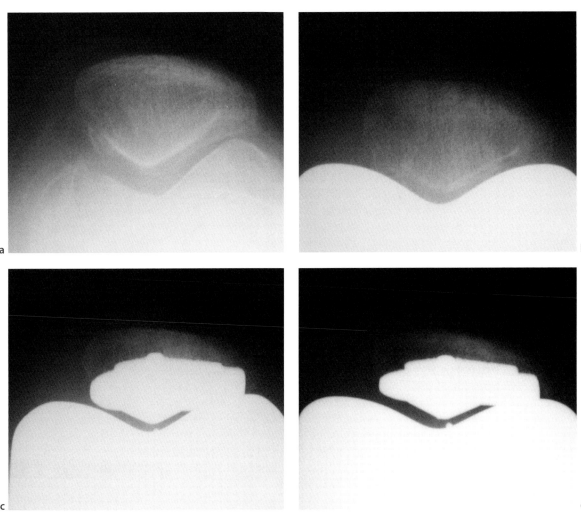

Fig. 3.7a–d. Skyline view radiographs. a Preoperative status of an osteoarthritis case. b Eight months postoperatively. Patient has anterior knee pain and painful range of motion, despite good patellar tracking both radiographically and clin- ically. c Radiographs showing status post secondary resurfac- ing of patella due to anterior knee pain. d Persistent anterior knee pain 4 years after patella resurfacing. Patellofemoral tracking unchanged

had no improvement after secondary resurfacing. In- cidental resurfacing at revision for other failure mechanisms was carried out in 20 (1.1%) cases. Patel- la resurfacing for any reason (worst-case scenario) was 2.2%. There were no reoperations for patella maltracking.

Patella Tracking: Radiographic Analysis

Patellofemoral alignment was studied in 200 cases with the longest follow-up (100 cases in each centre) via a method of radiographic skyline view analysis. The mean follow-up was 9.2 years. Clinical scores in this subgroup improved from 57 points preoperative-

ly to 85 at the latest evaluation. Two cases with poor scores had satisfactory patella tracking radiographi- cally. Radiographic analysis focused on patella track- ing congruency and patella tilt with comparable pre- and postoperative skyline radiographs (Fig. 3.8). Tracking improvement based on alignment of the femoral trochlear sulcus and the tip of the patella was measured in mm of lateral deviation on comparable pre- and postoperative skyline views (Fig. 3.9). Radio- graphic assessment revealed perfectly congruent tracking in 97% of the cases (Figs. 3.10 and 3.11). There was improved tracking from 2.0 mm (mean) lateral deviation to 0 mm perfect tracking in these cases. Six (3%) cases had less than perfect congruent contact postoperatively, but clinical scores remained

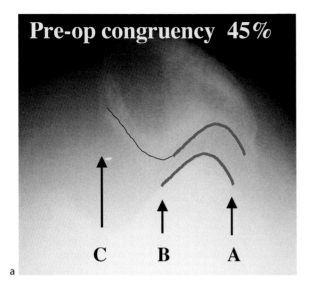

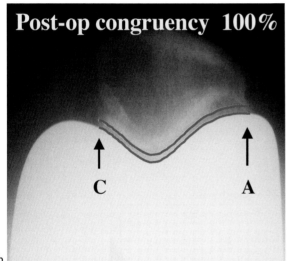

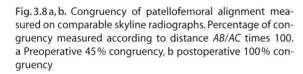

Fig. 3.8 a, b. Congruency of patellofemoral alignment measured on comparable skyline radiographs. Percentage of congruency measured according to distance *AB/AC* times 100. a Preoperative 45% congruency, b postoperative 100% congruency

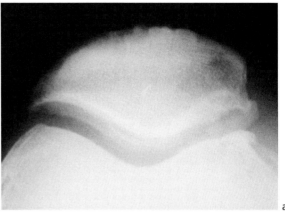

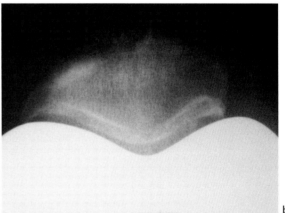

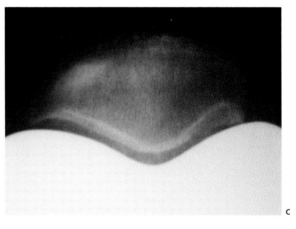

excellent or good in those cases. None of these cases had lateral deviation over 6 mm. There were no subluxations. Three (1.5%) cases showed a deteriorated patella tile angle with a lift off at the medial femoral condyle. Remodelling (mirroring the femoral component shape) of the patellar bone structure occurred in 16 (8%). Decreased height and sclerosis of the lateral facet was seen in 5 (2.5%) cases. Sixteen (9%) patellae had one or more osteolytic cysts within the patella bone. None of these patella changes was correlated with clinical symptoms.

Fig. 3.9 a–c. Patella skyline view radiographs (Schulthess Clinic). a Preoperative patient with osteoarthritis. b Immediate postoperative radiographs using LCS components and patelloplasty procedure, demonstrating normal patellofemoral tracking with 100% congruency. c Same case 10 years postoperatively. Patient had excellent result (modified HSS score 93)

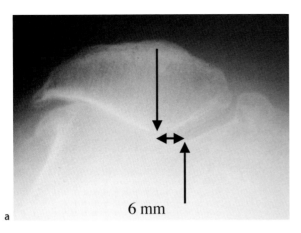
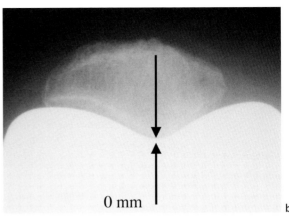

Fig. 3.10a, b. Method of measurement of lateral patella orientation/subluxation. Improvement of lateral patella subluxation postoperatively. **a** Preoperatively mild subluxation of more than 6 mm, **b** postoperatively perfect tracking

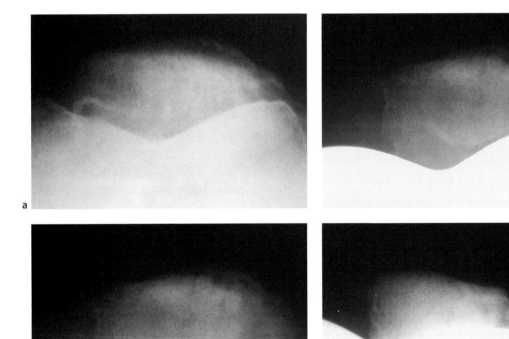

Fig. 3.11a–d. Patient with osteoarthritis showing patella remodelling of lateral facet without deterioration of clinical symptoms. **a** Preoperative skyline view, **b** 1 year postoperatively, **c** 7 years postoperatively, **d** 9 years postoperatively. Patient had an excellent result and no anterior knee pain

Discussion

Patella and patellofemoral problems remain a major cause of failure in TKA secondary to anterior knee pain, symptomatic maltracking (subluxation or dislocation), patella tendon rupture, and a multiplicity of patella resurfacing problems including aseptic loosening, prosthetic dissociation and polyethylene wear. Early failure rates attributed to the non-resurfaced patella ranged from 25 to 50% in some series and led to the development of patella resurfacing by Aglietti et al. (1975). Patella problems were reduced significantly, with early reports of a reduction from 25 to 6%, but increased again with various TKA designs in the 1980s and to date. Although TKA complications have decreased significantly, the patella still accounts for approximately 50% of TKA failures requiring reoperation.

The all-polyethylene cemented dome-shaped patella has remained the norm for most tricompartmental TKA systems. During the late 1970s and early 1980s, fine points of surgical technique, such as sizing, component positioning, and especially the concept of the tibiofemoral rotation relationship to patella tracking were less well understood. The most significant technical misdirection was the concept of femoral component positioning based on the posterior femoral condyles, which placed the femoral component internally rotated in most cases. Femoral designs, usually non-anatomic and non-conforming, led to high contact stress areas, which were accentuated by the addition of metallic backing and thinner polyethylene at the periphery.

Reported results on patella outcomes in TKA frequently fail to define the technical details of patella management. Despite design changes, many TKA failures in the 1980s and early 1990s were related to the resurfaced patella. Little attention was directed to femoral rotation or specific femoral design in the vast literature citing patella failures. Many designs and approaches accentuated extensor mechanism problems at the patellofemoral joint, which led to an increased number of problems of the resurfaced patella. Some designs were more prone to failures at the patellofemoral joint and have gone through corrective changes with improved outcomes. Many have failed and are no longer on the market. The surviving TKA systems appear to have adapted the design to a more condylar femoral shape and anatomic patellar groove.

Patellofemoral management in TKA is as key to successful outcome as is femorotibial management. First-generation non-constrained designs, such as the Geomedic, UCI, duocondylar or medial/lateral unicompartmental approach, retained the anterior patellofemoral anatomy. Failures of these devices were usually related to the femorotibial side and not the patellofemoral joint. Long-term follow-up was not available in large numbers, as most of these devices became obsolete. Further TKA designs in the late 1970s, such as kinematic condylar, total condylar, stabilocondylar, and posterior stabilised Insall-Bernstein type added an anterior femoral flange, initially with less than anatomic designs and often to accommodate the dome-shaped patellar component. The patella, when left unresurfaced in these designs, had higher failure rates. Failures due to increased anterior knee pain and functional restriction with activities such as stair climbing were attributed to the non-resurfaced patella rather than other factors such as design, subtle maltracking, poor femorotibial kinematics, etc. The question of biological tissues such as cartilage and bone articulating against metal prosthetic components raised the issue of potential complications and was of concern.

Insall et al. in 1976 reported initial experience with four different TKA designs, including geomedic and duocondylar, without accommodation for patella resurfacing. Patella-related problems (pain/subluxation) accounted for up to 60% of failures, often treated by partial or complete patellectomy. Subsequent experience with the total condylar knee revealed 26% patella failures when the patella was left unresurfaced. The majority of authors who evaluated patella resurfacing found superior results in their patella-resurfaced TKA. Braakman et al. (1995), Smith et al. (1989) and Figgie et al. (1986) reported higher complication rates with non-resurfaced patellae with different fixed bearing non-constrained and semi-constrained prosthetic designs. Barrack et al. (2001) noted that patellofemoral pain was more common in patients with "severe" OA, RA and obesity. On the basis of these experiences, at least in the USA, resurfacing of the patella was recommended as a routine, because of: (1) a lack of objective criteria for patella retention; (2) variation in surgical technique and soft tissue management; (3) variation in TKA femoral design, and (4) lack of long-term non-resurfaced TKA results in large series.

Patella-resurfaced TKA problems increased in the 1980s, during which time femoral component designs varied from condylar to less anatomical types (often box-like or flat), and metal-backed patella components (which required thinner polyethylene) became more commonly used. Since the mid-1980s, patella-resurfaced TKA failures became a well-recognised and most common cause for reoperation. The option of not resurfacing the patella re-emerged as a practical and safer alternative in many centres, especially with improved femoral component designs and surgical technique. Recent publications have suggested that results of TKA without patella resurfacing can be equally satisfactory. Fern et al. (1992) reported excellent to good results in rheumatoid knees without resurfacing. Shoji et al. (1989) compared rheumatoid patients with and without resurfacing of the patella in the same patient and did not advocate routine resurfacing in RA, since there were similar results in the unresurfaced knee. Keblish and Greenwald (1990) found no significant difference of resurfaced versus non-resurfaced patellae (same patient) in a prospective study utilising LCS knees including patients with RA. Improved clinical results in the non-resurfaced group, excluding RA as a primary diagnosis, were observed and reported by Bourne et al. (1995).

The patella has been analysed in many excellent studies, from normal to diseased states, as well as in TKA. Scientific support of patella non-resurfacing includes several biomechanical studies, which show significant alteration of patella forces following TKA. Patella forces have been measured at up to seven times body weight, potentially increasing with TKA, whether resurfaced or retained. Control of these forces is influenced by many factors, including quadriceps–hamstring balance, the biomechanical axis (extremity), cruciate competence, joint status, and others. Matsuda et al. (2000), in a cadaver study, demonstrated that patellofemoral contact stresses were less in the non-resurfaced as compared to dome-shaped anatomic (fixed bearing) resurfaced patellae. Reuben et al. (1991) have shown that patella thickness reduced to less than 14 mm can decrease tensile strength by as much as 50 %, which increases the likelihood of patella fractures and/or patella dissociation. Multiple problems of patella resurfacing, such as fracture of the patella or polyethylene bearing, quadriceps-patella-tendon rupture, component fracture/loosening, bearing edge wear, increased incidence of traction osteophytes and combinations have been reported. If the surgical technique is less than optimal (i.e. overresection, malresection, maltracking), potential problems are increased further. These potential complications are decreased/eliminated if the patella is left unresurfaced.

As noted, key factors in patella outcomes include femoral component design, rotational positioning, femorotibial positioning and treatment of the extensor mechanism and patella (if left unresurfaced). Designs vary from non-anatomic trochlear grooves that are too flat to others that are too constrained and not favourable for patella retention. The LCS femoral component was designed to the natural patella shape and contour with a common generating curve and deep trochlear groove, which best accommodates the unresurfaced patella. Tibial bearing position also affects patella tracking. Malpositioning of a fixed bearing tibial component is not uncommon, especially with more constrained designs. Moveable bearings minimise or eliminate this problem and allow for optimal patellofemoral alignment and patella tracking. Soft tissue techniques to enhance patella tracking, as described, are also important factors.

Femoral rotation positioning as a primary determinant of patellofemoral tracking, until recently, has been ignored or not appreciated in many systems. Eyeballing techniques and reference from the posterior condyles place the femoral component in internal rotation, which increases risks for lateral soft tissue tension, patella maltracking, and anterior knee pain. Femoral rotational references most commonly used today include the transepicondylar axis, the Whiteside Line, or an arbitrary 3 degrees of external rotation. The other method is a system based on the tibial axis and a balanced flexion gap (Fig. 3.12). This method places the femoral component in the appropriate rotational position and allows for optimum patella tracking to adapt to anatomic variation between patients. This step has been consistent for implantation with the LCS system since 1979 (prior to description of the other methods) and is felt to be a major technical factor in excellent patella results with or without resurfacing.

Our clinical results in this two-centre long-term TKA study without resurfacing of the patella have shown excellent to good scores in 94.6 % of all cases and 98.9 % survivorship of the non-resurfaced patella (97.8 % worst-case scenario). Retaining the patella in TKA has shown excellent results and an acceptable reoperation rate in both OA and RA patients, which compares favourably with results of patella resurfacing TKA reported in the literature. True patella failures due to anterior knee pain, which were subsequently resurfaced, were noted in 19 (1.1 %) of 1,777 cases, none of which was related to maltracking. Including those patellae that were incidentally resurfaced (20 cases) would give a worse-case scenario with 39 (2.2 %) of 1,777 patella complications in this study.

Patella tracking (or absence of maltracking) is the common denominator of patella outcomes in TKA. Therefore, radiographic evaluation of the patellofemoral articulation with skyline views is important

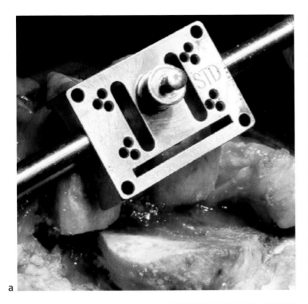

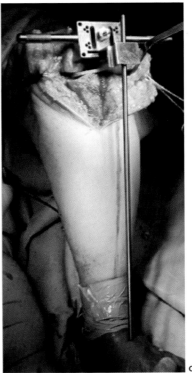

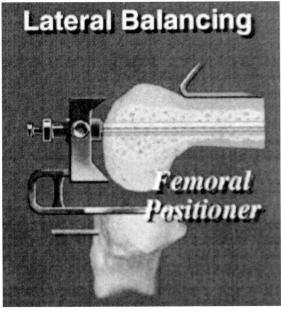

Fig. 3.12 a–c. Tibial axis (LCS) method of determining femoral rotation. Following soft tissue release (in extension with fine tuning in flexion) and a perpendicular mediolateral tibial resection: a a properly sized femoral resection block is selected. b The rotationally unconstrained block is connected to an instrumented IM rod, which is drilled parallel to the anterior cortex. A "flexion tension" spacer guide is set flush onto the tibial resection and connects parallel with the block. c The spacer guide establishes a balanced quadrolateral space (flexion gap) and automatically sets the correct femoral rotational position. The alignment rod double checks the tibial resection, which must be perpendicular to the tibial axis (best referenced proximally to the tibial crest and distally to the lateral edge of the tibialis anterior tendon)

in any study. Radiographic evaluation of the patella in 200 cases with the longest follow-up (mean 9.2 years) focused on pre- to postoperative correction of Q-angle, patella subluxation, patella tilt, and congruent patella contact areas, as described in the literature. Normal tracking of the patella was observed in 97%, and less than perfect congruent contact (0–6 mm lateral deviation) noted in six (3%) cases. None of these mild maltracking cases required reoperation. There was no patella subluxation or dislocation in either series.

Patella maltracking will result in ultimate failure with or without resurfacing. The surgeon should evaluate the pros and cons of patella resurfacing with consideration of prosthetic design, literature reports, and personal experience. The option of not resurfacing the patella in a given TKA system is felt to be important in that it is practical, economical, and can decrease the downside risk of patella-resurfaced catastrophes reported in the literature. All systems may not share similar results, and should be studied thoroughly if a recommendation for patella non-resurfacing in TKA is appropriate.

Acknowledgements. We thank U. Munzinger MD and T. Drobny, Schulthess Clinic, for clinical data and support, and Carol Varma, BS, Lehigh Valley Hospital, Allentown, Pennsylvania, USA, for illustrations.

Bibliography

Abd-el Wahab M, Szepesi K, Szucs G, Farkas C, Csernatony Z (1998) Functional improvement after knee arthroplasty without resurfacing of patella. Acta Chir Hung 37:59–66

Abraham W, Buchanan JR, Daubert H, Greer RB 3rd, Keefer J (1988) Should the patella be resurfaced in total knee arthroplasty? Efficiency of patellar resurfacing. Clin Orthop 236: 128–134

Aglietti P, Baldini A, Buzzi R, Indelli PF (2001) Patella resurfacing in total knee replacement: functional evaluation and complications. Knee Surg Sports Traumatol Arthrosc 9 [Suppl 1]:S27–S33

Aglietti P, Insall JN, Walker PS, Trent P (1975) A new patella prosthesis. Design and application. Clin Orthop 107:175–187

Arnold MP, Friederich NF, Widmer H, Muller W (1998) Patellar substitution in total knee prosthesis – is it important? Orthopade 27:637–641

Badalamente MA, Cherney SB (1989) Periosteal and vascular innervation of the human patella in degenerative joint disease. Semin Arthritis Rheum 18:61–66

Barrack RL, Wolfe MW (2000) Patellar resurfacing in total knee arthroplasty. J Am Acad Orthop Surg 8:75–82

Barrack RL, Wolfe MW, Waldman DA, Milicic M, Bertot AJ, Myers L (1997) Resurfacing of the patella in total knee arthroplasty. A prospective, randomized, double-blind study. J Bone Joint Surg Am 79A:1121–1131

Barrack RL, Bertot AJ, Wolfe MW, Waldman DA, Milicic M, Myers L (2001) Patellar resurfacing in total knee arthroplasty. A prospective, randomized, double-blind study with five to seven years of follow-up. J Bone Joint Surg Am 83A:1376– 1381

Berend ME, Ritter MA, Keating EM, Faris PM, Crites BM (2001) The failure of all-polyethylene patellar components in total knee replacement. Clin Orthop 388:105–111

Bizzini M, Boldt J, Munzinger U, Drobny T (2003) Rehabilitation guidelines after total knee arthroplasty. Orthopade 32(6):527–534

Boldt JG, Munzinger UK, Zanetti M, Hodler J (2004) Arthrofibrosis associated with total knee arthroplasty: gray-scale and power Doppler sonographic findings. AJR Am J Roentgenol 182(2):337–340

Boldt J, Munzinger U, Keblish P (2004) Comparison of isokinetic strength in resurfaced and retained patellae in bilateral TKA. J Arthroplasty 19(2):264

Bourne RB, Rorabeck CH, Vaz M, Kramer J, Hardie R, Robertson D (1995) Resurfacing versus not resurfacing the patella during total knee replacement. Clin Orthop 321:156–161

Boyd AD Jr, Ewald FC, Thomas WH, Poss R, Sledge CB (1993) Long-term complications after total knee arthroplasty with or without resurfacing of the patella. J Bone Joint Surg Am 75A:674–681

Braakman M, Verburg AD, Bronsema G, van Leeuwen WM, Eeftinck MP (1995) The outcome of three methods of patellar resurfacing in total knee arthroplasty. Int Orthop 19:7–11

Buechel FF (1982) A simplified evaluation system for the rating of the knee function. Orthop Rev 11:9

Buechel FF, Rosa RA, Pappas MJ (1989) A metal-backed, rotating-bearing patellar prosthesis to lower contact stress. An 11-year clinical study. Clin Orthop 248:34–49

Buechel FF, Pappas MJ, Makris G (1991) Evaluation of contact stress in metal-backed patellar replacement. A predictor of survivorship. Clin Orthop 273:190–197

Cameron HU (1991) Comparison between patellar resurfacing with an inset plastic button and patelloplasty. Can J Surg 34:49–52

Crites BM, Berend ME (2001) Metal-backed patellar components: a brief report on 10-year survival. Clin Orthop 388: 103–104

Enis JE, Gardner R, Robledo MA, Latta L, Smith R (1990) Comparison of patellar resurfacing versus nonresurfacing in bilateral total knee arthroplasty. Clin Orthop 260:38–42

Ewald FC (1989) The Knee Society total knee arthroplasty roentgenographic evaluation and scoring system. Clin Orthop 248:9–12

Feller JA, Bartlett RJ, Lang DM (1996) Patellar resurfacing versus retention in total knee arthroplasty. J Bone Joint Surg Br 78B:226–228

Fern ED, Winson IG, Getty CJ (1992) Anterior knee pain in rheumatoid patients after total knee replacement. Possible selection criteria for patellar resurfacing. J Bone Joint Surg Br 74B:745–748

Figgie HE 3rd, Goldberg VM, Heiple KG, Moller HS 3rd, Gordon NH (1986) The influence of tibial-patellofemoral location on function of the knee in patients with the posterior stabilized condylar knee prosthesis. J Bone Joint Surg Am 68A: 1035–1040

Freeman MA, Swanson SA, Todd RC (1973) Total replacement of the knee using the Freeman-Swanson knee prosthesis. Clin Orthop 94:153–170

Freeman MA, Samuelson KM, Elias SG, Mariorenzi LJ, Gokcay EI, Tuke M (1989) The patellofemoral joint in total knee prostheses. Design considerations. J Arthroplasty 4 [Suppl]:S69–S74

Furia JP, Pellegrini VD Jr (1995) Heteroscopic ossification following primary total knee arthroplasty. J Arthroplasty 10: 413–419

Hirano A, Fukubayashi T, Ishii T, Ochiai N (2001) Relationship between the patellar height and the disorder of the knee extensor mechanism in immature athletes. J Pediatr Orthop 21:541–544

Ikejiani CE, Leighton R, Petrie DP (2000) Comparison of patella resurfacing versus non-resurfacing in total knee arthroplasty. Can J Surg 43:35–85

Insall J, Tria AJ, Scott WN (1979) The total condylar knee prosthesis: the first 5 years. Clin Orthop 145:68–77

Insall JN, Ranawat CS, Aglietti P, Shine J (1976) A comparison of four models of total knee-replacement prosthesis. J Bone Joint Surg Am 58A:754–765

Kawakubo M, Matsumoto H, Otani T, Fujikawa K (1997) Radiographic changes in the patella after total knee arthroplasty without resurfacing the patella. Comparison of osteoarthritis and rheumatoid arthritis. Bull Hosp Joint Dis 56:237–244

Keblish PA (1991) The lateral approach to the valgus knee. Surgical technique and analysis of 53 cases with over two-year follow-up evaluation. Clin Orthop 271:52–62

Keblish PA, Greenwald AS (1990) Patella retention versus patella resurfacing in total knee arthroplasty. AAOS Scientific Exhibit, New Orleans, LA

Keblish PA, Stiehl JB, Varma CL (2000) The tibial axis as a determinant of femoral rotational alignment in TKA. AAOS Scientific Exhibit, Orlando, FL

Kim BS, Reitman RD, Schai PA, Scott RD (1999) Selective patellar nonresurfacing in total knee arthroplasty. 10 year results. Clin Orthop 367:81–88

Kulkarni SK, Freeman MA, Poal-Manresa JC, Asencio JI, Rodriguez JJ (2001) The patello-femoral joint in total knee arthroplasty: is the design of the trochlea the critical factor? Knee Surg Sports Traumatol Arthrosc 9 [Suppl 1]:S8–S12

Larson CM, Lachiewicz PF (1999) Patellofemoral complications with the Insall-Burstein II posterior-stabilized total knee arthroplasty. J Arthroplasty 14:288–292

Laskin RS (2001) Lateral release rates after total knee arthroplasty. Clin Orthop 392:88–93

Laurin CA, Dussault R, Levesque HP (1979) The tangential x-ray investigation of the patellofemoral joint: x-ray technique, diagnostic criteria and their interpretation. Clin Orthop 144:16–26

Levai JP, McLeod HC, Freeman MA (1983) Why not resurface the patella? J Bone Joint Surg Br 65B:448–451

Levistsky KA, Harris WJ, McManus J, Scott RD (1993) Total knee arthroplasty without patellar resurfacing. Clinical outcomes and long-term follow-up evaluation. Clin Orthop 286:116–121

Liebau C, Pap G, Nebelung W, Merk H, Neumann HW (1998) Comparison of functional outcome in implantation of Natural Knee knee prostheses with and without patellar resurfacing. Z Orthop Ihre Grenzgeb 136:65–69

Marcacci, M, Iacono F, Zaffagnini S, Visani A, Petitto A, Neri MP, Kon E (1997) Total knee arthroplasty without patella resurfacing in active and overweight patients. Knee Surg Sports Traumatol Arthrosc 5:258–261

Matsuda S, Ishinishi T, White SE, Whiteside LA (1997) Patellofemoral joint after total knee arthroplasty. Effect on contact area and contact stress. J Arthroplasty 12:790–797

Matsuda S, Ishinishi T, Whiteside LA (2000) Contact stresses with an unresurfaced patella in total knee arthroplasty: the effect of femoral component design. Orthopedics 23:213–218

Merchant AC, Mercer RL, Jacobsen RH, Cool CR (1974) Roentgenographic analysis of patellofemoral congruence. J Bone Joint Surg Am 56A:1391–1396

Muller W, Wirz D (2001) The patella in total knee replacement: does it matter? 750 LCS total knee replacements without resurfacing of the patella. Knee Surg Sports Traumatol Arthrosc 9 [Suppl 1]:S24–S26

Munzinger UK, Petrich J, Boldt JG (2001) Patella resurfacing in total knee arthroplasty using metal-backed rotating bearing components: a 2- to 10-year follow-up evaluation. Knee Surg Sports Traumatol Arthrosc 9 [Suppl 1]:S34–S42

Olcott CW, Scott R (2000) A comparison of 4 intraoperative methods to determine femoral component rotation during total knee arthroplasty. J Arthroplasty 15:22–26

Picetti GD 3rd, McGann WA, Welch RB (1990) The patellofemoral joint after total knee arthroplasty without patellar resurfacing. J Bone Joint Surg Am 72A:1379–1382

Reilly DT, Martens M (1972) Experimental analysis of the quadriceps muscle force and patello-femoral joint reaction force for various activities. Acta Orthop Scand 43:126–137

Reuben JD, McDonald CL, Woodward PL, Hennington LJ (1991) Effect of patella thickness on patella strain following total knee arthroplasty. J Arthroplasty 6:251–258

Schroeder-Boersch H, Scheller G, Fischer J, Jani L (1998) Advantages of patellar resurfacing in total knee arthroplasty. Two-year results of a prospective randomized study. Arch Orthop Trauma Surg 117:73–78

Scott RD, ReWy DT (1980) Pros and cons of patellar resurfacing in total knee replacement. Orthop Trans 4:328

Shoji H, Yoshino S, Kajino A (1989) Patellar replacement in bilateral total knee arthroplasty. A study of patients who had rheumatoid arthritis and no gross deformity of the patella. J Bone Joint Surg Am 71A:853–856

Singerman R, Gabriel SM, Maheshwer CB, Kennedy JW (1999) Patellar contact forces with and without patellar resurfacing in total knee arthroplasty. J Arthroplasty 14:603–609

Smith SR, Stuart P, Pinder IM (1989) Nonresurfaced patella in total knee arthroplasty. J Arthroplasty 4 [Suppl]:S81–S86

Soudry M, Mestriner LA, Binazzi R, Insall JN (1986) Total knee arthroplasty without patellar resurfacing. Clin Orthop 205:166–170

Stiehl JB, Cherveny PM (1996) Femoral rotational alignment using the tibial shaft axis in total knee arthroplasty. Clin Orthop 331:47–55

Stiehl JB, Voorhorst PE, Keblish P, Sorrells RB (1997) Comparison of range of motion after posterior cruciate ligament retention or sacrifice with a mobile bearing total knee arthroplasty. Am J Knee Surg 10:216–220

Stiehl JB, Komistek RD, Dennis DA, Keblish PA Kinematics of the patellofemoral joint in total knee arthroplasty. J Arthroplasty (in press)

Tanzer M, McLean CA, Laxer E, Casey J, Ahmed AM (2001) Effect of femoral component designs on the contact and tracking characteristics of the unresurfaced patella in total knee arthroplasty. Can J Surg 44:127–133

Thompson NW, Ruiz AL, Breslin E, Beverland DE (2001) Total knee arthroplasty without patellar resurfacing in isolated patellofemoral osteoarthritis. J Arthroplasty 16:607–612

Wasilewski SA, Frankl U (1989) Fracture of polyethylene of patellar component in total knee arthroplasty, diagnosed by arthroplasty. J Arthroplasty 4 [Suppl]:19–22

Windsor RE, Scuderi GR, Insall JN (1989) Patellar fractures in total knee arthroplasty. J Arthroplasty 4 [Suppl]:63–67

Wojtys EM, Beaman DN, Glover RA, Janda D (1990) Innervation of the human knee joint by substance-P fibers. Arthroscopy 6:254–263

3.3 Isokinetic Strength in Resurfaced and Retained Patellae

Jens G. Boldt, Mario Bizzini, Urs K. Munzinger

Patella management in total knee arthroplasty (TKA) still remains controversial. The influence of non-resurfacing or resurfacing the patella in TKA on the extensor and flexor mechanisms of the knee is not well understood, and few data about instrumented muscle strength measurement are available in the literature. This retrospective double-blinded study aimed to evaluate the extensor and flexor strength in patients with bilateral TKA, with patella resurfacing in one side and patelloplasty procedure at the contralateral side.

Out of a large cohort of over 3,000 TKAs, 35 patients with bilateral osteoarthritis underwent bilateral low contact stress (LCS) TKA within a 12-month period. One side received a tricompartmental TKA with patella resurfacing utilising a metal-backed rotating platform patella component and the other side was treated without patella resurfacing, but with a patelloplasty procedure including partial rim denervation, contouring cheilectomy, and vastus lateralis filet decompression as needed. All study patients had no known musculoskeletal problems or operations of hips, knees, ankle, or lumbar spine. All surgeries were

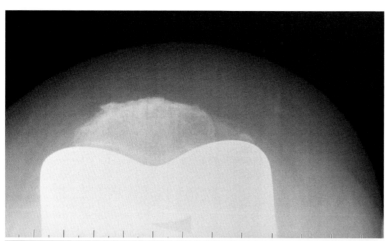
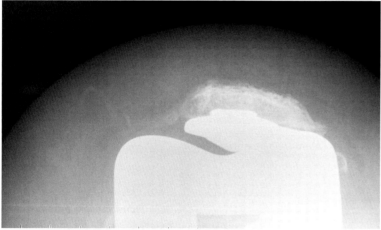

Fig. 3.13. Clinical example of bilateral TKA with and without patella resurfacing. The non-resurfaced patella was significantly stronger (higher isokinetic extension strength)

performed by two senior lower extremity orthopaedic surgeons between 1989 and 1996. Of the 35 patients with bilateral TKA, three were excluded because of deep infection and one patient underwent revision surgery for tibial component failure; three patients died of reasons independent of TKA prior to 5-year follow-up examination. Four patients out of 26 were lost to follow-up, leaving 22 (85%) patients that entered the study, 18 women and four men with a mean age of 77.3 years (48–88). Mean follow-up time was 7.4 years (5–10). There was no significant difference in time post surgery between tricompartmental (7.4 years) and bicompartmental TKA (7.5 years).

Preoperative varus deformity was noted in four patients and neutral leg alignment in 18 patients; no patient had valgus deformity in either leg. All patients received the identical femoral LCS component that has a patella-friendly design and rotational alignment placed perpendicular to the tibial shaft axis. In 17 patients, both tibial components were identical and five patients had different mobile bearing polyethylene bearings, a rotating platform in one knee and meniscal bearings in the other.

All isokinetic strength measurements were double blinded, since neither the patient nor the independent examiner was aware of the patella status post TKA. Isokinetic strength measurements were performed utilising a Biodex unit with five maximal repetitions at 180 degrees per second. A detailed radiographic analysis in anteroposterior, lateral and patella axial views (in defined 40 degrees of flexion) was performed by another independent orthopaedic surgeon. Measurement criteria included patella height, baja or alta position, lateral deviation, lateral tilt angle and patellofemoral congruency. The Cheltenham anterior knee pain questionnaire was administered for all patients, and the Knee Society Score (KSS) was obtained for both TKAs. Statistical analyses included analysis of variance testing for repeated measures and Stat View statistical software. Statistical significance level was set at a p value less than 0.05.

The mean extension strength for unresurfaced patellae in TKA was significantly ($p<0.0001$) stronger (40.2 Nm) compared with resurfaced patellae in the opposite TKA (37.9 Nm) (Fig. 3.13). Standard deviations were comparable in both TKA, 10.3 Nm versus

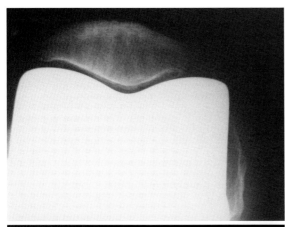

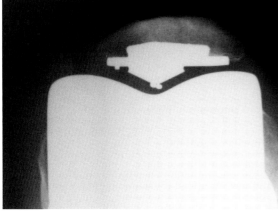

Fig. 3.14. Clinical example demonstrating perfect tracking of non-resurfaced patella and lateral maltracking plus tilt of resurfaced patella

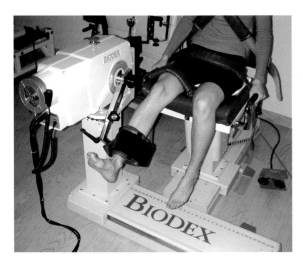

Fig. 3.15. Biodex isokinetic strength set-up. All patients were warmed up for 10 minutes on a stationary bike followed by three courses of five repetitive maximal knee extension and flexion

11.3 Nm. Mean flexion strength was also significantly ($p<0.0001$) stronger in the unresurfaced TKA compared with the resurfaced TKA (22.8 Nm versus 19.9 Nm). Mean patella congruent contact was significantly ($p<0.034$) better in all unresurfaced TKA (100%) compared with all resurfaced TKA (89%). Lateral tilt angle was significantly ($p<0.035$) better in the unresurfaced patellae (0 degrees) compared with resurfaced patellae (1.8 degrees tilt angle). There was a statistical trend ($p<0.083$) for better lateral patella tracking with unresurfaced patellae (0 mm lateral deviation) compared with resurfaced patellae (1.5 mm lateral deviation) (Fig. 3.14). There was no statistical difference in mean patella length (25.0 mm versus 23.4 mm) and patella (baja) position (22 mm each). The mean Cheltenham anterior knee pain score was significantly ($p<0.001$) better in the unresurfaced group (23 points) compared with resurfaced patellae (20 points). Overall clinical outcomes were statistically ($p=0.55$) comparable and had a mean KSS score of 83 points in the unresurfaced group compared with 82 points in the resurfaced group (Figs. 3.15 and 3.16).

Patella and patellofemoral problems remain a major cause of failure in TKA secondary to anterior knee pain, symptomatic maltracking, patella tendon rupture, and a multiplicity of patella resurfacing problems, including aseptic loosening, prosthetic dissociation, polyethylene wear, etc. Early failure rates attributed to the non-resurfaced patella ranged from 25 to 50% in some series and led to the development of patella resurfacing by Aglietti et al. (1975). Patella problems were reduced significantly, from early reports of 25% to 6%, but increased again with various TKA designs in the 1980s. Although TKA complications have decreased significantly, the patella still accounts for approximately 50% of TKA failures requiring reoperation.

The all-polyethylene cemented dome-shaped patella has remained the norm for most tricompartmental TKA systems. During the late 1970s and early 1980s, fine points of surgical technique, such as sizing, component positioning, and especially the concept of the tibiofemoral rotation relationship to patella tracking were less well understood. The most significant technical misdirection was the concept of femoral component positioning based on the posterior femoral condyles, which placed the femoral component internally rotated in most cases. Femoral designs, usually non-anatomic and non-conforming, led to high contact stress areas, which were accentuated by the addition of metallic backing and thinner polyethylene at the periphery.

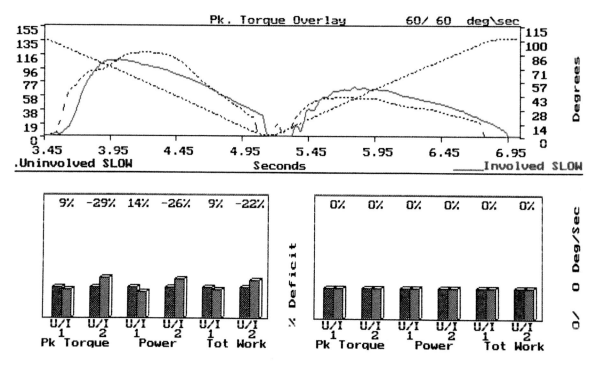

Fig. 3.16. Peak torque isokinetic strength showing faster acceleration and higher peak torque of the non-resurfaced patella TKA

Reported results on patella outcomes in TKA frequently fail to define the technical details of patella management. Despite design changes, many TKA failures in the 1980s and early 1990s were related to the resurfaced patella. Little attention was directed to femoral rotation or specific femoral design in the vast literature citing patella failures. Many designs and approaches accentuated extensor mechanism problems at the patellofemoral joint, which led to an increased number of problems of the resurfaced patella. Some designs were more prone to failures at the patellofemoral joint and have gone through corrective changes with improved outcomes. Many have failed and are no longer on the market. The surviving TKA systems appear to have adapted the design to a more condylar femoral shape and anatomic patellar groove.

Patellofemoral management in TKA is as key to successful outcome as is femorotibial management. First-generation non-constrained designs, such as the Geomedic, UCI, duocondylar or medial/lateral unicompartmental approach, retained the anterior patellofemoral anatomy. Failures of these devices were usually related to the femorotibial side and not the patellofemoral joint. Long-term follow-up was not available in large numbers since most of these devices became obsolete. Further TKA designs in the late 1970s, such as kinematic condylar, total condylar,

stabilocondylar, and posterior stabilised Insall-Bernstein type, added an anterior femoral flange, initially with less than anatomic designs and often to accommodate the dome-shaped patellar component. The patella, when left unresurfaced in these designs, had higher failure rates. Failures due to increased anterior knee pain and functional restriction with activities such as stair climbing were attributed to the non-resurfaced patella rather than other factors such as design, subtle maltracking, and poor femorotibial kinematics. The question of biological tissues such as cartilage and bone articulating against metal prosthetic components raised the issue of potential complications and was of concern.

On the basis of early experiences, at least in the USA, resurfacing of the patella was recommended as a routine, because of: (1) a lack of objective criteria for patella retention; (2) variation in surgical technique and soft tissue management; (3) variation in TKA femoral design, and (4) lack of long-term non-resurfaced TKA results in large series. Patella-resurfaced TKA problems increased in the 1980s, during which time femoral component designs varied from condylar to less anatomical types, and metal-backed patella components with thinner polyethylene bearings became more commonly used. Since the mid-1980s, patella-resurfaced TKA failures became a well-recognised and most common cause for reoperation.

The option of not resurfacing the patella re-emerged as a practical and safer alternative in many centres, especially with improved femoral component designs and surgical technique. Recent publications have suggested that results of TKA without patella resurfacing can be equally satisfactory.

Key factors in patella outcomes include femoral component design, rotational positioning, femorotibial positioning and treatment of the extensor mechanism and patella treatment. Designs vary from non-anatomic trochlear grooves that are too flat to others that are too constrained and not favourable for patella retention. The LCS femoral component was designed to the natural patella shape and contour with a common generating curve and deep trochlear groove, which best accommodates the unresurfaced patella. Tibial bearing position also affects patella tracking. Malpositioning of a fixed bearing tibial component is not uncommon, especially with more constrained designs. Moveable bearings minimise or eliminate this problem and allow for optimal patellofemoral alignment and patella tracking. Soft tissue techniques to enhance patella tracking, as described, are also important factors. Femoral rotation positioning as a primary determinant of patellofemoral tracking is felt to be a major technical factor in excellent patella results with or without resurfacing.

This study showed better strength values, anterior knee pain scores and x-ray findings in the non-resurfaced patella TKA. This is to our knowledge the first paper with a detailed analysis of the isokinetic strength characteristics in TKA with and without patella resurfacing within the same patient. Only Bourne et al. (1995), in a prospective study, showed that patients with non-resurfaced patella TKA had a significant better knee flexion torque than those with resurfaced patella TKA (for the extension torque only a trend for the non-resurfaced patellae was observed). The KSS scores at 2 years postoperative were slightly better in the non-resurfaced group. In the past decades the surgical trend in TKA has moved from patella resurfacing (1980s) to the balanced view (1990s) and in 2000 towards the tendency for non-resurfacing the patella (in non-USA countries).

Detailed analysis of all axial patella radiographs shows significant better patella tracking and congruency in the non-resurfaced patella. The outcome of patella resurfacing is dependent upon femoral component design, femoral rotation and patelloplasty procedure. Patella resurfacing represents a potentially difficult operation, which can finally lead to patella maltracking and poor patellofemoral congruency. Interestingly, the knees with the non-resurfaced patella TKA also had a significantly better Cheltenham score than those with resurfaced patella: maltracking and bad congruence of the patella prosthesis can be among the causes of anterior knee pain.

This TKA outcome study indicates an advantage in not resurfacing the patella, if compared to a metal-backed rotating anatomic LCS patella component in a long-term follow-up. Surgery for resurfacing the patella, by definition, implicates potential technical errors of position, fixation, resection, as well as femoral rotation and extensive soft tissue alignment and balance. Therefore one should question routinely resurfacing the patella in TKA. The results of this objective and subjective study indicate that mean isokinetic strength of both knee flexion and extension was significantly stronger in non-resurfaced LCS TKA. Non-resurfacing in TKA is easier, safer and may offer better outcome results. However, clinical scores did not show any differences or a patient preference.

Bibliography

Aglietti P, Insall JN, Walker PS, Trent P (1975) A new patella prosthesis. Design and application. Clin Orthop 107:175–187

Barrack RL, Matzkin E, Ingraham R, Engh G, Rorabeck C (1998) Revision knee arthroplasty with patella replacement versus bony shell. Clin Orthop 356:139–43

Berman AT, Bosacco SJ, Israelite C (1991) Evaluation of total knee arthroplasty using isokinetic testing. Clin Orthop 271:106

Berry DJ, Rand JA (1993) Isolated patellar component revision of total knee arthroplasty. Clin Orthop 286:110–115

Bizzini M, Boldt J, Munzinger U, Drobny T (2003) Rehabilitation guidelines after total knee arthroplasty. Orthopade 32(6):527–534

Boldt JG, Bezzini M, Keblish PA, Munzinger UK (2004) Isokinetic strength in resurfaced and retained TKA. Scientific exhibition, AAOS annual meeting, San Francisco, USA, Mar 2004

Boldt JG, Keblish PA, Drobny T, Munzinger UK Patella non-resurfacing in LCS mobile bearing TKA. Evaluation of 1777 cases with 2 to 15 year follow-up

Boldt JG, Keblish PA, Munzinger UK (2003) Bone graft options during TKA in patellectomized knes. ISTA, San Francisco, USA

Boldt JG, Keblish PA, Munzinger UK (2003) Patella bone graft reconstruction in patellectomized knees undergoing primary TKA. Scientific poster, AAOS annual meeting, New Orleans Febr 2003, USA

Boldt J, Munzinger U, Keblish P (2004) Comparison of isokinetic strength in resurfaced and retained patellae in bilateral TKA. J Arthroplasty 19(2):264

Boldt JG, Munzinger UK (2003) Patella resurfacing in LCS mobile bearing TKA. A 2 to 12 year evaluation. EFORT, Helsinki, Finland

Boldt JG, Munzinger UK, Zanetti M, Hodler J (2004) Arthrofibrosis associated with total knee arthroplasty: gray-scale and power Doppler sonographic findings. AJR Am J Roentgenol 182(2):337–340

Bourne RB, Rorabeck CH, Vaz M, Kramer J, Hardie R, Robertson D (1995) Resurfacing versus not resurfacing the patella during total knee replacement. Clin Orthop 321:156–161

Björkström S, Goldie IF (1980) A study of the arterial supply of the patella in the normal state, in chondromalacia patellae and in osteoarthrosis. Acta Orthop Scand 51:63–70

Buechel FF (1982) A simplified evaluation system for the rating of knee function. Orthop Rev 11:9

Buechel FF (1991) Patellar tendon bone grafting for patellectomized patients having total knee arthroplasty. Clin Orthop 271:72–78

Buechel FF Sr, Buechel FF Jr, Pappas MJ, D'Alessio J (2001) Twenty-year evaluation of meniscal bearing and rotating platform knee replacements. Clin Orthop 388:41–50

Buechel FF Sr, Buechel FF Jr, Pappas MJ, Dalessio J (2002) Twenty-year evaluation of the New Jersey LCS rotating platform knee replacement. J Knee Surg 15:84–89

D'Lima DD, Poole C, Chadha H, Hermida JC, Mahar A, Colwell CW Jr (2001) Quadriceps moment arm and quadriceps forces after total knee arthroplasty. Clin Orthop 392:213–220

Elia EA, Lotke PA (1991) Results of revision total knee arthroplasty associated with significant bone loss. Clin Orthop 271:114–121

Ewald FC (1989) The Knee Society total knee arthroplasty roentgenographic evaluation and scoring system. Clin Orthop 248:9

Huang CH, Cheng CK, Lee YT, Lee KS (1996) Muscle strength after successful total knee replacement: a 6- to 13-year followup. Clin Orthop 328:147–154

Hungerford DS (1994) Management of extensor mechanism complications in total knee arthroplasty. Orthopedics 179:843–844

Hanssen AD (2001) Bone-grafting for severe patellar bone loss during revision knee arthroplasty. J Bone Joint Surg Am 83A:171–176

Hirano A, Fukubayashi T, Ishii T, Ochiai N (2001) Relationship between the patellar height and the disorder of the knee extensor mechanism in immature athletes. J Pediatr Orthop 21:541–544

Hsu HC, Luo ZP, Rand JA, An KN (1996) Influence of patellar thickness on patellar tracking and patellofemoral contact characteristics after total knee arthroplasty. J Arthroplasty 11:69–80

Jiang CC, Chen CH, Huang LT, Liu YJ, Chang SL, Wen CY, Liu TK (1993) Effect of patellar thickness on kinematics of the knee joint. J Formos Med Assoc 92:373–378

Joshi AB, Lee CM, Markovic L, Murphy JC, Hardinge K (1994) Total knee arthroplasty after patellectomy. J Bone Joint Surg Br 76:926–929

Kim BS, Reitman RD, Schai PA, Scott RD (1999) Selective patellar nonresurfacing in total knee arthroplasty. 10 year results. Clin Orthop 367:81–88

Larson KR, Cracchiolo A 3rd, Dorey FJ, Finerman GA (1991) Total knee arthroplasty in patients after patellectomy. Clin Orthop 264:243–254

Lennox DW, Hungerford DS, Krackow KA (1987) Total knee arthroplasty following patellectomy. Clin Orthop 223:220–224

Leopold SS, Greidanus N, Paprosky WG, Berger RA, Rosenberg AG (1999) High rate of failure of allograft reconstruction of the extensor mechanism after total knee arthroplasty. J Bone Joint Surg Am 8111:1574–1579

Kang JD, Papas SN, Rubash HE, McClain EJ Jr (1993) Total knee arthroplasty in patellectomized patients. J Arthroplasty 85:489–501

Marmor L (1987) Unicompartmental knee arthroplasty following patellectomy. Clin Orthop 218:164

Martin SD, Haas SB, Insall JN (1995) Primary total knee arthroplasty after patellectomy. J Bone Joint Surg Am 77:1323–1330

Munzinger UK, Petrich J, Boldt JG (2001) Patella resurfacing in total knee arthroplasty using metal-backed rotating bearing components: a 2- to 10-year follow-up evaluation. Knee Surg Sports Traumatol Arthrosc 9 [Suppl 1]:S34–S42

Paletta GA Jr, Laskin RS (1995) Total knee arthroplasty after a previous patellectomy. J Bone Joint Surg Am 77:1708–1712

Rand JA, Trousdale RT, Ilstrup DM, Harmsen WS (2003) Factors affecting the durability of primary total knee prostheses. J Bone Joint Surg Am 85A:259–265

Railton GT, Levack B, Freeman MA (1990) Unconstrained knee arthroplasty after patellectomy. J Arthroplasty 5:255–257

Parvizi J, Seel MJ, Hanssen AD, Berry DJ, Morrey BF (2002) Patellar component resection arthroplasty for the severely compromised patella. Clin Orthop 397:356–361

Ritter MA, Keating EM, Faris PM (1989) Clinical, roentgenographic, and scintigraphic results after interruption of the superior lateral genicular artery during total knee arthroplasty. Clin Orthop 248:145

Ritter MA, Herbst SA, Keating EM, Faris PM, Meding JB (1996) Patellofemoral complications following total knee arthroplasty. Effect of a lateral release and sacrifice of the superior lateral geniculate artery. J Arthroplasty 11:368–372

Stiehl JB, Komistek RD, Dennis DA, Keblish PA (2001) Kinematics of the patellofemoral joint in total knee arthroplasty. J Arthroplasty 166:706–714

Tabutin J (1998) Osseous reconstruction of the patella with screwed autologous graft in the course of repeat prosthesis of the knee. Rev Chir Orthop Reparatrice Appar Mot 84: 363–367

Wendt PP, Johnson RP (1985) A study of quadriceps excursion, torque, and the effect of patellectomy on cadaver knee. J Bone Joint Surg 67A:726–732

Walker PS, Haider H (2003) Characterizing the motion of total knee replacements in laboratory tests. Clin Orthop 410:54–68

Watkins MP, Harris BA, Wender S, Zarins B, Rowe CR (1983) Effect of patellectomy on the function of the quadriceps and hamstrings. J Bone Joint Surg 65A:390–395

3.4 Total Knee Arthroplasty in Isolated Patellofemoral Arthritis

N.W. Thompson, A.L. Ruiz, E. Breslin, D.E. Beverland

Isolated patellofemoral arthritis has been reported to occur in approximately 5% of patients with arthritis of the knee (Laskin and van Steijn 1999). Patients with patellofemoral arthritis are often severely debilitated and in particular have marked difficulty ascending or descending stairs, arising from chairs and riding comfortably in a car. Anterior knee pain and a history of recurrent "giving way" of the knee due to the patella locking or sticking in its groove are the usual clinical features (Amis 1999). The management of isolated patellofemoral arthritis remains a challenge for the orthopaedic surgeon due to the complexity of patellofemoral joint biomechanics and the difficulties that have been encountered with patello-femoral joint replacement. This retrospective study was undertaken to evaluate the efficacy of knee arthroplasty without patellar resurfacing in this subset of patients. We present our results to date.

We reviewed 31 patients (33 knees) with isolated patellofemoral arthritis who underwent low contact stress (LCS) total knee arthroplasty (TKA) (LCS, De-Puy, Leeds, UK) without patellar resurfacing. All patients were referred to the senior author (D.E.B.) with moderate to severe symptoms arising from their patellofemoral joint. All patients had radiological evidence of patellofemoral osteoarthritis, with minimal tibiofemoral disease as seen on the anteroposterior and lateral radiographs. The radiographic findings were confirmed intraoperatively on inspection of the tibiofemoral compartments. Patients were evaluated preoperatively and at each review using a standard proforma to assess their mobility, knee pain and the presence of night pain. Range of movement was measured at each visit using a hand-held goniometer.

Standard radiographs included an anteroposterior, lateral and patellar skyline view of the symptomatic knee. The degree of patellofemoral arthritis was graded in severity (0–4) according to the classification of Sperner et al: grade 0, no degenerative changes; grade 1, definite subchondral sclerosis with minimal osteophytes on the patella; grade 2, definite osteophytes on the patella; grade 3, narrowing of the patellofemoral joint space, osteophytes on the patella and femoral condyles; grade 4, tight joint space and large osteophytes with a deformed patella. Lateral patellar tilt was measured according to the method described by Gomes et al. (1988) on both the preoperative and postoperative skyline views. Patellar congruency was measured on both the preoperative and postoperative skyline views using the method described by Keblish et al. (1994).

All operations were performed by the senior author (D.E.B.) using a cementless-LCS cruciate sacrificing prosthesis under tourniquet control in a laminar flow environment. Perioperative antibiotics (cephamandole) and dextran 70 as an antithrombotic medication were used in all patients. In all cases the patellar fat pad was resected and any peripheral patellar osteophytes were excised. In patellae with distortion of the lateral facet due to the presence of a large traction osteophyte (Figs. 3.17–3.19), a saw was used to recreate the normal keel-shape of the patella ("patellar contouring"). If after contouring the patella continued to maltrack, a lateral patellar release was performed. Patellae that did not require contouring but failed to track satisfactorily had a lateral patellar

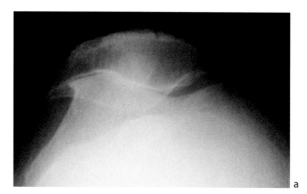

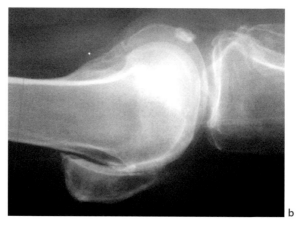

Fig. 3.17. Preoperative and skyline (a) and lateral (b) view demonstrating grade 4 patellofemoral arthritis with large lateral traction osteophyte

release. Postoperatively, all patients were mobilised on the day after surgery and received daily inpatient physiotherapy. Patients were referred for further physiotherapy following discharge at the discretion of the physiotherapist.

Of the 31 patients (33 knees), 26 were female and five were male (two females had bilateral TKA). Average age was 73 years (range 58–89 years). The patients had their surgery between July 1996 and May 1999. During the same period 720 total knee replacements were performed and thus these patients represent 4.6% of the senior author's patient population.

All patients had preoperative knee pain, with 21 patients (22 knees) reporting sleep disturbance due to their knee pain. Preoperatively, 21 patients (23 knees) required the use of some form of walking aid, most commonly one walking stick. Of note, seven patients had knee joint injections preoperatively without benefit and one patient had surgery 22 years previously for recurrent patellar dislocation. Average preoperative range of motion (ROM) was 108 degrees (range 80–125).

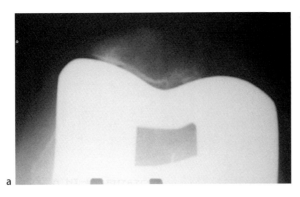

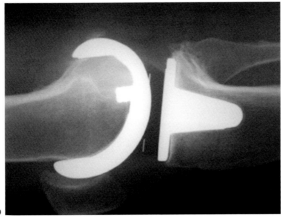

Fig. 3.18. Postoperative skyline (a) and lateral (b) view following patellar contouring and lateral patellar release

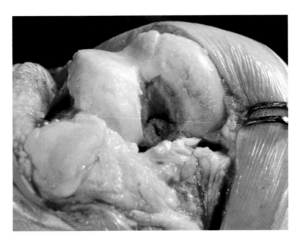

Fig. 3.19. Intraoperative site demonstrating gross wear of the patellar and trochlear articulating surfaces

According to the classification by Sperner et al, 19 knees were grade 4, ten knees were grade 3 and four knees were grade 2. Average preoperative patellar tilt was 10 degrees (range 1–29) and average preoperative patellar congruency was 73% (range 17–95). No intra-operative complications were encountered; however, early in the postoperative period, one patient developed atrial fibrillation, one patient developed a lower respiratory tract infection and two patients had superficial wound infections. All these patients were treated successfully.

At 3-monthly review, 14 knees were pain-free and patients reported an improvement in their pain in 17 knees. Two patients felt that their knee pain was worse than before. However, at latest review (average 20 months), 21 knees were pain-free, with12 knees only having mild discomfort on occasion. Of the two patients who failed to improve at 3 months, both reported that their pain had improved with time. Two patients continue to have night discomfort.

At latest review (average 20 months), only ten patients required the use of a walking aid compared with 21 patients preoperatively. Of note, five of the ten patients had problems with other joints (ipsilateral hip and/or knee, contralateral hip and/or knee, and low back pain). One patient required a stick because of restricted mobility due to Parkinson's disease, and one patient was able to walk a distance of one mile without difficulty while using a stick.

Range of movement at 3 months was on average 99 degrees (range 75–125). Average ROM at latest review (average 20 months) was 104 degrees (range 70–135). Of note, in 11 knees ROM improved on average by 15 degrees (range 5–35), while four knees regained their preoperative ROM. The remaining 18 knees had a ROM less than their preoperative measure by 18 degrees on average (range 5–40), with only three knees exhibiting a ROM greater than the average value of 104 degrees. Patellar tilt improved by an average of 7 degrees in 27 knees (range 1–26) and 30 knees had an improvement in patellar congruency averaging 18% (range 3–63) (Table 3.1).

Patellofemoral osteoarthritis commonly exists as a component of generalised knee arthritis. In our patient population, isolated patellofemoral osteoarthritis represented 4.6% of patients having knee replacement. This figure compares well with that reported by Laskin and van Steijn (1999), who found an incidence of 5%. A precise incidence is, however, difficult to quantify, as many individuals are asymptomatic. In addition, the condition is frequently underdiagnosed, as skyline views are often not routinely requested.

Table 3.1. Summary of clinical data (figures reflect number of knees affected) before surgery, at 3-monthly review and at latest follow-up (average, 20 months)

Parameter	Preoperative	3-month review	Latest review
Knee pain	33	14 pain-free; 17 pain improved; 2 pain worse	21 pain-free; 12 only occasional pain
Mobility (walking aid required)	23	14	10
Night pain	21	2	2
Average ROM	108°	99°	104°

Patellofemoral arthritis is primarily a disease of the older patient. Laskin and van Steijn (1999), in their series of 53 patients with isolated patellofemoral arthritis, found the average age of these patients to be 67 years. No significant age difference was noted when compared with patients with tricompartmental knee arthritis. This is a similar finding in our practice, with the average age in our series being 73 years compared with 72 years for patients with generalised knee arthritis. Younger patients are, however, not exempt, with seven patients in our series being 65 years or less.

Patellofemoral arthritis may occur secondary to a prior patellar fracture or severe long-standing extensor mechanism malalignment (Laskin and van Steijn 1999). However, it would appear that the majority of patients have no history of previous patellar trauma or patellar symptoms before the onset of the symptoms of osteoarthritis (Laskin and van Steijn 1999). In our series, only one patient had previous patellar pathology.

Anteroposterior and lateral radiographs, in those patients with isolated patellofemoral arthritis, often have a relatively benign appearance. Radiographic changes are best seen on the skyline patellar view. These can include joint space narrowing, periarticular osteophyte formation, lateral patellar tilt and lateral translation of the patella.

Often in severe patellofemoral osteoarthritis, the patellar and trochlear surfaces are distorted, which prevents normal patellar tracking. Frequently, the lateral facet of the patella is elongated and distorted by the presence of a large traction osteophyte, which closely embraces the lateral femoral condyle. In this situation, the patella, which has lost its keel-shape, will not track centrally within the patellar groove (patellar maltracking). Both maltracking and malalignment have been reported to be major determinants of anterior knee pain (Smith et al. 1989).

Treatment options for patellofemoral arthritis include conservative measures such as exercise and oral and intra-articular medications. However, for those with more debilitating symptoms, surgery becomes an option.

Unfortunately, results to date have been disappointing with some of the more conservative approaches such as extensor mechanism alignment and patellar debridement procedures (Harvey et al. 1993). Patellectomy, while removing a worn patellar surface, does not address the worn trochlear groove and a high failure rate has been reported (Laskin and Paletta 1995). In addition, patellectomy increases the risk of extensor mechanism dislocation (Amis 1999) and has been shown to compromise the results of subsequent TKA (Laskin and Paletta 1995). Patellar hemiarthroplasty, performed by resurfacing the patella as opposed to the trochlea, has also proved disappointing, as revealed by the efforts of Insall et al (1980), Levitt (1973) and Worrell et al. Patellofemoral arthroplasty, where both joint surfaces are replaced, also has not proven to be effective in the majority of patients (Argensen et al. 1995, Cartier et al. 1990).

Laskin and van Steijn (1999) compared the results of 53 patients with isolated patellofemoral arthritis who underwent tricompartmental TKA with those of a concomitant series of patients with generalised knee arthritis. They found that the patellofemoral group had significantly better postoperative mean flexion and knee scores (122 versus 117 degrees, 96 versus 88 points respectively). Residual anterior knee pain was present in approximately 7% of patients in both groups.

Laskin and van Steijn (1999) concluded that tricompartmental TKA resulted in better outcomes for older patients with patellofemoral arthritis as compared with patellofemoral replacement, debridement procedures and patellectomy.

From our results, we agree that total knee replacement is the most suitable option for older patients with debilitating patellofemoral arthritis; however, in our practice we do not resurface the patella.

We feel that our approach has been successful for two important reasons. First, we ensure that patellar maltracking and malalignment are corrected by employing the technique of "patellar contouring" as described, with or without lateral release. Second, conventional knee arthroplasty is a "tried and tested" procedure, which we know from experience has excellent results (Beuchal and Pappas 1989, Keblish 1991). Perhaps also removing the patellar fat pad may play a part, as it has been shown to be one of the most pain-sensitive structures within the knee joint (Dye et al. 1998).

There are at least three potential criticisms of this work. First, although these patients had isolated patellofemoral arthritis, it is possible that a proportion of their pain may have arisen from minimal tibiofemoral compartment wear and that by replacing these joint surfaces this site of pain activity has been abolished. Second, while our results to date have been encouraging, we appreciate that the duration of follow-up is relatively short. However, in this study we were more interested in early outcome measures such as relief of pain and improved mobility. Third, we replace the healthy tibiofemoral compartment without patellar resurfacing, for what is essentially isolated patellofemoral disease. Our approach seems to work, however, and since there are no satisfactory prostheses for replacing the patellofemoral joint at present, we are further encouraged to continue to apply our technique. In conclusion, we propose knee arthroplasty without patellar resurfacing as an option in older patients with isolated patellofemoral arthritis and emphasise the importance of correcting patellar maltracking. We look forward to presenting our longer-term results at a later date.

Bibliography

Amis AA (1999) Patello-femoral joint replacement. Current Orthop 13:64
Argensen JN, Guillaume JM, Aubaniac JM (1995) Is there a place for patellofemoral arthroplasty? Clin Orthop 321:162
Beuchal FF, Pappas MJ (1989) New Jersey low contact stress knee replacement system: ten year evaluation of meniscal bearings. Orthop Clin North Am 2:147
Cartier P, Sanoviller JL, Grelsamer RP (1990) Patellofemoral arthroplasty. J Arthroplasty 5:49
Dye SF, Vaupel GL, Dye CC (1998) Conscious neurosensory mapping of the internal structures of the human knee without intraarticular anaesthesia. Am J Sports Med 6:773
Gomes LSM, Bechtold JE, Gustilo RB (1988) Patellar prosthesis positioning in total knee arthroplasty. A roentgengraphic study. Clin Orthop 236:72
Harvey IA, Barry K, Kirby SPJ, Johnson R, Elloy MA (1993) Factors affecting the range of movement of total knee arthroplasty. J Bone Joint Surg 75A:950
Insall JN, Tria AJ, Aglietti P (1980) Resurfacing of the patella. J Bone Joint Surg 62A:933
Keblish P (1991) Results and complications of the LCS (Low Contact Stress) knee system. Acta Orthop Belg 2:124
Keblish PA, Varma AK, Greenwald AS (1994) Patellar resurfacing or retention in total knee arthroplasty: a prospective study of patients with bilateral replacements. J Bone Joint Surg Br 76B:930
Laskin RS, Paletta G (1995) Total knee replacement in the patient who has undergone patellectomy. J Bone Joint Surg 77A:1708
Laskin RS, van Steijn M (1999) Total knee replacement for patients with patello-femoral arthritis. Clin Orthop 367:89
Levitt RL (1973) A long-term evaluation of patellar prostheses. Clin Orthop 97:153
Schroeder-Boersch H, Scheller G, Fischer J, Jani L (1998) Advantages of patellar resurfacing in total knee arthroplasty: two year results of a prospective randomised study. Arch Orthop Trauma Surg 117:73
Smith SR, Stuart P, Pinder IM (1989) Nonresurfaced patella in total knee arthroplasty. J Arthroplasty 4 [Suppl]:581

3.5 Long-Term Outcomes Utilizing LCS Mobile Bearing TKA

Jens G. Boldt

The low contact stress (LCS) total knee arthroplasty (TKA) was designed in the late 1970s to overcome problems in TKA including mechanical loosening due to polyethylene wear debris, as observed in fixed bearing TKA, and to improve knee biomechanics. Particulate debris developed from increased contact stress of usually flat bearing designs. Fixed bearing prostheses with a more congruent shape and large contact areas had increased shear forces at the implant–bone interface, thus leading to early mechanical loosening despite screw fixation or cementing. The LCS femoral and mobile bearing shape represents an optimum for maximal contact area and minimal constraint forces. Advantages of this knee system include: near anatomical biomechanics during full range of motion, minimal aseptic mechanical loosening, minimal wear synovitis, and minimal periprosthetic osteolysis.

Fig. 3.20. Distribution of TKA cases that entered the study

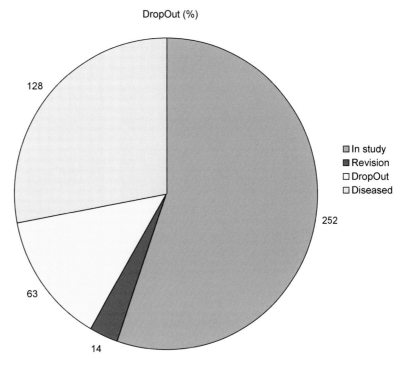

DropOut (%)

128

252

63

14

☐ In study
■ Revision
☐ DropOut
☐ Diseased

The femoral component design has been unchanged for 25 years. It has an anatomic patellar groove requiring a box resection at the anterior femur. This patella-friendly design has proven to produce minimal contact stress and minimal constraint forces, is self centering and difficult to deviate laterally. The patella may articulate with or without resurfacing. Two different patella components are available: an all-polyethylene anatomic patella for cement fixation and a metal-backed rotating patella component for cementless fixation. Three different tibial platforms were available at that time: (1) bicruciate retaining, (2) posterior cruciate ligament (PCL) sacrificing (MB) design, and (3) bicruciate retaining design, (4) the newer LCS complete system combines the rotating platform for PCL retention or sacrifice, but was not available in this study. The latter tibial component has a three-fin design and all other designs a large tibial cone for fixation.

Outcome studies in TKA do not depend on knee design alone, but also on surgical technique, balanced flexion and extension gaps, as well as soft tissue appreciation when restoring the overall mechanical axes. This surgical factor is difficult to exclude in outcome studies, but a recent worldwide multicenter study of the LCS knee that included both average and specialist surgeons showed little differences. Another important factor is the patient's preoperative knee pathology. Varus or valgus deformities, bone deformities, malalignments, contractures, or instabilities

play a vital role in postoperative results. Further problems may occur with regards to bone and ligament quality and quantity. Younger and more active patients will put higher demand on the prosthesis than older, less active or rheumatoid patients.

The purpose of this study was to evaluate the outcome of 266 primary LCS mobile bearing TKA, both MB and RP. All data were evaluated from one major joint replacement center and all cases were performed by consultants or under their direct supervision. All patients were routinely invited for follow-up at 6 weeks, 6 months, 1 year, 2 years, 5 years and 10 years, or when complications were encountered. A specific knee joint follow-up and evaluation questionnaire was performed and fed online into a digital databank (IDES system, see Sect. 5.2). Preoperative diagnosis, age, gender, range of motion, clinical scores, and device configurations were encountered. Surgical approach and technique points are intensively discussed throughout this book. Failure analysis included body mass index, general health impediments, wound problems and prosthetic-related complications. Survivorship analysis was calculated utilizing Kaplan-Meier curves. Component-related complications were separated into specific component (femur, tibia, and patella) aseptic loosening, bearing problems, patella problems, and instability.

There were 457 cases operated before December 1991. There were 128 deaths and 63 were lost to follow-up, leaving 266 (86.2%) entering the study (Fig. 3.20).

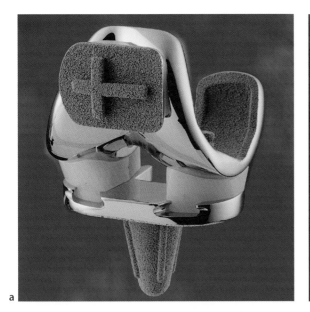

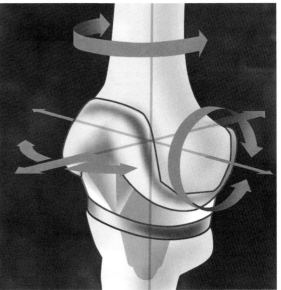

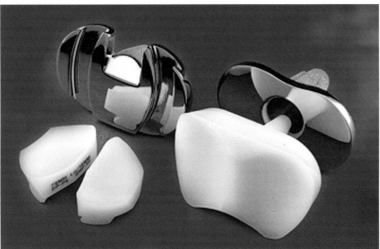

Fig. 3.21. a LCS mobile bearing knee prosthesis with meniscal bearings for PCL retention and cementless fixation, **b** six directions of motion allowed by prosthetic components, **c** alternatively, a rotating-only platform for PCL sacrifice is available

Mean follow-up was 11 years (range 10–13). Demographics included 76% females and 8% patients with rheumatoid arthritis. There were 60% PCL retaining MB and 40% PCL sacrificing RP components (Fig. 3.21). The patella was unresurfaced in 79% and 96% were cementless. One hundred and fifty-eight TKAs were approached laterally and 299 medially. In 182 TKAs, RP bicruciate sacrificing mobile bearing devices were used and 275 TKAs had meniscal PCL retaining bearings. Mean age was 68 years at time of surgery.

Clinical scores were excellent or good in 89%, fair in 9% and poor in 2%. The mean Knee Society Score (KSS) improved from 35.4 to 81.8 points (max 100 points) and the mean function KSS score improved from 38.3 to 74.4. The range of motion improved significantly ($p<0.001$) from 97 to 109 degrees of flexion. Extension deficit of 7.5 degrees improved significantly ($p<0.001$) to 0 degrees (full extension) on average. Total survivorship was 86.8% (Fig. 3.22).

Complications were most commonly bearing wear related and included: nine MB, eight tibial loosening (six MB, two RP), and six metal-backed patella. There were 16 patella resurfacings secondary to anterior knee pain or incidental to revision for other reasons. There were three RP spinouts, two requiring reoperation. One femoral component became aseptically loose. Bearing exchange was successful in 14 MB and five RP. Tibial revision was required in eight cases, seven because of loosening and one because of platform fracture (Tables 3.2, 3.3).

Table 3.2. Complications

Anterior knee pain	27
Hematoma	14
Arthrofibrosis	13
Ligament instability	12
Wound problems	9
Infection (micro+)	8
Synovitis	6
Infection (micro-)	2
Fracture tibia	1
Avulsion tuberositas tibiae	1
Vascular	1

Table 3.3. Treatment of complications

Hematoma debridement	22
Synovectomy	16
Revisions	14
Arthrolysis	7
Arthrodesis	2
Soft tissue releases	1
Hoffa resection	1

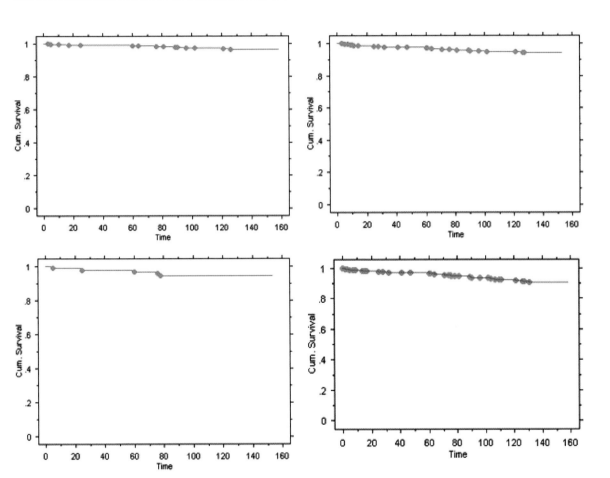

Fig. 3.22 a–d. Kaplan-Meier survival curves **a** of the femoral component with 96.7% after 11 years, **b** of the tibial component with 94.3% after 11 years, **c** of the patella component with 94.7% after 11 years, and **d** of all-polyethylene bearing components with 91.2% after 11 years

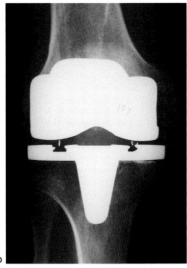
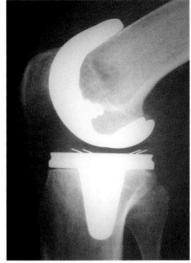
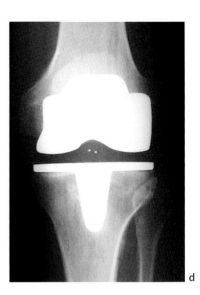

a–b

d

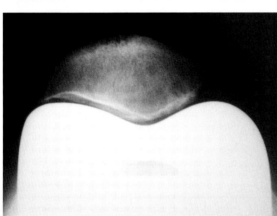

c

Fig. 3.23. a, b Radiographic example of a meniscal bearing PCL retaining LCS knee with 12 years follow-up and excellent clinical results. c Note perfect patellofemoral congruency and tracking without patella resurfacing. d Anteroposterior view of a rotating platform cementless TKA after 11 years

Buechel et al. (2001, 2002) reported his personal LCS series in a number of follow-up studies, including 83% survival rate for MB after 16 years and 97.7% for cemented RP, and 98.3% for cementless RP after 18 years. Jordan et al. (1997) reported 94.6% LCS survival rate after 8 years. Sorrels et al. (2001) described LCS survival of 88% at 14 years. Callaghan et al. (2000) studied 114 cemented LCS knees with 100% survival at 11 years follow-up. The clinical performance of the LCS remains exemplary based on long-term studies.

Initial concerns of mobile bearing knee prostheses included bearing spinout, progressive ligament instability, post-traumatic cases, severe deformity, the multiply operated knee and soft tissue balancing. Successful use, however, stimulated the improvement and understanding of soft tissue techniques, rotational alignment of both components, extension and flexion gap balancing, wear mechanics, and patella management. Three advantages of mobile bearing prostheses with RP should be highlighted: decreased contact stress (wear) and increased congruency (stability), improved knee joint biomechanics, and rotationally forgiving implantation of the tibial component to best anatomical fit (Fig. 3.23).

Patella results had higher scores and complications were less critical (at times catastrophic) when not resurfaced. Not resurfacing the patella, however, does not necessarily mean that the patella is left untouched. The patelloplasty procedure includes peripheral patella rim denervation, cheilectomy, removal of loose cartilage, lateral facet remodeling, and (if required) an in-to-out partial lateral rim release. Optimal patella tracking throughout the entire range of motion must be ensured prior to closure. Further details are discussed in both chapters on the patella.

Evaluation of initial experience of the original LCS mobile bearing TKA (primarily cementless) utilizing first-generation instrumentation resulted in satisfactory long-term outcome at a mean of 11.0 years. Excellent long-term outcomes up to 20 years have been reported with the LCS knee system. Clinical results

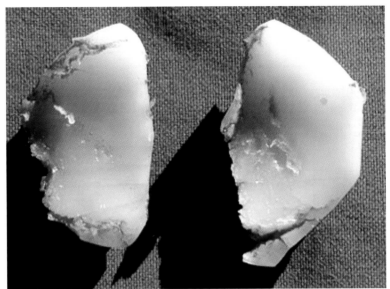

Fig. 3.24. Meniscal bearings demonstrated more wear than rotating platform polyethylene. Most bearings revealed increased shelf life (up to 7 years) and poor sterilization technique (gamma in air)

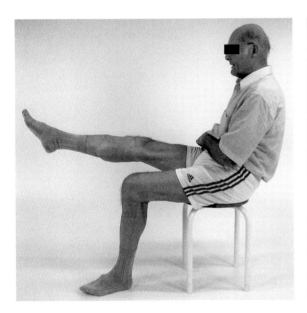
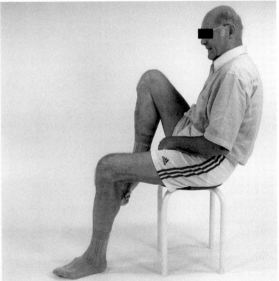

Fig. 3.25. Clinical example of a 73-year-old male patient 10 years postoperatively demonstrating full active extension and 160 degrees of flexion

showed a survivorship of over 85 % after 20 years. The femoral component performed uniquely best, followed by the tibial cone component and the RP. Meniscal bearing and metal-backed patella wear accounted for the majority of failures, which were associated with a long shelf life and gamma in air radiation for sterilization (Fig. 3.24). Patella resurfacing appeared to jeopardize successful long-term results and is, therefore, not recommended for routine use. Improved polyethylenes, surgical technique, and use of more durable RPs will further improve long-term outcomes.

The concept of the LCS mobile bearing knee was initiated in the late 1970s and appeared to be accepted in the late 1990s. This concept is now embellished in the new millennium. Numerous mobile bearing designs (40+) have emerged in the past 5 years; however, one should be cautious of untested variations and components that do not maintain the proven design of established knee systems. With unchanged design and surgical technique, the LCS mobile bearing TKA continues to perform well after 25 years. A tibial first approach, appropriate soft tissue balancing, proper component placement, and patelloplasty procedure without resurfacing are recommended for successful outcomes, whereas meniscal bearings and patella resurfacing jeopardize excellent long-term results (Fig. 3.25).

Acknowledgements. I thank Dr U. Munzinger MD, Schulthess Clinic, Zurich, Switzerland, for clinical data and support.

Bibliography

Berger RA, Rosenberg AG, Barden RM, Sheinkop MB, Jacobs JJ, Galante JO (2001) Long-term followup of the Miller-Galante total knee replacement. Clin Orthop 388:58–67

Boldt JG, Munzinger UK (2003) Longterm outcomes of LCS TKA with over 10 years follow-up. Oral presentation, EFORT, Helsinki, Finland, June 2003

Buechel FF (1998) Mobile-bearing joint replacement options in post-traumatic arthritis of the knee. Orthopedics 21:1027–1031

Buechel FF (2001) My platform moveth and that's all that's needed! Orthopedics 24:890–892

Buechel FF (2002) Knee arthroplasty in post-traumatic arthritis. J Arthroplasty 17 [Suppl 1]:63–68

Buechel FF Sr (2002) Long-term followup after mobile-bearing total knee replacement. Clin Orthop 404:40–50

Buechel FF Sr, Buechel FF Jr, Pappas MJ, D'Alessio J (2001) Twenty-year evaluation of meniscal bearing and rotating platform knee replacements. Clin Orthop 388:41–50

Buechel FF Sr, Buechel FF Jr, Pappas MJ, Dalessio J (2002) Twenty-year evaluation of the New Jersey LCS Rotating Platform Knee Replacement. J Knee Surg 15:84–89

Buechel FF Sr, Buechel FF Jr, Pappas MJ, Dalessio J (2002) Twenty-year evaluation of the New Jersey LCS Rotating Platform Knee Replacement. J Knee Surg 15:84–89

Callaghan JJ, Squire MW, Goetz DD, Sullivan PM, Johnston RC (2000) Cemented rotating-platform total knee replacement. A nine to twelve-year follow-up study. J Bone Joint Surg Am 82:705–711

Hartford JM, Hunt T, Kaufer H (2001) Low contact stress mobile bearing total knee arthroplasty: results at 5 to 13 years. J Arthroplasty 16:977–983

Jordan LR, Olivio Jl, Voorhorst PE (1997) Survivorship analysis of cementless meniscal bearing TKA. CORR 338:119–123

Khaw FM, Kirk LM, Gregg PJ (2001) Survival analysis of cemented Press-Fit Condylar total knee arthroplasty. J Arthroplasty 16:161–167

Kim YH, Kook HK, Kim JS (2001) Comparison of fixed-bearing and mobile-bearing total knee arthroplasties. Clin Orthop 392:101–115

Mancuso CA, Sculco TP, Wickiewicz TL, Jones EC, Robbins L, Warren RF, Williams-Russo P (2001) Patients' expectations of knee surgery. J Bone Joint Surg Am 83A:1005–1012

Ranawat CS, Luessenhop CP, Rodriguez JA (1997) The press-fit condylar modular total knee system. Four-to-six-year results with a posterior-cruciate-substituting design. J Bone Joint Surg Am 79:342–348

Rodriguez JA, Bhende H, Ranawat CS (2001) Total condylar knee replacement: a 20-year followup study. Clin Orthop 388:10–17

Rosenberg N, Henderson I (2001) Medium term outcome of the LCS cementless posterior cruciate retaining total knee replacements. Follow up and survivorship study of 35 operated knees. Knee 8:123–128

Schai PA, Thornhill TS, Scott RD (1999) Total knee arthroplasty with the PFC system. Results at a minimum of ten years and survivorship analysis. J Bone Joint Surg Br 81:558–559

Sorrels RB (2000) The rotating platform mobile bearing total knee arthroplasty. Surg Technol Int IX:245–251

Sorrells RB, Stiehl JB, Voorhorst PE (2001) Midterm results of mobile-bearing total knee arthroplasty in patients younger than 65 years. Clin Orthop 390:182–189

Spicer DD, Pomeroy DL, Badenhausen WE, Schaper LA Jr, Curry JI, Suthers KE, Smith MW (2001) Body mass index as a predictor of outcome in total knee replacement. Int Orthop 25:246–249

Stiehl JB (2002) World experience with low contact stress mobile-bearing total knee arthroplasty: a literature review. Orthopedics 25 [Suppl 2]:s213–s217

Stiehl JB, Dennis DA, Komistek RD, Keblish PA (1997) In vivo kinematic analysis of a mobile bearing total knee prosthesis. Clin Orthop 345:60–66

Stiehl JB, Dennis DA, Komistek RD, Keblish PA (2000) In vivo kinematic comparison of posterior cruciate ligament retention or sacrifice with a mobile bearing total knee arthroplasty. Am J Knee Surg 13:13–18

Stiehl JB, Komistek RD, Dennis DA, Keblish PA (2001) Kinematics of the patellofemoral joint in total knee arthroplasty. J Arthroplasty 16:706–714

3.6 Early Outcomes of INNEX Mobile Bearing TKA

Yaw Jakobi, Thomas Guggi, Urs K. Munzinger

This study evaluated early outcomes and complications encountered with a new mobile bearing knee prosthesis (INNEX, Centerpulse, Winterthur, Switzerland) in one large joint replacement centre (Schulthess Clinic, Zurich, Switzerland). The first INNEX total knee arthroplasty (TKA) was implanted in April 1996 and 1,133 TKAs were performed by study cut-off date in December 2002. Different types of polyethylene platforms were used: 63 (6%) posterior stabilised, 105 (9%) cruciate retaining, and 953 (85%) ultra-congruent only rotating (UCOR). There were only 16 (1.4%) patellae resurfaced in 688 women and 328 men. The average age of the patient at the time of surgery was 69 years (range 31–92), mean body mass index was 28 kg/m^2 (range 15.8–47.1) and 117 procedures were bilateral. Preoperative diagnoses were osteoarthritis in 1,015 knees (90%), inflammatory arthritis in 72 knees (6%), post-traumatic arthritis in 27 knees (2%), aseptic necrosis in 11 knees (1%), and arthritis of other origins in eight knees (1%). Osteoarthritis was tricompartmental in 47%, unilateral medial in 28%, unilateral lateral in 6% and bicompartmental in

17 %. At time of operation, the severity of arthritis was grade II (33 %) or III (32 %) of the Ahlback osteoarthritis classification. Knees with unicompartmental arthritis were operated at an earlier stage (II) than those with bi- or tricompartmental arthritis (III). Knee axis deformity was varus in 556 (49 %) cases and valgus in 419 (37 %) cases. One hundred and fifty-eight cases (14 %) had a physiological valgus. One or more previous knee operations had been performed in 528 (47 %) knees. Of these knees, 278 (53 %) had a previous partial meniscectomy, 141 (27 %) a tibial osteotomy, 29 (5 %) a femoral osteotomy, 33 (6 %) a fracture osteosynthesis, 31 (6 %) a cruciate ligament reconstruction, 28 (5 %) a synovectomy, nine (2 %) a patella realignment, one a patellectomy, and 56 (11 %) other operations.

Mean operation time was 80 minutes (range 60–120). Spinal anaesthesia was performed in 889 (78 %) operations; 130 (11 %) had epidural, 88 (8 %) general, and 26 (2 %) combined anaesthesia. The standard approach was a medial capsulotomy in 938 knees (83 %). In 195 (17 %) cases the lateral approach was used mostly in combination with an osteotomy of the tibial tuberosity (167 knees, 86 %). For most of the 195 knees with valgus deformity, the lateral approach (159 knees, 82 %) was used, usually in combination with an osteotomy of the tibial tuberosity (134 knees, 84 %) (Fig. 3.26). The tibial component was cemented in 1,096 cases (97 %) and in 644 (57 %) knee replacements cement was used for fixation of the tibial as well as the femoral component. Cement was not used in 32 (3 %) cases.

Clinical and radiographic assessment was performed preoperatively, postoperatively, and at most recent follow-up using the IDES documentation system. The Knee Society Score (KSS) was used. Two different scores were assigned: a knee score with maximum 100 points (knee pain, range of motion, and stability) and a function score with maximum 100 points (duration of walking and stair-climbing ability). Radiographic evaluation was performed using a modification of the Knee Society Roentgenographic Evaluation and Scoring System. It was used to determine the overall mechanical alignment of the knee, the relative position of the prosthetic components with respect to the bones, and to define the zones for radiolucencies and osteolytic lesions at the cement–bone interface.

During the first year, the patient was seen by the surgeon himself. Further follow-up was organised via a specific outpatients clinic. Two doctors examined all patients at 1, 2 and 5 years postoperatively. The contact with the patient was administered automati-

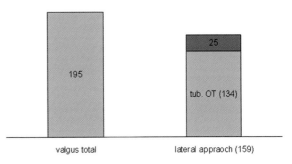

Fig. 3.26. Valgus deformity was approached laterally in 159 cases, 134 of which were in combination with an osteotomy of the tibial tuberosity (*tub. OT*)

cally through our ReCallOne software system. The average time of last follow-up was 20 months (range 8–73) after the INNEX TKA. Of the original 1,016 patients (1,133 knees), three died (three knees), seven (eight knees) were infirm and non-ambulatory secondary to systemic disease and seven (seven knees) were under external follow-up. Nineteen cases (1.7 %) were lost to follow-up as they refused further clinical control or were not contactable. Survivorship analysis was performed using the actuarial life table method. Component revision was defined as endpoint. The mean preoperative score according to the KSS (max. 100) for the patients was 38 (range 0–95) and 57 (25–100) for the function score (max. 100). At the time of latest follow-up, the average knee score had improved to 90 (25–100) and the function score to 81 (70–100). The pain score (max. 50) improved from 12 to 47 (0–50). After the operation, 79 % (preoperative 1 %) had no or occasional mild pain, 10 % (preoperative 0 %) had mild pain during climbing stairs, 3 % (preoperative 11 %) had mild pain during walking and climbing stairs, 0 % (preoperative 28 %) had occasional moderate pain, and 0 % (preoperative 68 %) had occasional moderate or severe pain. Patients were asked to state their personal opinion about the outcome of the knee replacement on a 4-point scale. Forty-seven per cent of patients found the result to be excellent, 49 % good, and 4 % fair. There were no dissatisfied patients.

Postoperatively, the average tibiofemoral angle was 5 degrees valgus (range 0–10). On the anteroposterior radiographs, the femoral alignment was 95 degrees (range 88–104). The mean alignment of the tibial component was 93 degrees (84–101). The lateral radiographs revealed an average femoral component flexion of 88 degrees (79–96). The average tibial component flexion measured 86 degrees (79–93).

PostOP   Tibiofemoral angle   5° (0-10°)

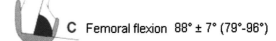

A   Femoral alignment   95° ± 6° (88°-104°)

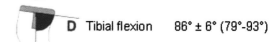

B   Tibial alignment   93° ± 7° (84°-101°)

C   Femoral flexion   88° ± 7° (79°-96°)

D   Tibial flexion   86° ± 6° (79°-93°)

a

Femur	%	total	ant	post	dist	med	lat
anterior	none	96.8	94.9	96.9	98.6	-	-
distal	>2 mm	0.1	0.3	0.0	0.0	-	-
posterior	1 mm	2.7	4.4	2.4	1.4	-	-
	2 mm	0.3	0.3	0.7	0.0	-	-
Tibia	none	98.3	97.3	99.3	-	98.3	97.3
lateral medial	>2 mm	0.0	0.0	0.0	-	0.0	0.0
anterior posterior	1 mm	1.2	1.7	0.7	-	1.4	2.0
	2 mm	0.5	1.0	0.0	-	0.3	0.7

b

Fig. 3.27 a, b.
Radiographic results
at time of last follow-up.
a Axis, component
alignment,
b percentages
and size of radio-
lucencies

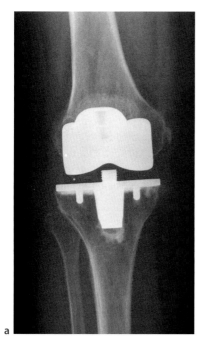

a

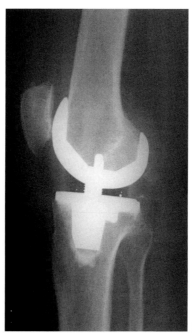

b

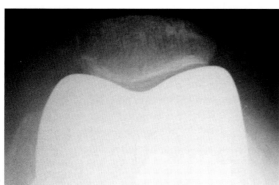

c

Fig. 3.28 a–c. INNEX UCOR
a anteroposterior,
b lateral, and
c axial radiographs at 4 years follow-up

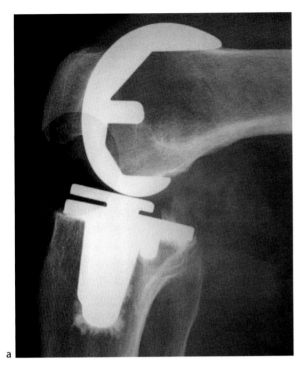

a

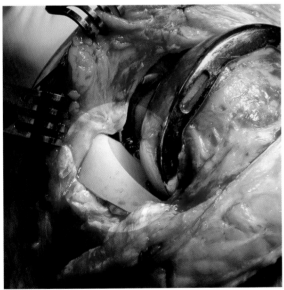

b

Fig. 3.29. a Revision due to impingement of Hoffa fat pad by the polyethylene. **b** The cruciate retaining insert was exchanged for UCOR

The radiological evaluation of INNEX TKA with a minimum follow-up of 2 years (n=294) showed no complete radiolucent lines and none of the components was radiographically loose at the latest follow-up. The size of the radiolucencies averaged 1 mm, and the largest measured 2 mm. In 3.2 %, radiolucencies of one region were found in the femoral component. In 1.7 %, the tibial component showed radiolucencies of one region. The percentages of radiolucencies per region and heights are specified in Fig. 3.27. Radiographs at 4 years follow-up are shown in Fig. 3.28.

Complications

Eighteen of 1,133 INNEX TKAs required revision surgery. Revision was performed on average after 13 months (range 0–30) after the primary joint replacement. Four knees were revised as a result of an infection. Three of these were early infection more than 3 months after operation, and one was late infection after 30 months. Instability was the cause for reoperation in three cases, all of which required further releases and a higher insert. In three cases, anterior knee pain was caused by ventral impingement of the Hoffa fat pat by the insert during flexion (fat pat impingement) and required exchange of insert (Fig. 3.29). Arthrofibrosis occurred in two cases and was treated with arthrolysis and exchange of insert. Both cases were associated with internal malrotation of the femoral component and were subsequently exchanged. One tibial component was exchanged because of aseptic loosening. One case required realignment of the extension mechanism and secondary patella resurfacing. One polyethylene platform had to be exchanged because of spinout (Fig. 3.30). One patient had a flexion deficit as a result of an interaction of the cruciate retaining platform with the posterior cruciate ligament and was without any further deficit after a polyethylene exchange (UCOR).

Survival Rate

The 2-year survival rate with revision as the endpoint was 97.8 % and at 5 years 95.9 % (Fig. 3.31). After 5 years the average annual failure rate was 0.08 %. The cumulative survival rates for each INNEX type at 2 years are as follows: cruciate retaining 93.5 %, posterior stabilised 98.3 %, Fix 100 %, UCOR 98.7 % (Table 3.4).

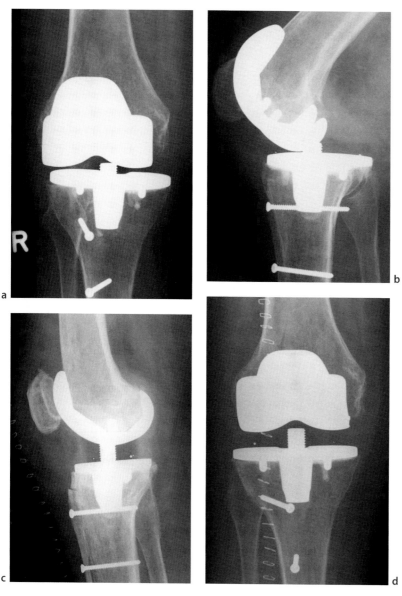

Fig. 3.30 a–d. Revision due to polyethylene spinout. Polyethylene exchange from UCOR-12.5 to UCOR-15 (pre- and postoperative radiographs)

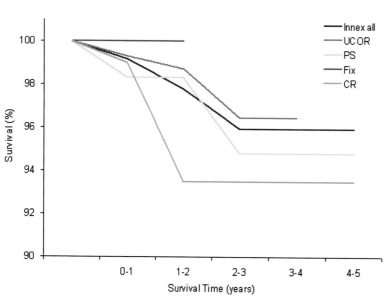

Fig. 3.31. Survival analysis for all INNEX TKA and the different INNEX types with revision as endpoint

Table 3.4. Cumulative survival rates listed separately for all components

Follow-up interval since operation (years)	Number of knees at start of interval	Withdrawn	Failure, revision	Number of knees at risk	Predicted annual percentage of Failures	Survival	Cumulative survival	Confidence interval 95% Lower	Higher
Innex total									
0–1	1031	343	7	859.5	0.0081	0.9919	0.9919	98.3	99.6
1–2	681	368	7	497	0.0141	0.9859	0.9779	96.1	98.8
2–3	306	190	4	211	0.019	0.981	0.9593	92.3	97.9
3–4	112	46	0	89	0	1	0.9593	89.6	98.5
4–5	66	66	0	33	0	1	0.9593	83.2	99.1
UCOR									
0–1	860	337	5	691.5	0.0072	0.9928	0.9928	98.3	99.7
1–2	518	345	2	345.5	0.0058	0.9942	0.9987	96.9	99.5
2–3	171	168	2	87	0.023	0.977	0.9643	90.2	98.8
3–4	1	1	0	0.5	0	1	0.9643	10.7	100.0
PS									
0–1	60	1	1	59.5	0.0168	0.9832	0.9832	91.1	99.7
1–2	58	0	0	58	0	1	0.9832	90.9	99.7
2–3	58	5	2	55.5	0.036	0.964	0.9478	85.5	98.2
3–4	51	21	0	40.5	0	1	0.9478	83.3	98.5
4–5	30	30	0	15	0	1	0.9478	72.1	99.2
Fix									
0–1	10	2	0	0	0	1	1	70.1	100.0
1–2	8	8	0	0	0	1	1	51.0	100.0
CR									
0–1	101	3	1	99.5	0.0101	0.9899	0.9899	94.5	99.8
1–2	97	15	5	89.5	0.0559	0.9441	0.9346	86.3	97.0
2–3	77	17	0	68.5	0	1	0.9346	85.0	97.3
3–4	60	24	0	48	0	1	0.9346	82.8	97.7
4–5	36	36	0	18	0	1	0.9346	72.9	98.7

UCOR ultracongruent only rotating, PS posterior stabilised, CR cruciate retaining

Bibliography

Ahlback S (1969) Osteoarthrosis of the knee. A radiographic
    investigation. Acta Radiol [Suppl] 277:1–72
Armitage P (1994) Statistical methods in medical research, 3rd
    edn. Blackwell Scientific, Oxford, pp 468–492
Ewald CF (1989) The Knee Society total knee arthroplasty ro-
    entgenopraphic evaluation and scoring system. CORR 248:
    9–12
Insall NJ (1989) Rational of the knee Society clinical rating sys-
    tem. CORR 248:13–14

3.7 Total Knee Arthroplasty in the Young and Active Population

Jens G. Boldt, Urs K. Munzinger

Young patients undergoing total knee arthroplasty (TKA) for knee arthritis are usually more active and naturally have a longer life expectancy. There are several questions and concerns in this group of patients, including the best type of prosthesis, implantation technique, soft tissue balancing, and patella treatment (resurfacing or not). The importance of optimizing kinematic function, minimizing wear, appropriate rehabilitation, and ongoing fitness with activities of daily living should not be underestimated. Active younger patients with post-traumatic arthritis usually present with higher demands and better knowledge/information regarding the status of their knee arthritis and treatment options. Juvenile rheumatoid arthritis patients are usually well informed but have lower functional demands.

Commonly, information is drawn from internet web pages, which recommend specific implant materials and designs, as well as operating techniques. Because of the complexity of knee arthritis and individual treatment options, this "over-information" can, at times, be more problematic than helpful for both the patient and the surgeon. There is still no consensus on information available for the patient (and the surgeon) with regards to the rehabilitation program and physical activities post-TKA in the physiologically younger population. Rehabilitation recommendations vary depending on disease process, type of prosthesis, fixation, and specific therapy directions, from conservative isometric exercise, walking and cycling to other extremes including high-impact sports activities such as squash, soccer, motor sports, or alpine skiing. Return to high-demand physical labor employment presents other issues regarding patients' goals, workmen's compensation risk assessment, etc. The surgeon's philosophy, confidence, and willingness to take responsibility will determine the direction in most cases.

In order to evaluate clinical outcomes and function, and to obtain in-depth information on physical, recreational, as well as sports activities in TKA patients younger than 55 years, an 80-topic questionnaire was designed and completed, of which 86% were retrieved. Questions included information on the patient's general health status, satisfaction with knee prosthesis, and in-depth information about activities. Rheumatoid and non-inflammatory cases were reviewed independently in this study. There was no interdiction, nor ban for any sports activity the patient wished to perform after TKA.

Non-inflammatory Osteoarthritis Group

From over 3,000 mobile bearing TKAs performed in patients with non-inflammatory knee arthritis, implanted from 1988 to 2000, a total of 228 low contact stress TKAs entered the study. Follow-up time was 2–11 years, mean total score was 95.2 points (out of 100). Sixty-one per cent of patients were currently in occupation and 39% were retired. There were 2% complications, which will be discussed in depth. Of the group, 89% participated in active exercises, with a mean of 475 min on 2.5 days per week. Average walking distance per day ranged from less than 1 km in 8% to more than 10 km in 10% of the group. Sports activities included: swimming 36%, fitness 18%, hiking 14%, cycling 11%, tennis 7%, jogging 7%, and alpine skiing 7%. Daily gardening and housework was encountered in 51%.

Rheumatoid Arthritis Group with TKA

There were 3.2 times more rheumatoid arthritis cases in this young group compared with the general patient profile in a cohort of over 3,000 TKAs. From the same cohort of one major joint replacement center, 79 rheumatoid patients younger than 55 years who had undergone mobile bearing TKA with at least 1 year follow-up were sent the questionnaire. Nine patients died since surgery and 57 (81%) cases replied to the questionnaire. Follow-up time was 1–11 years; mean total postoperative score was 81.5 points (out of 100). Twenty-one per cent were currently in active occupation. There were 9.5% complications, but these did not relate to the more aggressive rehabilitation and will be discussed. Of the group, 45% participated in regular active exercises, with a mean of

65 min/week on 2.5 days. Average walking distance per day ranged from less than 1 km to more than 10 km. Sports activities included: swimming, fitness, hiking, cycling, tennis, alpine skiing, and jogging. Daily gardening and housework was noted in over 50 %. Rheumatoid patients younger than 55 years perform better in general physical activity, work performance, and sports activities than older patients with rheumatoid arthritis. The quality of life after mobile bearing TKA observed in this group was significantly improved.

It is generally accepted that daily living activities, physical preferences, and recreational sports play a significant part in overall patient satisfaction and social integration. The pattern of postoperative rehabilitation and recreational activities following TKA surgery has changed dramatically in the past four decades, from a highly conservative and protecting approach to a more aggressive and active regimen. During the early years of TKA, postoperative patients were directed to protect the artificial knee prosthesis as much as possible. Recreational activities were mostly banned or at least considered to be associated with early and rapid failure of the implant. Complications such as severe polyethylene wear, patella component loosening, cement disease, and revision surgery were linked with overuse of the knee prosthesis and, therefore, patients were advised to modify any excessive activities. A 6-week non-weight-bearing regimen with a walker or two crutches, followed by gradual increased loading after TKA (cementless and/or cemented implantation) was routine practice. These rules were partly justified due to less confidence on the part of the surgeon with a newer operation plus concerns regarding poor high-constraint prosthetic designs, materials (polyethylene quality and thickness) and fixation methods.

Today, there appears to be a worldwide trend for early and more aggressive postoperative management and return to demanding labor and recreational activities. Recent studies indicate that early weight bearing and more aggressive rehabilitation management, including resumption of sports activities after TKA (and other joint replacements), are considered to be beneficial (or at least not harmful). The rehabilitation regimen in this group should allow for protected weight bearing to tolerance and active isometric/isokinetic exercises after 24 hours and recreational activities after the 6-week clinical and radiographic evaluation. No sports activity is generally banned, but individual recommendations are provided based on past patient profile. Patients who performed well in a specific sport and have proven lower extremity strength and dexterity are less likely to harm the knee prosthesis or risk general injury after returning to their sport. Patients who wish to learn a new sports activity or have a less athletic musculoskeletal physic are cautioned against new or risk-related activities. A 50-year-old established tennis player or alpine skiing instructor, for instance, will more likely perform well in his sport without risking excessive prosthetic stress. Inexperienced patients who commence a new sport activity are likely to load and stress their prosthesis more inappropriately and risk injury to other bones and joints.

The results of this intense questionnaire showed a high percentage of patient satisfaction with TKA, both in rheumatoid arthritis and osteoarthritis. Patients younger than 55 perform well after TKA with regards to physical activity, work performance, and sports activities, allowing a high proportion of patients to continue with their desired functional lifestyle. There was no increased risk of TKA complications, wear or failure in this young population when compared with the overall much older and less active cohort in this center. We, therefore, lowered our threshold for index TKA in this group and we have advised a rational postoperative rehabilitation program to satisfy their functional goals. Better quality of life, delayed retirement and/or resumption of their profession, and sports activities after mobile bearing TKA, as seen in our study, can be expected in physiologically younger patients.

Bibliography

Bizzini M, Boldt J, Munzinger U, Drobny T (2003) Rehabilitation guidelines after total knee arthroplasty. Orthopade 32(6):527–534
Bock P, Schatz K, Wurnig C (2003) Physical activity after total knee replacement. Z Orthop Ihre Grenzgeb 141:272–276
Boldt J, Munzinger U, Keblish P (2004) Comparison of isokinetic strength in resurfaced and retained patellae in bilateral TKA. J Arthroplasty 19(2):264
Boldt JG, Munzinger UK, Zanetti M, Hodler J (2004) Arthrofibrosis associated with total knee arthroplasty: gray-scale and power Doppler sonographic findings. AJR Am J Roentgenol 182(2):337–340
Botte MJ, Ezzet KA, Pacelli LL, Guzman MJ, Meyer RS, Meunier MJ, D'Lima DD, Colwell CW (2002) What's new in orthopaedic rehabilitation. J Bone Joint Surg Am 84A:2312–2320
Bradbury N, Borton D, Spoo G, Cross MJ (1998) Participation in sports after total knee replacement. Am J Sports Med 26:530–535
Buechel FF (2002) Knee arthroplasty in post-traumatic arthritis. J Arthroplasty 17 [Suppl 1]:63–68
Callaghan JJ, Insall JN, Greenwald AS, Dennis DA, Komistek RD, Murray DW, Bourne RB, Rorabeck CH, Dorr LD (2001)

Mobile-bearing knee replacement: concepts and results. Instr Course Lect 50:431–449

Chockalingam S, Scott G (2000) The outcome of cemented vs. cementless fixation of a femoral component in total knee replacement (TKR) with the identification of radiological signs for the prediction of failure. 0968–0160 7:233–238

Cirincione RJ (1996) Sports after total joint replacement. Md Med J 45:644–647

Hartford JM, Banit D, Hall K, Kaufer H (2001) Radiographic analysis of low contact stress meniscal bearing total knee replacements. J Bone Joint Surg Am 83A:229–234

Healy WL, Iorio R, Lemos MJ (2000) Athletic activity after total knee arthroplasty. Clin Orthop 380:65–71

Healy WL, Iorio R, Lemos MJ (2001) Athletic activity after joint replacement. Am J Sports Med 293:377–388

Heegaard JH, Leyvraz PF, Hovey CB (2001) A computer model to simulate patellar biomechanics following total knee replacement: the effects of femoral component alignment. Clin Biomech (Bristol, Avon) 16:415–423

Jorn LP, Johnsson R, Toksvig-Larsen S (1999) Patient satisfaction, function and return to work after knee arthroplasty. Acta Orthop Scand 70:343–347

Joshi AB, Gill G (2002) Total knee arthroplasty in nonagenarians. J Arthroplasty 17:681–684

Kuster MS, Stachowiak GW (2002) Factors affecting polyethylene wear in total knee arthroplasty. Orthopedics 25 [Suppl 2]:s235–s242

Kuster MS, Grob K, Gachter A (2000) Knee endoprosthesis: sports orthopedics possibilities and limitations. Orthopade 29:739–745

Kuster MS, Spalinger E, Blanksby BA, Gachter A (2000) Endurance sports after total knee replacement: a biomechanical investigation. Med Sci Sports Exerc 32:721–724

Lavernia CJ, Sierra RJ, Hungerford DS, Krackow K (2001) Activity level and wear in total knee arthroplasty: a study of autopsy retrieved specimens. J Arthroplasty 16:446–453

Lonner JH, Hershman S, Mont M, Lotke PA (2000) Total knee arthroplasty in patients 40 years of age and younger with osteoarthritis. Clin Orthop 380:85–90

Macario A, Schilling P, Rubio R, Bhalla A, Goodman S (2003) What questions do patients undergoing lower extremity joint replacement surgery have? BMC Health Serv Res 3:11

Mallon WJ, Callaghan JJ (1993) Total knee arthroplasty in active golfers. J Arthroplasty 8:299–306

Mancuso CA, Sculco TP, Wickiewicz TL, Jones EC, Robbins L, Warren RF, Williams-Russo P (2001) Patients' expectations of knee surgery. J Bone Joint Surg Am 83A:1005–1012

McGrory BJ, Stuart MJ, Sim FH (1995) Participation in sports after hip and knee arthroplasty: review of literature and survey of surgeon preferences. Mayo Clin Proc 70:342–348

Mont MA, LaPorte DM, Mullick T, Silberstein CE, Hungerford DS (1999) Tennis after total hip arthroplasty. Am J Sports Med 27:60–64

Mont MA, Rajadhyaksha AD, Marxen JL, Silberstein CE, Hungerford DS (2002) Tennis after total knee arthroplasty. Am J Sports Med 30:163–166

Moran M, Khan A, Sochart DH, Andrew G (2003) Evaluation of patient concerns before total knee and hip arthroplasty. J Arthroplasty 18:442–445

Moran M, Khan A, Sochart DH, Andrew G (2003) Expect the best, prepare for the worst: surgeon and patient expectation of the outcome of primary total hip and knee replacement. Ann R Coll Surg Engl 853:204–206

Nicholls MA, Selby JB, Hartford JM (2002) Athletic activity after total joint replacement. Orthopedics 25:1283–1287

Ranawat CS, Ranawat AS, Mehta A (2003) Total knee arthroplasty rehabilitation protocol: what makes the difference? J Arthroplasty 18 [Suppl 1]:27–30

Ries MD, Philbin EF, Groff GD, Sheesley KA, Richman JA, Lynch F Jr (1996) Improvement in cardiovascular fitness after total knee arthroplasty. J Bone Joint Surg Am 78:1696–1701

Roos EM (2003) Effectiveness and practice variation of rehabilitation after joint replacement. Curr Opin Rheumatol 15:160–162

Scholz R, Freiherr von Salis-Soglio G (2002) Sports fitness after prosthetic joint replacement. Orthopade 31:423–430; quiz 430–431

Schroder HM, Berthelsen A, Hassani G, Hansen EB, Solgaard S (2001) Cementless porous-coated total knee arthroplasty: 10-year results in a consecutive series. J Arthroplasty 16:559–567

Schroder HM, Berthelsen A, Hassani G, Hansen EB, Solgaard S (2001) Cementless porous-coated total knee arthroplasty: 10-year results in a consecutive series. J Arthroplasty 16:559–567

Sorrells RB (2002) The clinical history and development of the low contact stress total knee arthroplasty. Orthopedics 25 [Suppl 2]:s207–s212

Sorrells RB, Stiehl JB, Voorhorst PE (2001) Midterm results of mobile-bearing total knee arthroplasty in patients younger than 65 years. Clin Orthop 390:182–189

Stiehl JB (2002) World experience with low contact stress mobile-bearing total knee arthroplasty: a literature review. Orthopedics 25 [Suppl 2]:s213–s217

Tanzer M, McLean CA, Laxer E, Casey J, Ahmed AM (2001) Effect of femoral component designs on the contact and tracking characteristics of the unresurfaced patella in total knee arthroplasty. Can J Surg 44:127–133

Walsh M, Woodhouse LJ, Thomas SG, Finch E (1998) Physical impairments and functional limitations: a comparison of individuals 1 year after total knee arthroplasty with control subjects. Phys Ther 78:248–258

Weiss JM, Noble PC, Conditt MA, Kohl HW, Roberts S, Cook KF, Gordon MJ, Mathis KB (2002) What functional activities are important to patients with knee replacements? Clin Orthop 404:172–188

Yip J (2003) The CPM challenge. Rehab Manag 16:44–47

CHAPTER 4

Urs K. Munzinger · Peter A. Keblish · Jens G. Boldt
Tomas K. Drobny · David Beverland
Jean-Louis Briard · Thomas Henkel

Operating Technique

4.1 Planning, Implant Selection, and Preparation

Urs K. Munzinger (Concept by K. A. Krackow)

Two different alignment schemes are extensively used by total knee arthroplasty (TKA) surgeons today: classical arthroplasty alignment and anatomic arthroplasty alignment.

Classical Arthroplasty Alignment

The goal is to create a prosthetic joint line perpendicular to the tibial shaft as this shaft axis coincides with the mechanical axis. The distal femoral cut is made perpendicular to the femoral mechanical axis, and has an orientation with respect to the femoral shaft axis, which differs by an angle of 5–7 degrees.

Anatomic Arthroplasty Alignment

The goal is reproduction of the joint line angulation with respect to the mechanical axis in which the joint line is parallel to the ground during two-legged stance in the frontal plane (feet approximated and parallel to the ground during gait). The distal femoral cut is 8–9 degrees valgus and the proximal tibial cut is 2–3 degrees varus. Both yield the same tibiofemoral angle but produce a slightly different joint line orientation (Fig. 4.1).

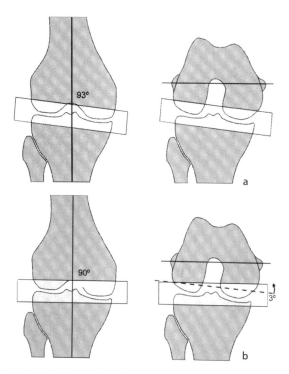

Fig. 4.1. a Anatomic arthroplasty alignment. The cut at the upper tibia is 3 degrees varus. To recreate a proper tibiofemoral angle leading to a mechanical axis that is centered through the joint, it is necessary to perform a distal femoral cut of 93 degrees. b Classical arthroplasty alignment. The goal is to create a prosthetic joint line perpendicular (90 degrees) to the mechanical axis. The transepicondylar line is parallel to the cut at the upper tibia

Preoperative Radiographic Analysis

The discussion in this section is devoted to developing an understanding of deformity as determined radiographically, planning the position of the major bone cuts, and establishing bony landmarks and other features of orientation that will facilitate use of instrument systems. The element provided by the long, weight-bearing x-ray film, is the picture of overall tibiofemoral and hip–knee–ankle alignment.

Normal Knee Alignment

The conditions of axial and rotational alignment, as they relate to the normal and pathologic knee, are analyzed preoperatively on routine x-ray films and by physical examination. There appears to be a consensus on most aspects of "normal" knee alignment. Such normal alignment involves restoration of the proper mechanical axis and joint line orientation. Figure 4.2 depicts a state of normal alignment with the mechanical axis passing from the center of the femoral head through the center of the knee and on to the center of the ankle. The amount of varus or valgus deformity may be quantified. Drawing one line from the center of the femoral head through the center of the knee and beyond indicates the position that would normally be assumed by the tibia. Comparing this projected line to the existing tibial shaft axis indicates the degree of angular deformity present. The "normal" tibiofemoral angle relates to the geometry of the femur. This angle is derived as a function of the length of the femoral shaft, the length of the femoral neck, the version of the neck, and the valgus/varus orientation. The second condition that must be met for normal knee joint alignment is the orientation of the joint line. The joint line orientation with respect to the ground depends on the position of the lower extremity in space. Two independent analyses of presumably normal subjects indicate that the "average normal" alignment appears as indicated in Fig. 4.2. The knee is centered on the mechanical axis, and the joint line forms an angle that is only approximately perpendicular to the mechanical axis, differing on average by 2–3 degrees. If one considers the top of the tibia as describing a plane and recalls that this plane has a posterior slope of 5–10 degrees and that weight bearing during the midstance phase of gait occurs on a flexed knee, then it appears that the joint may be close to parallel to the ground in the sagittal plane as well.

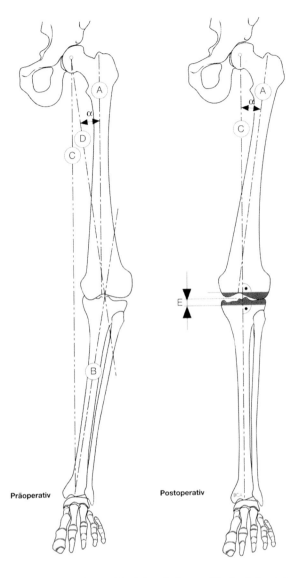

Präoperativ   Postoperativ

Fig. 4.2. The radiographic deformity is quantified as follows. A line is drawn from the center of the femoral head to the center of the knee, the mechanical axis of the femur. A second line, the tibial shaft axis, is drawn from the center of the knee to the center of the talus. The angle formed between these two lines represents the angular deformity

Deformity

The radiographic varus or valgus deformity is quantified as follows. A line is drawn from the center of the femoral head to the center of the knee and beyond; defining the mechanical axis of the femur. A second line, the tibial shaft axis, is drawn from the center of the knee to the ankle. The acute angle formed between these two lines represents the angular deformity. The definition of the center of the knee is a problem. The line that represents best the femoral shaft axis may not intersect the femoral axis at the center of the knee. The single point used at the distal extent of the femoral mechanical axis, also the femoral shaft axis, and the proximal extent of the tibial shaft axis is defined as follows: a point midway between the medial and lateral margins of the joint line is chosen as the center of the knee. This point is lined to the center of the femoral head to define the femoral mechanical axis and then to the center of the ankle joint to define the tibial shaft axis. At the proximal aspect of the femur we choose the midpoint of a line drawn transversely across the femur at the upper border of the lesser trochanter.

Extra-articular Bone Deformity

When significant deformity (especially near the joint line) exists, consideration of corrective osteotomy must be a part of preoperative planning (Fig. 4.3). The potential impact of significant shaft deformity altering the distal femoral or proximal tibia resection lines in their relationship to the ligament attachments must be determined so as not to compromise TKA stability. The amount of such deformity, or its impact on the knee, is proportional to its proximity to the joint, for example shaft angulation of 10 degrees located at the midpoint of the femur or tibia will lead to 5 degrees angulation of the femoral or tibial side of the joint. If an osteotomy is performed in addition to a total knee replacement, its timing should be carefully planned so that postoperative requirements of each do not interfere with those of the other.

Fig. 4.3 a–h. Extra-articular femoral deformity due to previous fracture (a, b) treated with correcting osteotomy (c, d) and stemmed femoral component (e, f).
d–f. see p. 142

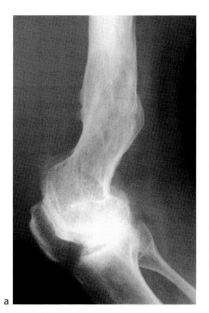
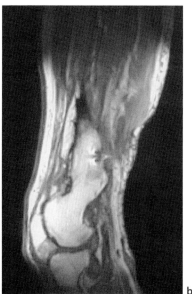

a

b

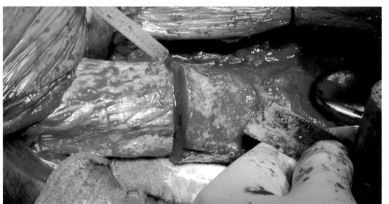

c

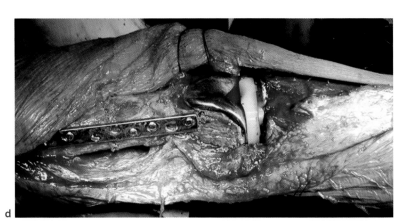

Fig. 4.3 d–f.

d

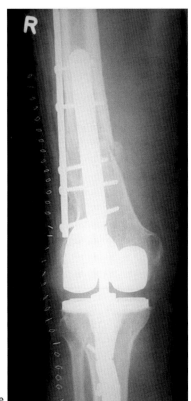

e

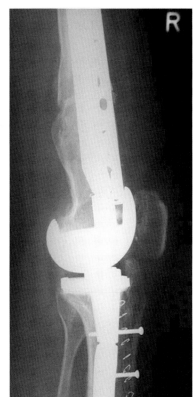

f

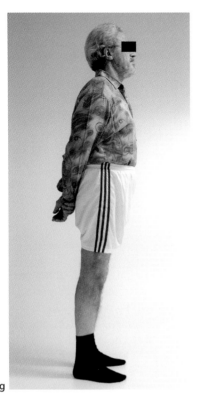

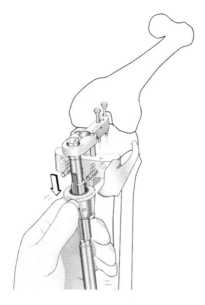

Fig. 4.4. The tibia is usually resected 10 mm below the highest point of the intact compartment. If necessary, the resection level can be adjusted to suit the anatomical conditions

Selection of Proximal Tibial and Distal Femoral Resection Lines

When asymmetrical bone loss is not present and the projected resection is nearly parallel to the existing tibial joint line, the bone can be marked at a level corresponding to a minimum thickness resection appropriate to the knee systems being used. When asymmetrical bone loss exists, two extremes span the range of options. One can draw a resection line that represents a minimum thickness resection of the less worn compartment or a maximum thickness resection, i.e. one extending to the level of the more worn compartment (Fig. 4.4). Alternatively, some intermediate, compromise resection levels can be selected. The depth of resection will be influenced by the concave release correction. It is important to appreciate the distal femoral margins as well. Drawing the distal femoral resection line, or at least indicating its orientation, provides useful information. There is a direct relationship between the relative amounts of bone actually resected and the projected amounts indicated on the x-ray film. This double-checking helps to assure that the angle of distal femoral resection is correct, minimizing any instrument errors and potential major malresections.

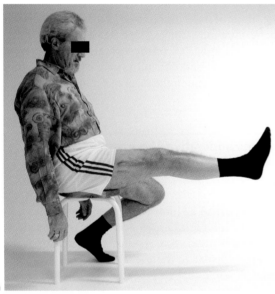

h

Fig. 4.3 g–h. Note postoperative correction and clinical outcome (g, h)

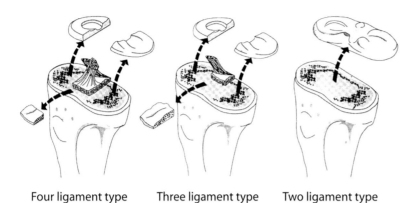

Fig. 4.5. Placement of a two-ligament collateral stabilized prosthesis with excision of anterior and posterior cruciate ligaments can be expected to be technically easier than implantation of a four-ligament sparing less constrained prosthesis

Four ligament type   Three ligament type   Two ligament type

Prosthetic Implant Selection and Fixation

Currently, there is still significant controversy concerning the issue of cemented versus uncemented fixation. Among the popular cemented prostheses, the major distinguishing fixation features are seen on the tibial side. The metal backing may be smooth, coarsely textured, or porous coated. Within the category of "uncemented" prostheses, many different features relate to the issue of fixation. Most have significant areas of porous coating for bone/tissue osseointegration. Prostheses have carrying types of stems, fins, multiple pegs, and a wide variety of screw fixation techniques to hold the tibial component securely against the tibial bone. Well-designed prostheses with anatomic features and mobile bearings have established track records and should be utilized. When in doubt, tibial components should be cemented.

Constraint describes the freedom of movement of a particular prosthesis. The overall degree and type of constraint provided by a prosthesis involves an interaction between tibial and femoral joint shape in terms of conformation, as well as the presence of intra-articular posts, rotating stems, fixed axes, and even entrapped ball-and-socket mechanisms. The claims regarding stability provided by the various different degrees of design constraint are relatively straightforward. A large proportion of primary TKAs are performed using three-ligament posterior cruciate sparing designs, collateral stabilized two-ligament models, or two-ligament sparing or posterior cruciate ligament sacrificing posterior stabilized designs and/or rotating platform designs.

The choice between the posterior stabilized and the two-ligament and three-ligament options is often not clear. There appears to be an implicit notion that preservation of more of the natural ligament stability or maximizing preservation of natural stability will consequently minimize undesirable interfacial forces. In support of the two-ligament collateral stabilized design, rather than a three-ligament one, are the general arguments that these approaches are technically easy and clinically seem to work as well as the less constrained prostheses (Fig. 4.5).

There is widespread agreement that use of the simple hinge and minimal-selective use of the rotating hinge should be reserved for extreme, low-demand situations. Clinical experience with these prostheses has indicated relatively high rates of loosening, infection, and difficulties achieving satisfactory salvage treatment in the form of revision or fusion.

4.2 Intraoperative Alignment and Instrumentation
Urs K. Munzinger

In the classical alignment, the goal is the establishment of a joint line perpendicular to the reconstituted mechanical axis. As a result, the proximal tibial cut is perpendicular to the overall tibial shaft axis. The distal femoral cut is perpendicular to the femoral portion of the mechanical axis; it is oriented at an angle of approximately 6 degrees relative to the femoral shaft axis. Understanding these angles and drawing them accurately on preoperative radiographic films is helpful, as it is necessary to judge the accuracy of instrument placement. Regardless of the ultimate depth of a distal femoral or proximal tibial cut, the angular orientation selected by the instrumentation system should be reproducible (within 1–2 degrees) to the angles outlined on the planning radiographs.

Fig. 4.6. The tibial alignment jig is fixed centrally in the region of the intercondylar eminence. Rotation refers to the axis of the intercondylar eminence

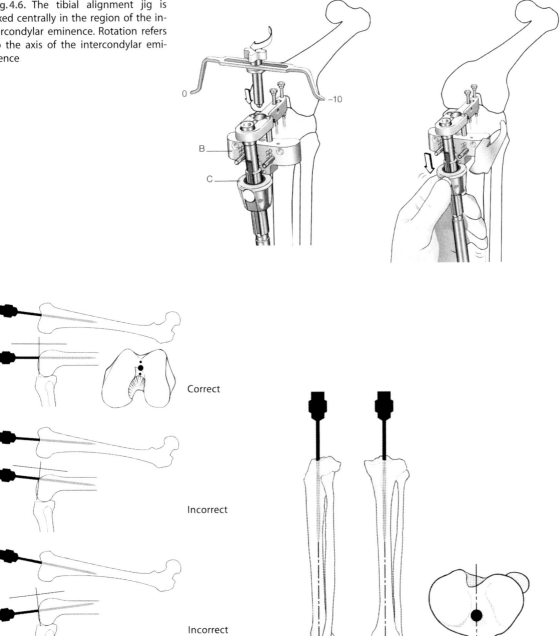

Fig. 4.7 a, b. The site of insertion for the intramedullary guide rod can be determined from the anteroposterior and lateral x-ray pictures on both femur and tibia

Tibia Axial Alignment

The instrumented guides are an extramedullary alignment from the center of the knee to the center of the ankle and an intramedullary system. One should be cautious about the accuracy of mediolateral place-

ment of such guides. Erroneous lateral positioning at the ankle moves the instrument to a varus error and vice versa. The aim of the placement at the ankle is the center of the talus, which corresponds to the outer border of the tibialis anterior tendon at the level of the ankle joint (Figs. 4.6–4.10).

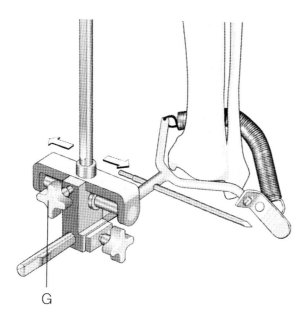

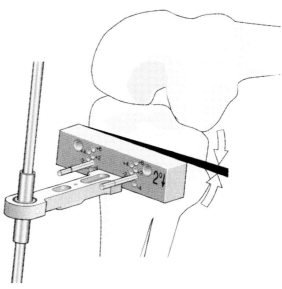

Fig. 4.8. The tendon of the anterior tibial muscle or extensor halucis longus is a suitable reference for determining the center of the ankle. At the level of the ankle the lateral edge of the tendon is the reference point to the center of the ankle

Fig. 4.10. Checking the axis: if the guide-rod shows a deviation from the center of the ankle, the position of the tibial resection block must be corrected

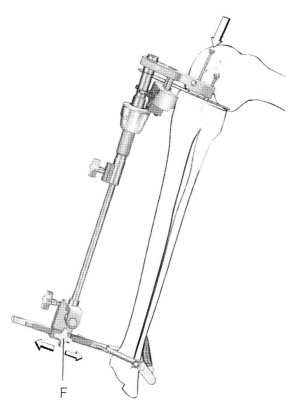

Femoral Axial Alignment

Current instrumentation approaches to establishing proper varus or valgus orientation at the distal femur cut involve three different techniques: intramedullary alignment rods, extramedullary alignment rods, which are meant to parallel the femoral shaft, and extramedullary alignment, which is intended to point towards the femoral head. Each of these approaches has its sources of error, which should be understood and the magnitude of potential errors appreciated. At the hip, medial displacement leads to valgus change, whereas lateral displacement leads to varus change.

With the use of an intramedullary alignment rod, it may be argued that uncertainty about the position of the proximal tip of the rod is minimized. This is true as long as the rod achieves an accurate position in the neighborhood of the femoral isthmus and the rod does not bend. Difficulties may occur in a femur with a relatively narrow canal. The resulting direction of this rod is significantly different from the true overall axis of the femur. A cutting block oriented relative to this rod would lead to a significant varus error. To avoid this error, the entry point for the pilot hole is chosen lateral to the intercondylar notch (see Sect. 4.1, preoperative planning). If any discrepancy becomes apparent, an extramedullary check, with reference to the femoral head, should avoid any major malresection. Tensors, half-spacers, and trac-

Fig. 4.9. The angle for the posterior slope is adjusted in accordance with the preoperative planning of the physiological slope of the proximal tibia. A dorsally inclined tibial resection improves the ability of the knee to bend and prevents excessive tension of the ligaments during flexion

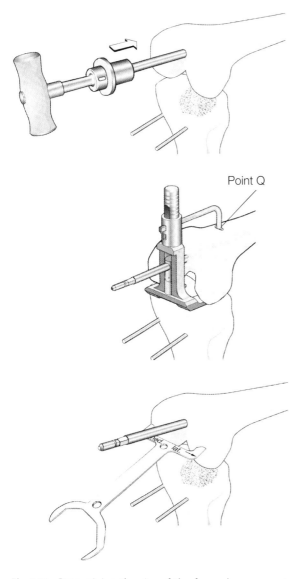

Fig. 4.11. Determining the size of the femoral component. The anteroposterior dimension is determined by means of the femur measuring device. The correct mediolateral dimension is checked using the femur template. If the reading is between two sizes, the smaller size is chosen.

Fig. 4.12. In order to obtain an optimal anterior resection, the hip of the femoral calliper must be placed on the ventral femoral cortex at the previously selected point *Q*

tion should confirm a parallel cut to the tibial resection.

In addition to the varus or valgus errors inherent in malpositioning any form of alignment rod, one must also consider the accurate placement of the cutting jig. If the jig is a separate component, there may be mechanical varus or valgus play as it interlocks. If it is to be stabilized by any pins or drill bits, any displacement or "wandering" of these pins as they perforate bone will lead to some degree of varus or valgus error (Figs. 4.11, 4.12).

Rotation at the Femur

Two main general approaches have been concerned with establishment of rotation of the femoral component. The issue is achievement of proper balance of external and internal rotation (i.e. rotation about a longitudinal axis). The first approach is to orient the anterior and posterior femoral cuts in a rotational sense so that the flexion space is approximately rectangular (Insall/Pappas). The second approach involves specific referencing from the posterior femoral condyles or, alternatively, from any other fixed aspect of femoral geometry (i.e. epicondylar line). The primary goal of both approaches is to re-establish normal rotation of the femur in relationship to the tibia. With varus deformity, the femur appears to be in internal rotation with the knee in flexion and to be in external rotation when valgus deformity is present (Figs. 4.13–4.15). During surgery, if the tibia is held in a straight neutral vertical position, the femur will rotate in a compensatory internal position for most varus cases and into a position of external rotation for some valgus cases. For the knee in extension, the non-anatomic (perpendicular, not two to three physiologic varus) cut made on the proximal tibia is offset by a corresponding non-anatomic asymmetric

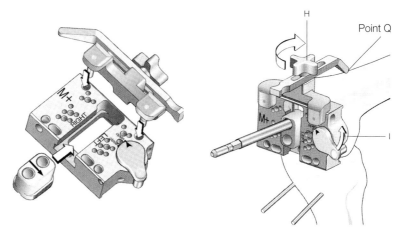

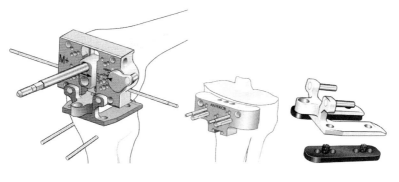

Fig. 4.13. Determination of rotation and ligament tension. The correct axial rotational alignment is obtained through the correct balance and tension of the ligaments. The rotation is checked by means of two Steinmann pins, inserted into the side of the anteroposterior resection block. The pins must be parallel to the Steinmann pins at the epicondyles

Fig. 4.14. A check with the resection device will prevent the anterior femoral resection from notching when making the posterior femoral resection; care must be taken to ensure that the collateral and cruciate ligaments are not damaged

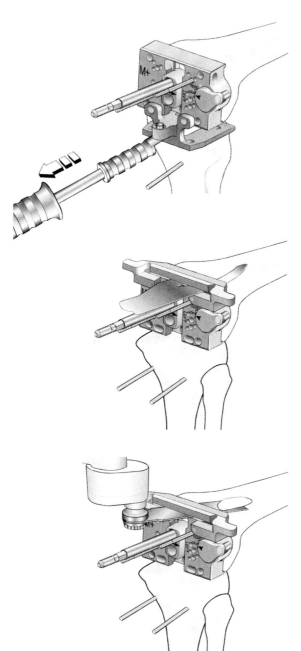

resection for the distal femur. In other words, a perpendicular proximal tibial cut can be expected to remove more lateral tibia than medial tibia, and this is balanced in extension by the fact that the distal femoral cut removes more bone medially than laterally.

This non-anatomic orientation of the proximal tibial cut affects alignment and ligament balance in flexion and extension. Posterior femoral resection should be parallel to proximal tibial resection, which removes more bone from the posterior medial condyle and less from the posterior lateral condyle. For establishing the femoral rotation, a combination of the method with condylar, epicondylar, and trochlear anatomy and the rectangle based on the tibial resection cut is preferable. In varus cases, quite commonly, the flexion gap is wider laterally than medially. If, after tibial resection, the preliminary flexion gap is wider laterally, the ligament (flexion tension–rectangular flexion gap) based technique leads to greater resection of posterior femur from the medial side. A posterior femoral resection line parallel to the tibial cut represents a position of relative external rotation. Therefore, the femoral component would be relatively externally rotated on an internally rotated femur, which is the most common clinical situation (Stiehl, Whiteside, Berger, Boldt, Jerosch).

Fig. 4.15. The femur has a tendency to be in apparent internal rotation with the knee in flexion in cases with varus deformity. (Reprinted with permission of K. A. Krackow)

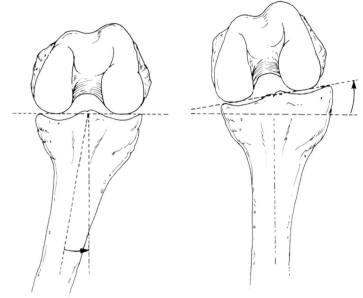

Flexion with neutral femoral rotation

Flexion with vertical tibial orientation and internal femoral rotation

Tibial Rotation

When analyzing tibial rotation, the overall appearance of the proximal joint surface of the tibia has to be considered. Bone loss, osteophyte formation, remodeling and general anatomic variability must be evaluated pre- and intraoperatively. The normal configuration of the posterior cortex extends further posteriorly on the medial than on the lateral side (Fig. 4.16). Another important anatomic structure is the patellar–tibial tuberosity, which typically lies lateral to an anterior midline. The tibial crest lies in the midline and is useful for correct placement of the tibial component. Another landmark is the intermalleolar axis.

Final consideration for referencing tibial rotation might be the position established by the soft tissues. This technique involves acceptance of the tibial rotation defined by the soft tissue attachments. The position of the tibia is marked to parallel that of the femur in extension when longitudinal tension is applied across the joint (Fig. 4.17). The rotation position of the tibia is taken to be the natural resting position, which is achieved during this tension stress testing.

Flexion–Extension Ligament Balance

The terminology flexion–extension ligament balance refers to the issue of providing ligament stability throughout a functional range of motion (i.e. good

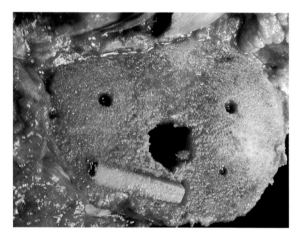

Fig. 4.16. The overall appearance of the proximal joint surface of the tibia has to be considered. The normal configuration of the posterior cortex extending further posteriorly on the medial than on the lateral side can be augmented by autologous bone grafting

stability throughout the entire flexion cycle and at full extension). Utilizing the tibial axis/ligament tension technique, the cut of reference is the proximal tibial cut (tibia first approach). A posterior femoral cut is then made based on a distraction gap with the knee at 90 degrees of flexion. The knee is then brought to full extension, and a distal femoral resection is performed to create an extension gap of appropriate size to match that of the gap in flexion. The measured resection technique is a process by which a

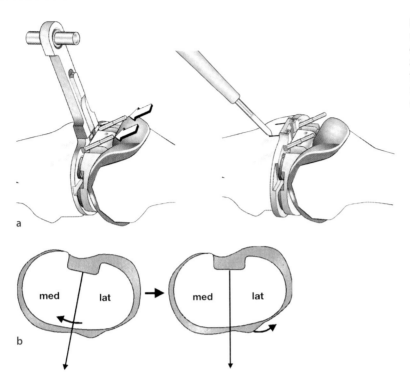

Fig. 4.17. **a** The position of the tibia is marked to parallel that of the femur in extension when longitudinal tension is applied through the joint. **b** Optimal tibial rotational alignment must be ensured, particularly when fixed bearing designs are utilized

predetermined thickness of distal femoral bone is excised, as well as a specific measure of each posterior condyle. The resected pieces of bone are replaced by corresponding thicknesses of distal and posterior femoral component. The rationale behind this approach can be viewed as a re-creation of the prosthetic femoral joint surface in proper spatial relationship to the origin of the collateral ligaments and posterior cruciate ligament. The tibial resection in this approach is basically independent of the femoral resection. Enough tibial bone is removed to make room for the thinnest tibial spacer. One can imagine various combinations of femoral first approaches. It is possible to measure from the posterior condyle and begin to establish the size and anteroposterior position of the femoral component. Alternatively one can measure the size of the flexion gap, take the knee to 0 degrees, and resect the distal femur to lead to an extension gap that matches.

Femoral Component Positioning: Flexion–Extension Component Position

The normal femur has an overall anterior bow, which is most prominent in its midsection. This bow produces an overall flexion–extension axis that differs by 2–5 degrees from the flexion–extension axis that is apparent at the distal metaphyseal area. As one directs a femoral component in a neutral position, there is a tendency to create an anterior notch (Fig. 4.18). For a femoral component placed in flexion, the relative position of the tibial and femoral components is actually one of hyperextension. If excessive, this position leads to inappropriate articulation with the distal aspect of the trochlear notch abutting on the anterior plastic bearing area. When placed in extension, collateral ligament tension is altered and extension may be restored.

Tibial Component Positioning: Flexion–Extension Position

It is important to note that the tibia, as well as the femur, has a relative anterior bow. This implies that any intramedullary rod would need to enter anteriorly if it is to describe an overall neutral flexion–extension position. Using an external rod or an ankle clamp arrangement, one must not be misled by drapes, by the bow in the tibia, tuberosity location or inaccurate positioning at the joint level or at the ankle. The bony anterior crest reference to an alignment rod or the fibula lateral view are consistent landmarks. Attempt to reconstitute the patient's given posterior slope (usually 5–7 degrees).

Fig. 4.18. The femoral bow implies that an overall flexion–extension axis will differ by 2–5 degrees from the flexion–extension axis that is apparent at the distal 25%. If one directs a femoral component in a neutral position, there is a tendency to create an anterior notch

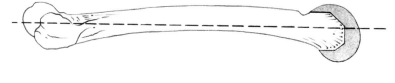

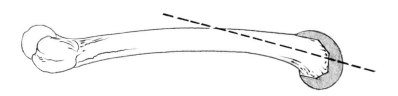

Tibia: Extension – Anterior Slope

Extension cuts (prosthetic positioning) lead to a cascade of problems including the tendency for anterior loading. As flexion proceeds, to the degree that femoral rollback occurs, it leads to the development of ligament tightness in flexion. The anterior bone is weaker, therefore anteroposterior rocking, lift off and prosthetic fixation failure are more likely to occur.

Tibia: Flexion – Posterior Slope

The advantages of a posterior slope include increased range of flexion and more symmetric removal of the tibial surface. However, several potential disadvantages exist if the slope is excessive. To the degree that femoral rollback during flexion does occur, ligament tension may tend to decrease during flexion, with development of flexion instability. With a deeper cut posteriorly, more care is necessary to protect the posterior cruciate ligament. If there is any question, posterior cruciate ligament sacrificing and more constraint prostheses should be used.

Tibia Anteroposterior Positioning

Ideally, the tibial component covers the entire area. If it does not, the surgeon must make his own judgement. It may depend on variation in bone quality, as well as on the relative position the tibia assumes in relationship to the femur in flexion and extension.

Femur Anteroposterior Positioning

Movement of the femoral component anteriorly leads to diminution of ligament and soft tissue tension in flexion, and flexion contracture (extension block) if a thicker tibial component is selected to provide stability in flexion. In the other direction, inappropriate movement of the femoral component posteriorly leads to relative tightness of the knee in flexion, as well as a higher probability of anterior femoral notching.

Tibia Proximal Positioning

Alterations of cut level or joint line position on the tibial side have much less influence on flexion–extension ligament balance than comparable alterations on the femoral side. Movement of the femoral surface of the joint line changes the curvature of the femoral component in relationship to the axes for the centers of rotation. On the tibial side, for an already properly matched femoral joint surface, the tibial cut has essentially equal influence on joint line position in both flexion and extension.

Tibial bone density diminishes as one moves distally from the joint surface, i.e. the deeper the cut, the softer the bone. All total knee systems use tibial components that are at least 8–10 mm thick. While one would like to stay as proximal as possible with a tibial cut, the joint will be too tight, as the tibial resection affects both flexion and extension gaps. Surgical release (avoiding over-release) of the tight soft tissue sleeve at the concave side of the deformity leads to distal "migration" of the tibia. Therefore, the bone resection level, especially when dealing with large defects, is more accurately determined. Slight under-release, with fine tuning and trial reduction will allow for optimal balance. Then one is not inadvertently left with too large a space to fill. The techniques used by instrumentation systems to help the surgeon establish the tibial cut level include: (1) making a routine tibial resection with bone graft/shim fill of slope defects, (2) measuring a minimum thickness cut using a gauge or a "finger" for the degree of posterior slope, and (3) making a tibial cut level that has some relationship to the position of the femur with the tibia distracted from the femur.

Femur Distal Positioning

If there is a good preoperative range of motion and ligament imbalance without deformity, reconstitution of a "normally" positioned femoral joint surface would appear to be a reasonable goal. Where there are condylar or epicondylar deformities, bone loss, or fixed varus or valgus flexion contracture deformities, some compromise of the femoral component position may be necessary. The proximal, distal level of femoral resection is selected using either the measured resection or the flexion–extension gap technique. Distal positioning leads to ligament tightness in extension, which implies either production of a flexion contracture or relative laxity in flexion. An abnormally proximal position leads to relative ligament laxity in extension and is combined with either instability in extension or excessive tightness of ligaments in flexion. Proximal resection also creates or accentuates a distal patella position (baja or infera) by raising the joint line.

Patella Management and Alignment

Alignment of the patellar component has not presented many technical instrumentation problems, as most patellar components have been buttons or domes. This geometric shape requires no particular orientation. Because the patella tends to position itself laterally with subluxation problems, the patellar component can be placed relatively more medial. In the case of an asymmetrically worn patella, the superficial cortical surface of the patella and the articular plane are not parallel. Creation of a cut surface that does excise bone from the thinner facet, and is parallel to the cortical surface of the patella, would lead to a relatively thick cut from the opposite (usually medial) facet, resulting in an extremely thin bone

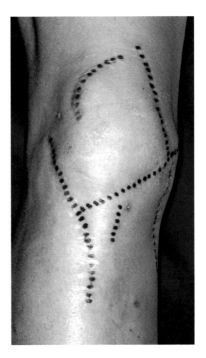

Fig. 4.19. All preoperative scars must be carefully identified and are best marked immediately prior to surgery. No scar must be crossed in less than 45 degrees and the most lateral scar should be chosen if more than one is available

bed with components not circularly symmetric, such as (1) those having a central groove, (2) an elliptical shape with offset central dome, or (3) quite constrained designs with sharp grooves or (4) rectangular cross-sections; several options can be considered as alignment landmarks. These include the position of the patellar ridge if visible before resection, the location of the midpoints of the quadriceps and patellar tendons, and the discernible position of the patella when it is turned back to a non-everted position and applied to the trochlear groove of the femoral component. If risk factors of patella resurfacing are significant, consider patelloplasty without patella resurfacing, which has proven to be satisfactory with patella-friendly condylar designs.

Surgical Technique

The aspects of surgical exposure with respect to placement of skin incision and also deeper capsular incision offer several alternatives. Of special importance is the presence of prior skin incisions, which may influence the particular incision line to be chosen (Figs. 4.19, 4.20).

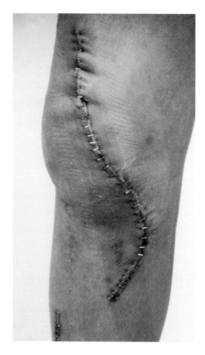

Fig. 4.20. Example of a curved skin incision when taking previous scars into account

Lateral Exposure

A detailed description of the lateral and alternative approaches is provided in Sects. 4.3 and 4.4. Lateral skin incision paired with a lateral parapatellar arthrotomy may be considered. This approach has many advantages for skin healing and skin innervation, and maintains both superior medial and inferior medial blood supply to the patella. It also preserves the general integrity of the medial tissues to obviate potential problems of lateral patellar subluxation. On the other hand, because of the relatively lateral position of the tibial tubercle, this exposure may not allow adequate access to the distal end of the femur and the proximal end of the tibia. In these situations, a lateral parapatellar incision should be combined with a tibial tubercle osteotomy. True lateral parapatellar approaches have a presumed advantage of effecting good lateral retinacular release, as well as providing direct exposure for deep concave side releases in a more stepwise fashion, preserving overall soft tissue stability.

Tibial Tubercle Osteotomy

A detailed description of the tibial tubercle osteotomy is given in Sect. 4.5. Osteotomy of the tibial tubercle for improved exposure offers the best access to the knee joint. It carries certain definite drawbacks, principally the concern of postoperative avulsion and/or failure of fixation. Efforts are made to achieve a suitably thick piece of bone without undermining the residual strength of the proximal tibial area. The bone fragment is made 8–10 cm long to provide room for two or three fixation screws. Conforming the bone proximally will impede proximal migration as long as the fragment remains opposed to the tibial base. The fragment is elevated using an osteotome or a bone saw. Fascia and muscle that attach to the fragment medially are maintained in as much continuity as possible. The fragment is reapplied with two 3.5 mm corticocancellous lag screws.

Medial Exposure

The knee joint incision for total knee arthroplasty may be performed through a variety of skin incisions. In obese patients, a strong point can be made for a straight midline incision or proximal lateral to distal medial midline incision because it is very difficult to evert the subcutaneous and skin tissue in these patients. Medial exposure may be divided into three types. One is a central type that involves midline or slightly medial incisions in both the quadriceps and patellar tendons. Next is a median parapatellar incision, and last is a more medial form of incision either as a mid-vastus approach or at the inferior border of the vastus medialis muscle (sub-vastus). Disadvantages of the mid- and sub-vastus approach include some tendency of less extensive exposure and potential damage to the muscle by traction. The median parapatellar approach gives relatively good and easy exposure even in more difficult cases. Its possible disadvantages include considerations of patellar circulation, especially if extensive lateral release is to be performed, potential for failure of the superior medial tendon–retinacular repair, and development of lateral patellar subluxation.

Exposure Details

Longer rather than shorter incisions avoid the trauma of stretching incisional margins. Incision is made to the level of the deep fascia over the quadriceps tendon and to the capsule medially. Exposure is carried deeper to the level of the quadriceps tendon, to the capsular tissue adjacent to the patella, and distally to the periosteum over the anteromedial flare of the tibia. The fascia is typically crossed at mid-aspect of the joint capsule. The fascia is divided; it remains with the subcutaneous fat and is retracted in the upper half of the wound and remains on the capsule in the lower half of the wound.

The incision is begun in the quadriceps tendon approximately at the junction of the central and medial one third. It proceeds distally, very close to the patella and sweeps around the proximal medial margin of the patella, preserving capsular and retinacular tissue for subsequent closure. The incision proceeds distally 1–2 cm medial and parallel to the patella tendon, again to ensure good tissue for suturing. This incision ends distal to the tibial tubercle.

Deep Exposure

Capsule and periosteal tissue are elevated medially. The attachments of the meniscotibial ligament are freed. It is relatively easy to perform a subperiosteal elevation just below the joint line and then, with the periosteal elevator, to clear soft tissue attachments right at the joint line itself and the inferior margin of the medial osteophytes. At the anterolateral aspect of the tibia, one is working deep to the patellar tendon. The vascular fat pad is a better periarticular tissue than fibrous tissue. In the interest of preserving blood supply to the patella, we leave at least half of the fat pat (removing the deepest synovial layer and part of the fat pad tissue). We perform a (conservative) anterior synovectomy if the synovium is seen to be inflamed, leaving the subsynovial fat as a natural interposition between the quadriceps muscle and tendon and the underlying femoral bone.

Once the knee is adequately flexed, dissection on the tibial side is carried past the posteromedial corner (level of the semimembranous insertion, pars reflexa, pars directa, and anterolaterally past Gerdy's tubercle). Instrumentation and bone resections can be accomplished. Careful inspection of the anterolateral mobility of the patella, as well as examination by palpation of the lateral patellar retinaculum from inside the joint, are other measures of adequate exposures.

Particular attention to the lateral patellar osteophytes is necessary, since they may be a remaining source of difficulty in achieving free patellar eversion. If they are, they should be removed early. Retraction of the everted patella is facilitated by dividing the lateral synovium. The remaining osteophytes on the periphery of the patella are removed. Lateral rim release, filet expansion of the vastus lateralis tendon, and patellofemoral ligament release improve exposure and patella tracking. A circular "denervation" of the patella is performed by electro-cauterization at this time or later. Dissection is carried out in the direction of the posterolateral corner to achieve exposure of the lateral collateral ligament and posterolateral capsular complex. The medial and lateral margin osteophytes are removed, with preservation of meniscal stability and integrity of soft tissues. Removal of the osteophytes of the intercondylar notch (notchplasty) and removal of the tibial spine provides a flat surface for instrumentation. The anterior cruciate ligament is resected and the tibia is retracted forwards for ease of instrumentation.

4.3 Alternative Medial Approaches
Peter A. Keblish

Surgical approaches in non-constrained mobile bearing total knee arthroplasty (TKA) should provide the best access for the specific deformity correction. Alternatives to the standard medial approach include medial mid-vastus, sub-vastus, and direct lateral approach, with or without tibial tubercle osteotomy or proximal rectus-snip. The direct lateral approach is a recommended alternative for fixed valgus knees, especially if there is lateral patellar subluxation and significant rotational deformity. The subvastus and mid-vastus medial approaches preserve quadriceps integrity/patella stability and are recommended for severely unstable knees in non-obese, non-fixed valgus, and medial unicompartmental knee replacement. Technique specifics of the three approaches are reviewed and illustrated.

The medial parapatellar approach remains the standard (utilitarian) method of accessing the arthritic knee when performing TKA. Since fixed varus is the most common deformity, this approach is most appropriate, especially in the obese patient with a normal quadriceps tendon mechanism. However, some complications can be related to the standard approach. When a lateral release is required, a portion of the blood supply may be compromised. Patel-

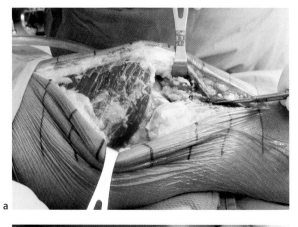
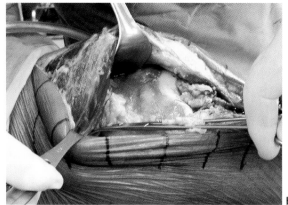
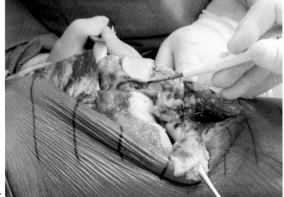
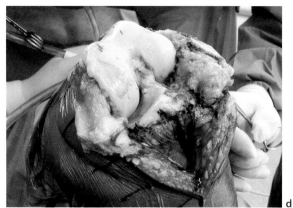

Fig. 4.21. a, b Sub-vastus exposure proximally along the medial border of the vastus medialis with partial detachment from the femur. **c, d** Quadriceps eversion allows for patella maltracking (tilt, edge loading, etc.), which is multi-factorial and often reported in TKA complications, may be related to subtle stretch-out or lack of complete integrity of the extensor mechanism with the standard medial retinacular incision/repair. Variables of deformity and anatomy, pre-existing incisions and ligament reconstruction may present challenges that are best treated with alternative surgical approaches to the standard medial parapatellar approach, which includes the medial sub-vastus, medial mid-vastus, and the direct lateral approaches. Tibial tubercle osteotomy, as advocated by Whiteside (1993) and Wolff et al. (1989) can be used in conjunction with any of the approaches for the stiff, complex/difficult, and/or revision TKA.

exposure and lateral rim release for detilting. Medial sleeve release allows for further exposure enhancement and release of fixed contracture

Medial Sub-vastus Approach

The indications for the medial sub-vastus approach are:

1. Unicompartmental knee replacement
2. Gross instability with easily mobilized quadriceps mechanism
3. Any knee with planned tubercle osteotomy.
   The contraindications are:
1. Obesity or large and short extremity
2. Rigid and stiff knee.

The medial sub-vastus approach or southern approach was described as early as 1929, but has not gained popularity in TKA (Fig. 4.21). Recent literature suggests a renewed interest in the approach because of advantages that allow for: (1) better preservation of the quadriceps mechanism and medial blood supply; (2) improved patellar tracking; (3) less need for lateral releases; and (4) more rapid rehabilitation. Patient preference of sub-vastus to the standard parapatellar approach has been reported in a comparison study. When utilized in TKA, patellar eversion is required; therefore, patient selection is important in that soft tissue compliance must allow for the extensive medial quadriceps mobilization to the lateral side. The sub-vastus approach is technically more demanding and should be performed by surgeons comfortable with the approach. The approach, with tibial tubercle osteotomy, has been advocated in TKA when femoral osteotomy (for extra-articular deformity) is performed at the same time, and should be considered whenever a tibial tubercle osteotomy is part of the preoperative planning.

Sub-vastus Technique Points

The midline incision is angulated proximal lateral to distal medial (off prominence of the tibial tubercle).

Distal arthrotomy begins distally 1 cm medial to the patella tendon and extends proximally to the inferior border of the vastus medialis oblique (VMO). The VMO is incised to the intramuscular septum with a sharp knife or electrocautery dissection, followed by a blunt finger-splitting dissection from the underlying capsule. Fibers of the medialis are released from the intramuscular septum proximally. Retraction of the quadriceps anteriorly and completion of the arthrotomy along the medial border of the vastus medialis, the patella tendon, and the tibial tubercle. Vessels should be controlled. Patella subluxation and eversion is performed beginning in extension with external tibial rotation followed by flexion that allows for satisfactory femoral–tibial exposure. Pre-cuts and tibial sleeve releases can enhance the exposure in difficult cases. A short sagittal incision of the inferior VMO tendon (0.5–1 cm) can be used to enhance patella mobilization further. Exposure is adequate for instrumentation/prosthetic insertion (Fig. 4.22). Trial/permanent prosthetic insertion shows that patella stability is superior when the majority of the vastus medialis remains intact. The VMO and medialis fall into place as shown. Closure begins proximally with suture of the synovial sheath. The distal–medial sleeve is advanced and secured to the medial corner of the VMO (just off the patella). The closure is completed distally from this point. Internal rotation of the tibia and closure in flexion allows for the most anatomic reattachment.

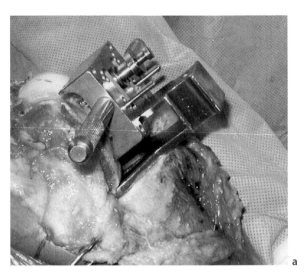
a

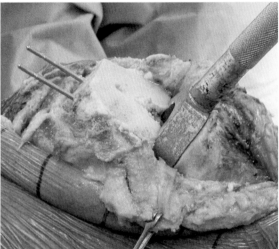
b

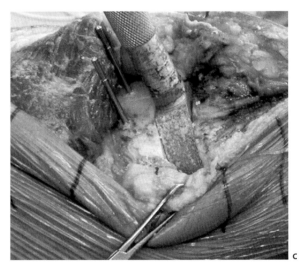
c

Fig. 4.22 a–c. Assessibility for instrumentation and flexion–extension gap balancing following femoral and tibial resections

Medial Mid-vastus Approach

The indications for the medial mid-vastus approach are:

1. Unicompartmental knee replacement
2. Varus deformity with normal soft tissue compliance
3. Short quadriceps tendon
4. Any knee with planned tubercle osteotomy.
   The contraindications are:
1. Obesity/large and short extremity
2. Rigid/stiff knee.

The medial mid-vastus approach, as described by Engh et al. (1997), is a compromise between the standard medial parapatellar and sub-vastus approaches (Fig. 4.23). The mid-vastus approach has similar advantages to the sub-vastus approach but is less difficult and can be utilized in most cases. Several authors have reported that the mid-vastus muscle-splitting approach provides excellent exposure in TKA. The approach has been evaluated in recent reports. Cited advantages include: (1) preservation of medial quadriceps integrity; (2) preservation of medial patellar blood supply; (3) easier joint exposure as compared to the sub-vastus approach; (4) better patellar control (tracking), which eliminates the need for excessive lateral releases; and (5) less pain and earlier return to function. The specifics of the approach have been described and the advantages/disadvantages noted. Cooper et al. (1999) described the anatomic variables (vascular/neurological) of the medial femoral neurovascular bundles and suggested that the mid-vastus splitting approach is secure and has a safety range regarding neurovascular compromise. Parentis et al. (1999) noted some denervation in the distal segment (electromyographic studies), but clinical results suggest that the vastus medialis remains intact, and the potential compromise of the distal segment of the VMO control may not be critical.

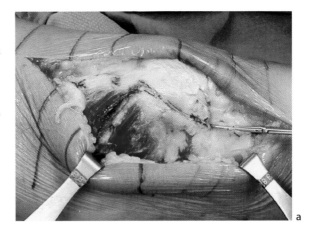

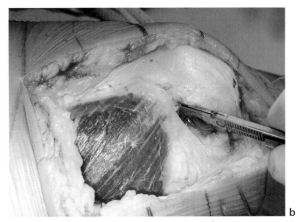

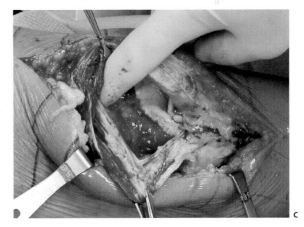

Fig. 4.23. a Mid-vastus exposure reveals skin incision and path of the medial retinacular incision. b Mid-vastus split to the upper medial border of the patella. c Sharp followed by blunt dissection along the natural muscle interval of the vastus medialis

Mid-vastus Technique Points

The midline incision is angulated proximal lateral to distal medial (off prominence of the tibial tubercle).

Distal arthrotomy begins distally 1 cm medial to the patella tendon and extends proximally to a point at the proximal medial patella border (between 10 and 11 o'clock). A muscle-splitting incision from this point is made with a sharp knife or electrocautery dissection, followed by a finger-splitting of the natural muscle separation proximally. Retraction of the quadriceps anteriorly and completion of the arthrotomy along the medial border of the vastus medialis, the patella tendon, and the tibial tubercle. Patella subluxation and eversion is performed beginning in extension with external tibial rotation followed by flexion that allows for satisfactory femoral–tibial exposure. Pre-cuts and tibial sleeve releases can enhance the exposure in difficult cases. Exposure is shown to be adequate for instrumentation/prosthetic insertion (Fig. 4.24). Closure begins proximally at the deep myofascia proximally and extends distally to include the medial retinacular sleeve. Internal rotation of the tibia and closure in flexion allows for the most anatomic reattachment and stability.

Dressings, Splints and Postoperative Care

Standard soft dressings (without construction) are utilized in the average patient with limited soft tissue.

When performing extensive soft tissue dissection in a high-risk rheumatoid-type (thin-skinned) patient, splinting in extension for 2–3 days should be considered. In general the rehabilitation is less intensive in this high-risk group. Supportive functional splinting should be considered in the fragile elderly patient if less than perfect stability has been achieved. Routine protocols with or without continuous passive motion devices vary between individual surgeons. The aggressiveness of therapy is guided by the patient disease process and extent of the soft tissue releases.

Soft tissue (interstitial) edema and subcutaneous dissection of blood/serum is more common with more extensive releases required. Suction drainage of both intra-articular and subcutaneous layers is advised. Achieving a good range of motion with an alternative approach is seldom a problem, since the extensor mechanism remains more intact. Avoid aggressive physical therapy programs (early) if there are any soft tissue concerns, especially with the lateral approach (Fig. 4.25).

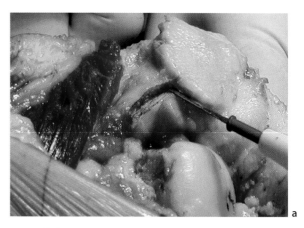

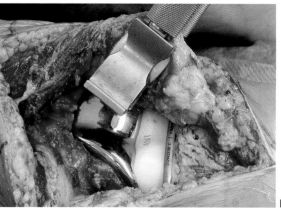

Fig. 4.24. a Patella eversion allows for patella eversion and appropriate releases for excellent joint exposure of all compartments. **b** Final prosthetic insertion showing adequate exposure for patella resurfacing

Bibliography

Bindelglass DF, Vince KG (1996) Patellar tilt and subluxation following subvastus and parapatellar approach in total knee arthroplasty. Implication for surgical technique. J Arthroplasty 11:507–511

Buechel FF (1990) A sequential three-step lateral release for correcting fixed valgus knee deformities during total knee arthroplasty. Clin Orthop 260:170–175

Cooper RE Jr, Trinidad G, Buck WR (1999) Midvastus approach in total knee arthroplasty: a description and a cadaveric study determining the distance of the popliteal artery from the patellar margin of the incision. J Arthroplasty 14:505–508

Dalury DF, Jiranek WA (1999) A comparison of the midvastus and paramedian approaches for total knee arthroplasty. J Arthroplasty 14:33–37

Engh GA, Parks NL (1998) Surgical technique of the midvastus arthrotomy. Clin Orthop 351:270–274

Engh GA, Parks NL, Ammeen DJ (1996) Influence of surgical approach on lateral retinacular releases in total knee arthroplasty. Clin Orthop 331:56–63

Osteoperiosteal Elevation

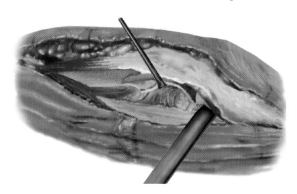 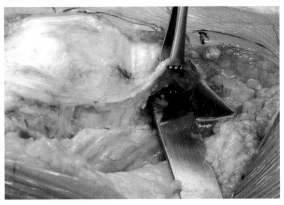

a

Tibial Tubercle Osteotomy

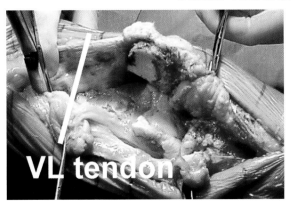 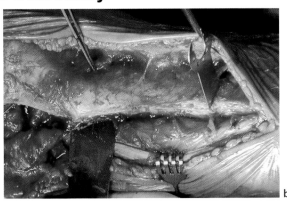

b

Fig. 4.25 a, b. Distal tubercle management options include an: a osteoperiosteal sleeve elevation, or b formal tibial tubercle osteotomy from lateral to medial

Engh GA, Holt BT, Parks NL (1997) A midvastus muscle-splitting approach for total knee arthroplasty. J Arthroplasty 12:322–331

Faure BT, Benjamin JB, Lindsey B, Volz RG, Schutte D (1993) Comparison of the subvastus and paramedian surgical approaches in bilateral knee arthroplasty. J Arthroplasty 8: 511–516

Hofmann AA, Plaster RL, Murdock LE (1991) Subvastus (Southern) approach for primary total knee arthroplasty. Clin Orthop 269:70–77

Keating EM, Faris PM, Meding JB, Ritter MA (1999) Comparison of the midvastus muscle-splitting approach with the median parapatellar approach in total knee arthroplasty. J Arthroplasty 14:29–32

Keblish PA (1991) The lateral approach to the valgus knee. Surgical technique and analysis of 53 cases with over two-year follow-up evaluation. Clin Orthop 271:52–62

Keblish PA (1985) Valgus deformity in TKR: the lateral retinacular approach. Orthop Trans 273:5–8

Lonner JH, Siliski JM, Lotke PA (2000) Simultaneous femoral osteotomy and total knee arthroplasty for treatment of osteoarthritis associated with severe extra-articular deformity. JBJS [Am] 82:342–348

Maestro A, Suarez MA, Rodriguez L, Guerra C, Murcia A (2000) The midvastus surgical approach in total knee arthoplasty. Int Orthop 24:104–107

Matsueda M, Gustilo RB (2000) Subvastus and medial parapatellar approaches in total knee arthroplasty. Clin Orthop 371:161–168

Moon MS, Kim JM, Woo YK (1997) Restoration of knee motion after total knee arthroplasty: subvastus approach and alternate flexion and extension splintage. Ryumachi 37:146

Ogata K, Ishinishi T, Hara M (1997) Evaluation of patellar retinacular tension during total knee arthroplasty. Special emphasis on lateral retinacular release. J Arthroplasty 12:651–656

Parentis MA, Rumi MN, Deol GS et al (1999) A comparison of the vastus splitting and median parapatellar approaches in total knee arthroplasty. Clin Orthop 367:107–116

Roysam GS, Oakley MJ (2001) Subvastus approach total knee arthroplasty: a prospective, randomized, and observer-blinded trial. J Arthroplasty 16:454–457

White RE Jr, Allman JK, Trauger JA, Dales BH (1999) Clinical comparison of the midvastus and medial parapatellar surgical approaches. Clin Orthop 367:117–122

Whiteside LA (1993) Correction of ligament and bone defects in total arthroplasty of the severely valgus knee. Clin Orthop 288:234–245

Wolff AM, Hungerford DS, Krackow KA, Jacobs MA (1989) Osteotomy of the tibial tubercle during total knee replacement. A report of twenty-six cases. JBJS [Am] 71:848–852

4.4 Lateral Retinacular Approach

Peter A. Keblish

Surgical approaches in total knee arthroplasty (TKA) should allow the surgeon to access the knee in the safest, most direct manner that allows for achievement of predictable stability at the patellofemoral and the femorotibial interfaces. Fixed contractures in valgus TKA require sequential releases that include the capsule, iliotibial band (I-TB), vastus lateralis (VL) tendon, lateral collateral ligament (LCL), and at times, the popliteus, lateral gastrocnemius, and inner aspect of the fibular head (preserving and lengthening the LCL). These releases are best addressed by the direct access using the lateral approach. The direct lateral approach is a technique that offers many advantages in correction of fixed valgus, as well as other challenges that confront the knee surgeon, primarily patella alignment and soft tissue considerations. It is less commonly used (and understood) than the standard medial approaches, but has been shown to improve stability and patella results in fixed valgus TKA.

This chapter will: (1) define the pathologic anatomy of the valgus knee; (2) define the technical problems and disadvantages of the medial approach in fixed valgus deformity; (3) illustrate the technique specifics and advantages of the direct lateral approach in fixed valgus deformity; and (4) discuss other indications for the lateral approach.

Pathologic Anatomy in Valgus Knee

Fixed valgus deformity is usually associated with femorotibial malrotation, resorption of the lateral femoral condyle and a relatively large more distal medial condyle (Fig. 4.26). Lateral structures are tight and the patella is frequently deformed and subluxed over the deformed lateral condyle. Valgus is most prevalent in females (9:1), and rheumatoid arthritis is more common and associated with flexion contracture. Prosthetic cover and joint seal can be a problem, as the skin and soft tissue are often deficient. Excessive undermining, increased tension, or lack of a soft tissue layer between skin and prosthesis can lead to skin necrosis, a potentially devastating complication of TKA. Understanding the anatomy is important.

Extra-articular Layer

The fascia lata extension envelops the quadriceps with attachment to the posterior aspect of the femur. The distal lateral confluence becomes the I-TB with distinct insertion into Gerdy's tubercle and the lateral tibial plateau. Transverse and oblique fibers extend to the patellar mechanism (lateral retinaculum), and longitudinal fibers attach to bone via Sharpey's fibers and extend to the fascia of the anterior compartment. The I-TB and the lateral retinaculum are deforming factors in the fixed valgus knee. The I-TB attachment to the upper tibia produces a valgus moment with external rotation (and sometimes flexion deformity), and the oblique and transverse extensions produce a lateral (subluxing) moment to the patella. The extra-articular (superficial) layer also includes the lateral hamstring, the fabello-fibular ligament, the lateral head of the gastrocnemius, and the popliteus (Fig. 4.27). These structures may be contracted secondary to long-standing valgus. Bony deformity may further increase concave side contractures.

The lateral superficial layer differs from the (compliant) medial oblique retinaculum of the vastus medialis in that the lateral retinaculum is relatively non-compliant. This non-compliant lateral fascial extension to the patellar mechanism, coupled with contractures of the deeper layer, becomes a major determinant of the soft tissue deformity in the valgus knee.

Intra-articular Deep Layer

The popliteus tendon, LCL, fabello-fibular ligament, arcuate ligament, and capsule form the posterolateral complex. Anteriorly, the VL inserts at the proximal patellar facet. The tendon of the VL is usually of substantial thickness and joins the lateral aspect of the central quadriceps (rectus tendon). This structure is covered by a capsular and/or synovial layer in the joint. The muscles, by definition, have an extra-articular origin. The LCL differs from the medial collateral ligament in that its distal insertion is at the fibular head. The deep anterior and posterior lateral soft tissue layers are usually contracted to different degrees, depending on factors such as the underlying pathology, longevity of the deformity, bony pathology, and others. Management of superficial and deep layer contractures in valgus TKA must be understood, and represents a key to correction of tibial rotation, centralization of the patella, and achieving proper flexion/extension gap balancing. In either case, the direct

Fig. 4.26. Valgus deformity involves bone and soft tissue. Deformities are graded from mild (<15 degrees) to severe (>30 degrees) and may be fixed, correctable or partially correctable. Type II valgus deformity implies incompetence of the medial collateral sleeve

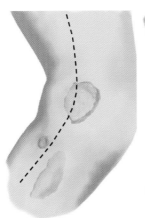
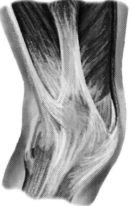
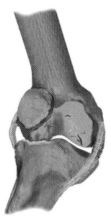

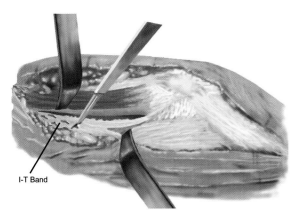

I-T Band

Fig. 4.27. Deep posterolateral structures are illustrated. Some or all are contracted, or abnormal with fixed valgus deformity

lateral approach enhances exposure and provides other advantages, which will be discussed in the technique section.

Medial Approach

The standard medial parapatellar and sub-vastus/mid-vastus variations are the most commonly used approaches in TKA. There is a general consensus that sequential releases should be performed from the femoral side prior to or after prosthetic insertion in fixed valgus. However, the medial approach in valgus TKA fails to address the pathologic anatomy directly and releases may be overdone, as exposure is limited following patella relocation and trial testing. Patella maltracking is more common, and there is increased potential for inaccurate flexion/extension gap balancing and less than optimum femorotibial stability.

Other technical disadvantages include: (1) external rotation of the tibia is increased; (2) access to the posterolateral corner is more difficult; (3) an extensive lateral release is still required; (4) joint seal and prosthetic soft tissue coverage is difficult; (5) vascularity to the quadriceps-patella-tendon (QPT) mechanism and lateral skin (beneath the extensive lateral release) is decreased; (6) it does not allow for optimal correction of the external rotation contracture of the tibia; and (7) it may encourage over-release of deep soft tissues.

Lateral Approach

The lateral approach in valgus deformity, by contrast, addresses the pathologic anatomy in a rational and sequential manner. The approach: (1) is direct; (2) accomplishes the extensive "lateral release" with the exposure; (3) decreases skin undermining; (4) internally rotates the tibia with improved access to the pathologic posterolateral corner; (5) allows for better titration of sequential releases based on flexion/extension gap balance requirements; (6) preserves vascularity because the medial side is untouched; (7) allows for planned soft tissue gap and prosthetic coverage; (8) centralizes the QPT mechanism, which optimizes patella tracking; (9) improves femorotibial alignment stability; and (10) rehabilitation is unimpeded because the medial quadriceps remains intact. This approach has not gained widespread use because it is less familiar and more demanding. The patella tendon/tibial tubercle presents an obstacle, and many surgeons associate tubercle osteotomy as a requirement for safe exposure. An in-depth illustration of the anatomy and approach (without tubercle osteotomy in the vast majority of cases) is presented to as-

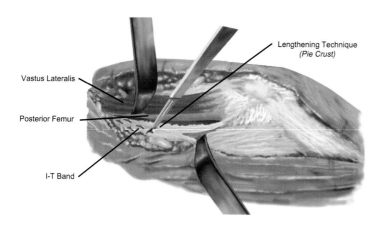

Vastus Lateralis

Posterior Femur

I-T Band

Lengthening Technique
(Pie Crust)

Fig. 4.28. Iliotibial band release is performed by stripping from the posterior femur and a "pie-crust lengthening" (while a varus stress is applied)

sist the TKA surgeon in addressing this most challenging deformity.

Surgical Technique

The surgical technique of the direct lateral approach differs substantially from the standard medial parapatellar approach. The surgeon is less familiar with the lateral side of the knee; orientation is reversed, and more careful handling of the soft tissues is required. The recommended skin incision in the virgin knee follows the Q-angle and is slightly lateral to the patella, lateral border of the patellar tendon, and the tibial tubercle. Long incisions are preferred, especially in short, large legs. It is important to avoid unnecessary undermining and the surgeon must respect layer 1 (superficial layer) and avoid dissecting between the skin and layer 1 as much as possible. In previously operated knees, the existing incision should be incorporated and extended proximally and distally. If multiple incisions are present, select the most direct or latest. A sham incision may be performed and consultation of a plastic surgeon considered since any lateral skin necrosis may be devastating. The approach will be described and illustrated. The skin incision should be atraumatic with identification of layer 1 in the plane of the prepatellar bursa medially. The lateral retinaculum is exposed with careful dissection to allow for the initial superficial (retinacular) incision.

Seven major steps are suggested as guidelines for the surgeon:

Step 1. Superficial longitudinal concave release: I-TB release/lengthening
Step 2. Lateral arthrotomy: transverse release: coronal plane Z-plasty
Step 3. Tibial sleeve release

Step 4. Patella dislocation – joint exposure
Step 5. Deep concave releases (Sect. 4.12)
Step 6. Instrumentation/prosthetic insertion
Step 7. Soft tissue closure deep to superficial layer.

Technique Points

Iliotibial Band Release/Lengthening

The I-TB is exposed proximally by separating the inner fascial sleeve from the VL muscle (Fig. 4.28). The VL is carefully retracted up to the linea aspera. The band is released from the posterior femur (linea aspera) and "finger stripped" to the posterolateral corner. A varus stress at the knee joint will "bowstring" the tight fascial bands, allowing for a multiple puncture "pie-crusting" lengthening (under visual and digital control) while paying attention to the most posterior fibers. The release is performed approximately 10 cm proximal to the joint line. The peroneal nerve can be palpated or explored, but this is seldom required and not recommended except in very severe cases.

Lateral Retinacular Incision (Superficial Layer)

The course of the lateral parapatella incision begins 2–4 cm lateral to the patella and extends distally into the midportion of Gerdy's tubercle (Fig. 4.29), preserving the fibrous layer, which joins with the patellar tendon sheath anteriorly. Proximally, the incision extends into the central quadriceps tendon. The lateral arthrotomy separates the superficial from the deep layers; therefore, proceed cautiously through the outer layers.

Lateral Arthrotomy (Deep Layer)

The superficial layer of the retinaculum is separated from the deep layer with a coronal plane Z-plasty, from superficial lateral to deep medial. Proximally, an oblique arthrotomy incision from the lateral to medial takes advantage of the laminated anatomy of the central quadriceps tendon. The VL tendon is nonyielding but substantially thick and allows for a horizontal (coronal) plane expansion release as well as a longitudinal expansion as shown. The VL tendon in-cision begins near the musculo-tendonous junction and ends distally at the midcoronal plane of the patella insertion. The midportion (lateral retinaculum) separates naturally from the deep capsule and fat pad. The capsule is incised from the patella rim. The fat pad incision continues obliquely to the intermeniscal ligament, retaining about 50% of the fat pad with the patella tendon and 50% with the lateral sleeve, which includes the lateral meniscus rim for increased soft tissue stability (Fig. 4.29).

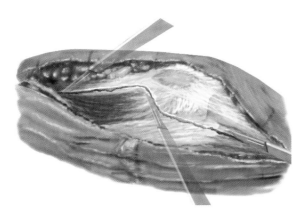

Fig. 4.29. Lateral arthrotomy is performed by separating the superficial and deep layers (coronal plane Z-plasty technique) to prepare the expanded soft tissue sleeve

Distal Tubercle Elevation or Osteotomy

The distal extension of the retinacular incision splits Gerdy's tubercle and continues distally into the anterior compartment fascia (Fig. 4.30). The osteoperiosteal sleeve release (utilizing a sharp osteotome) begins at mid-Gerdy's tubercle and extends anteriorly to, but stops at the tibial tubercle. As the osteoperiosteal sleeve is elevated, muscle fibers of the tibialis anterior are included and preserved in their natural plane. The elevation stops at the lateral border of the patella tendon, protecting the tendon insertion and dissipating stresses to the anterior compartment sleeve. A formal lateral to medial tibial tubercle osteotomy can be performed to enhance exposure in difficult cases or as the surgeon's choice.

Fig. 4.30. The distal elevation from mid-Gerdy's tubercle can be performed with an osteoperiosteal technique or a formal tibial tubercle osteotomy from lateral to medial

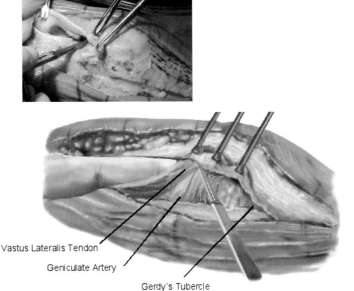

Vastus Lateralis Tendon

Geniculate Artery

Gerdy's Tubercle

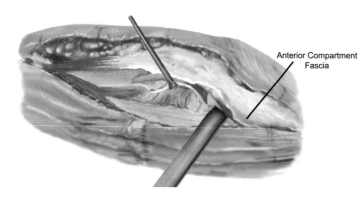

Anterior Compartment Fascia

Fig. 4.31. Lateral tibial sleeve release begins from mid-Gerdy's tubercle to the posterolateral corner. The release can begin in extension and is completed in flexion. Proximal and distal ligament integrity is preserved

Patella Dislocation – Joint Exposure

The patella is dislocated/everted medially as the knee is flexed with a varus stress. Grasping the patella with a towel clip may be helpful. Following patella eversion, a cobra-type retractor is placed medially through the periphery of the medial meniscus and over the medial cortical rim. Patella dislocation can be performed at this step or after the tibial sleeve release. Medial dislocation/eversion of the patella is more difficult than lateral dislocation. Methods to enhance exposure include: a long proximal incision to include a lateral to medial rectus snip (if indicated), osteophyte removal/downsizing of the patella/femur/tibia to normal peripheral anatomy, pre-cuts (measured) of the larger posterior medial and, at times, the distal medial femoral condyles, and pre-cuts of the tibial spine, including the posterior cruciate ligament (PCL). These maneuvers are usually adequate to allow for satisfactory exposure.

Tibial sleeve release

Tibial sleeve release is routinely performed. Osteoperiosteal release from mid-Gerdy's tubercle to the posterolateral tibia begins in extension (before joint exposure) and is completed in flexion, as shown in Fig. 4.31.

Osteophytes and posterior capsule are released and flexion/extension correction is checked with lamina spreaders. The PCL can be released at this time (if required because of non-correctable contractures) or as the surgeon's choice for PCL-substituting prostheses. If initial releases appear adequate, proceed with instrumentation and bone resection (Fig. 4.32).

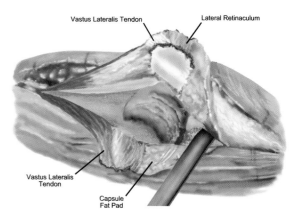

Vastus Lateralis Tendon   Lateral Retinaculum

Vastus Lateralis Tendon

Capsule Fat Pad

Fig. 4.32. Deep concave side release – distal option. If gap imbalance persists following appropriate level bone cuts, distal LCL lengthening is accomplished by excavating the fibular head and preserving the distal LCL insertion with the periosteum and outer fibular cortex. Note fibular fragmentation and excellent balance on postoperative x-ray

Instrumentation (Fine-tuning)/ Trial Reduction

Instrumentation with a flexion gap/femoral positioner allows for fine-tuning of soft tissue balancing (Fig. 4.33). Flexion and extension gaps are checked with appropriate spacer blocks. The distal femoral resection angle may vary from 4 to 60 degrees and should relate to the hip-knee-ankle axis. Some valgus is tolerable as patients' soft tissues and cosmetic appearance have adapted to this position over time. If stable gap balancing (in all planes) and/or failure to achieve full extension is not accomplished at this time, the more extensive femoral side releases will be required; these are described below.

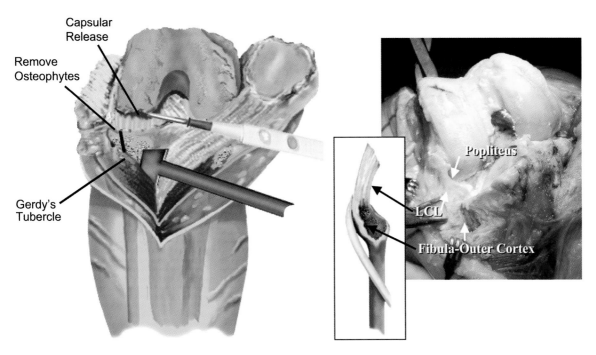

Fig. 4.33. Instrumentation with flexion/extension gap balancing. The deep distal concave lengthenings can be made prior to this step. However, the more extensive proximal osteotomies should be made following prosthetic insertion

Femoral Sleeve Release

In patients with more severe fixed valgus and/or extra-articular deformity, it may be necessary to lengthen or to slide the deep lateral structures and subsequently the posterior structures. Proximal and/or distal lengthening techniques can be used. The sleeve release is the more commonly recommended method, but it can lead to compromised ligament attachment and resultant instability. A proximal periosteal sleeve or limited osteotomy may not be very strong because of the absence of continuous soft tissue attachments. The sliding lateral condyle osteotomy will be discussed in Sect. 4.12 (Fig. 4.34).

Figure 4.35 shows an intraoperative example of trial reduction using a rotating platform prosthesis. Note the medial position of the tibial tubercle with correction of tibial rotation and natural patella tracking. The rotating bearing allows for self-adjustment at the femorotibial interface.

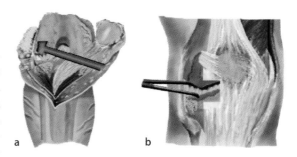

Fig. 4.34 a, b. Deep concave side release – proximal options. If the knee cannot be fully extended because of severe lateral contractures, proximal femoral release options include: a the more commonly performed soft tissue or small osteoperiosteal sleeve release with/without reattachment (especially with the medial approach); or b sliding lateral condyle osteotomy that preserves soft tissue attachments and allows for extensive correction without loss of stability. x-ray example of severe valgus correction with lateral and tibial tubercle osteotomy

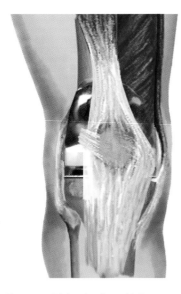

Fig. 4.35. Trial reduction with low contact stress rotating platform components in position showing excellent correction with adaptation of femorotibial and patellofemoral joints

Soft Tissue Sleeve Closure

Closure is accomplished in flexion. The expanded soft tissue closure is completed using sutures of choice proximally. The distal (bony) portion of the I-TB is reattached with trans-osseous sutures. Prosthetic joint seal can be accomplished in all cases (Fig. 4.36). The use of the fat pad may be required, especially in soft-tissue-deficient rheumatoid knees (Keblish 1991, 2002).

Tips and Pearls: Lateral Approach

The VL tendon must be carefully incised through the midcoronal plane to accomplish the lengthening release and subsequent closure at this most critical point. If the expansion release cannot be performed because of inadequate VL tendon thickness, the more compliant capsule/fat pad and/or hypertrophic (proximal) capsule can be mobilized to achieve the joint seal. The quadriceps tendon incision should proceed from superficial lateral to deep medial at an angle of approximately 30–45 degrees, which allows for a natural expansion of the laminated central quadriceps tendon fibers. If a thick, hypertrophic suprapatellar pouch is present, incising the capsule more medially will allow for a well-vascularized tissue mass that can be mobilized for incorporation into the lateral sleeve closure.

The main technical (instrument) problem is "working around" the prominent tibial tubercle when using an extramedullary tibial resection guide. A surgical option (to the osteoperiosteal technique) is the "formal" tibial tubercle osteotomy (lateral to medial), which allows for improved exposure, protection of the patella tendon, avoidance of proximal snip procedures, and ease of prosthetic removal in revision cases (Burki et al. 1999, Arnold et al. 1998). The osteotomized fragment must be large and long and the soft tissues must be preserved medially to allow the tubercle to rotate around this soft tissue hinge.

The depth of the medial tibial resection is less than usual in the valgus knee, especially in type II appearing (real or pseudo-laxity) deformities, which allows for presentation of the medial collateral ligament complex and improves stability. The lateral tibial release from mid-Gerdy's tubercle to the posterolateral corner can be performed before or after joint exposure. An osteoperiosteal technique with a sharp osteotome and/or electrocautery allows for exposure/release of the posterolateral corner and the posterior capsule. Release of the lateral gastrocnemius with the posterolateral capsule may also be required to achieve adequate lateral compartment space in extension.

If satisfactory correction is accomplished following the tibial sleeve, capsular/PCL releases, and downsizing maneuvers, proceed with bony resections and fine-tune the ligament releases at the time of trial reduction. If the lateral structures remain tight and do not allow for satisfactory varus/valgus balance, proceed with distal LCL lengthening (fibula or proximal lengthening femoral side).

When concave side releases of the LCL, popliteus, and secondary structures are required, they can be performed prior to or following trial reduction. Keep in mind that the LCL affects both the flexion and extension gap stability, while the popliteus tendon affects flexion and rotation stability. The more commonly recommended technique (with the medial approach) is a soft tissue release of the I-TB and posterolateral complex from the femur. The sliding lateral condyle osteotomy with a more extensive bone segment is a newer concept, which has the advantage of maintaining a strong proximal soft tissue ligament attachment.

When correcting a valgus deformity, distal femoral resection of 6–7 degrees is often acceptable because it allows for improvement of extension gap balancing and tensioning of "intact" medial structures. "Slight" residual valgus is cosmetically acceptable in the patient with long-standing valgus deformity.

Fig. 4.36. Soft tissue sleeve closure from superficial to deep layers. The iliotibial band is reattached with proper tension utilizing trans-osseous sutures

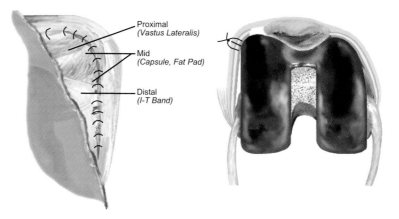

Proximal
(Vastus Lateralis)

Mid
(Capsule, Fat Pad)

Distal
(I-T Band)

Fixed valgus deformity presents a major challenge in TKA. The literature suggests that correction of fixed valgus deformities via the standard medial parapatellar approach leads to higher failure rates, primarily at the patellofemoral joint. A common factor in all reports is the medial surgical approach. Therefore, the surgeon should be familiar with and consider the direct lateral approach in challenging total knee replacements that include: (1) fixed valgus deformity with patella subluxation; (2) partially correctable valgus with lateral orientation and/or patella subluxation; (3) varus knee with severe tibial rotation, increased Q-angle, tight retinaculum, and I-TB with patella tilt and/or subluxation; (4) grossly unstable knee in a rheumatoid patient with expanded suprapatellar pouch; (5) previous lateral incisions in a multiply operated knee – when skin is at risk (with undermining); (6) lateral unicompartmental replacement; and (7) high tibial osteotomy conversion to TKA, especially if there is a lateral incision and/or retained metal.

Bibliography

Arnold MP, Friederich NF, Widmer H, Muller W (1998) Patellar substitution in total knee prosthesis – is it important? Orthopade 27:637–641

Buechel FF (1990) A sequential three-step lateral release for correcting fixed valgus knee deformities during total knee arthroplasty. Clin Orthop 260:170–175

Burki H, von Knoch M, Heiss C, Drobny T, Munzinger U (1999) Lateral approach with osteotomy of the tibial tubercle in primary total knee arthroplasty. Clin Orthop 362:156–161

Fiddian NJ, Blakeway C, Kumar A (1998) Replacement arthroplasty of the valgus knee. A modified lateral capsular approach with repositioning of vastus lateralis. JBJS [Br] 80:859–861

Insall JN, Scott WN, Keblish PA et al (1994) Total knee arthroplasty exposures and soft tissue balancing. In: Insall JN, Scott WN (eds) Videobook of knee surgery. Lippincott, Philadelphia

Keblish PA (1985) Valgus deformity in TKR: the lateral retinacular approach. Orthop Trans 9:28

Keblish PA (1991) The lateral approach to the valgus knee: surgical technique and analysis of 53 cases with over two-year follow-up evaluation. Clin Orthop 271:52–62

Keblish PA, Boldt J, Varma C, Briard JL (2002) Soft-tissue balancing in fixed valgus TKA: methods of achieving concave side releases. Presented at AAOS 2002 scientific exhibit, Dallas, Texas

Krackow KA, Jones MM, Teeny SM et al (1991) Primary total knee arthroplasty in patients with fixed valgus deformity. Clin Orthop 273:9–18

Lootvoet L, Blouard E, Himmer O, Ghosez JP (1997) Complete knee prosthesis in severe genu valgum. Retrospective review of 90 knees surgically treated through the anterio-external approach. Acta Orthop Belg 63:278–286

Merkow RL, Soudry M, Insall JN (1985) Patellar dislocation following total knee replacement. J Bone Joint Surg Am 67:1321–1327

Ranawat CS (1988) Total-condylar knee arthroplasty for valgus and combined valgus-flexion deformity of the knee. Tech Orthop 3:67–76

Scapinelli R (1967) Blood supply of the human patella. J Bone Joint Surg 49B:563

Tsai CL, Chen CH, Liu TK (2001) Lateral approach without ligament release in total knee arthroplasty; new concepts in the surgical technique. Artif Org 25:638–643

Whiteside LA (1993) Correction of ligament and bone defects in total arthroplasty of the severely valgus knee. Clin Orthop 288:234–245

Wolff AM, Hungerford DS, Krackow KA et al (1989) Osteotomy of the tibial tubercle during total knee replacement. J Bone Joint Surg Am 71:848–852

4.5 Tibial Tuberositas Osteotomy

Jens G. Boldt, Tomas K. Drobny

The standard surgical approach in total knee arthroplasty (TKA) at the Schulthess Clinic is the medial parapatellar retinacular approach. To date more than 3,500 mobile bearing TKAs have been implanted using this technique. However, some difficult knee arthropathies such as valgus knee deformities, arthrofibrosis, previously osteotomized knee joints, patella baja (infera) and revision situations require a more sophisticated surgical management, which includes a lateral approach with or without a tibial tubercle osteotomy (TTO). This technique has been used in this center with only slight changes for more than 15 years, with satisfactory results. Refixation of the tibial tubercle has been altered from wires to cancellous screws, but the principle of this approach remains unchanged.

Lateral retinacular releases are frequently performed after medial arthrotomy, particularly in cases with patellar maltracking, lateral subluxation, or tilt. These problems are frequent in fixed valgus knees as well as in varus knees with substantial external tibial rotation. A lateral release improves patellar maltracking. When the standard medial approach is used in combination with a lateral release, the vascularity of the patella and extensor mechanism might be compromised. Thus, the lateral approach to the knee, popularized by Keblish in the 1980s and published in 1991, uses a lateral release that forms an integral part of the surgical approach, and the vascularity is preserved because the medial side remains untouched.

Mechanical compromise of the tibial tendon insertion is a catastrophic complication in TKA. In our experience, a liberal and preoperatively planned TTO is a safe method to avoid this complication in TKA. An alternative osteoperiosteal elevation of the tubercle insertion has a higher risk of detachment and is, therefore, not used. Approaching the knee joint laterally with a TTO gains safe and wide access to the knee joint (open book) without stressing the entire extensor mechanism (Fig. 4.37). With this approach, flexion of the knee joint is facilitated, especially in knees with considerable fixed valgus and varus deformities, fixed flexion deformities, or other causes that may lead to a stiff and fibrosed joint. In these cases the patellar tendon insertion may be prone to spontaneous avulsion, when the knee is forcefully flexed during surgery (Figs. 4.38, 4.39).

Another advantage of this method is a reduced external rotation of the tibia, which facilitates further

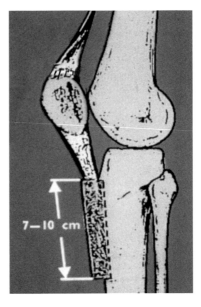

Fig. 4.37. The size of the tibial tubercle should be ideally 8–10 cm by 2–3 cm as demonstrated

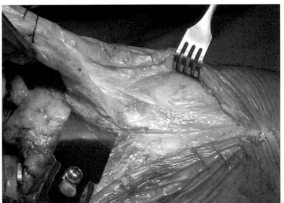

4.3

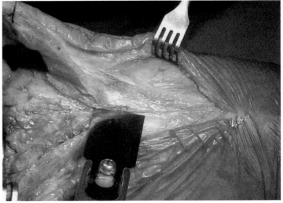

4.3

Figs. 4.38 and 4.39. Sharp osteotomes are preferably used, creating a hockey club type shape of the tibial tubercle. The distal cut is prepared prior to the proximal cuts in order to protect the middle third tibial from fracturing

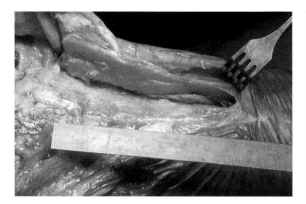

Fig. 4.40. Intraoperative view of the tubercle, which is carefully reverted. Care must be taken throughout the operation to preserve the medial periosteal sleeve

Figs. 4.41–4.43. Radiographs of a typical valgus knee deformity, which was approached using a lateral tibial tubercle osteotomy. After implantation of an unconstrained mobile bearing LCS total knee arthroplasty, the quest was reattached with three cortical lag screws   ▶

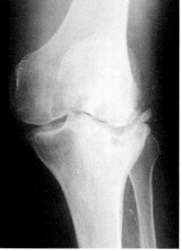

4.41

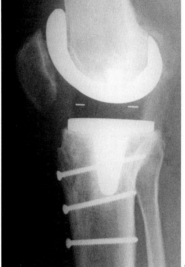

4.42

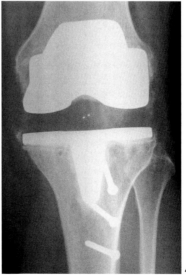

4.43

soft tissue releases and proper positioning of the tibial component. Patients with rheumatoid arthritis benefit from this procedure in particular, because of an increased incidence of valgus deformities, excessive synovitis, osteopenic bone stock and vulnerability of the extensor mechanism. Although Whiteside (1995) reported a tibial fracture post TTO, we could not confirm this complication in our series.

The rate of non-union or mal-union of the tibial tubercle after osteotomy is reported in the literature, but did not occur in our series. It appears vital for the success of this method to avoid undersizing of the osteotomized fragment. We recommend a length of no less than 7 cm and a width of no less than 2 cm at the proximal aspect. This leaves a large surface for comfortable handling and allows for sufficient refixation and vascularity of the avulsed tubercle with two or three cancellous lag screws. The medial periosteal tether should be carefully preserved throughout the entire operation. Using an osteotome instead of an oscillating saw is less traumatizing and devitalizing and is therefore preferred (Fig. 4.40). An illustration of a typical valgus knee is shown in Figs. 4.41, 4.42 and 4.43. Postoperative hematoma can develop in some cases and may be avoided with meticulous hemostasis. Compartment syndrome is another complication that is very hazardous. We, therefore, recommend routine anterior tibial fascia release by using several long incisions, when TTO has been performed.

Keblish (1991) reported that approaching the knee laterally is advantageous since it includes the lateral release that becomes mandatory in most cases with valgus knee, patella subluxation, external tibial rotation, or arthrofibrosis. Proper patellofemoral tracking as well as patella baja or alta can be alternatively achieved with lateral soft tissue releases or alteration of the tubercle refixation. The maneuver of moving the position of the tubercle proximally prior to fixation also allows for extensor mechanism lengthening in cases with limited flexion.

In order to evaluate the success of this method, we performed a prospective study, in which a conventional lateral approach was combined with an additional osteotomy of the tibial tuberosity in valgus knees and knees that had previous non-arthroplasty surgery. Between January 1993 and December 1995, 61 primary TKAs were performed in 51 patients at the Schulthess Clinic. In all cases, a direct lateral approach with tibial crest osteotomy from lateral to medial was performed. In a published prospective study, we evaluated both clinical and radiographical results of TKAs that included valgus knee deformities, high tibial correcting osteotomies and other non-arthroplasty procedures. The preoperative diagnosis was osteoarthritis in 78% and rheumatoid arthritis in 12%; the mean age was 63 years, with 73% being female. Valgus knee deformity was the predominant pathology, with 73% in this study. The preoperative score was 59.2 on a 100-point maximum scale (modified Hospital for Special Surgery score) and the mean preoperative range of motion was 92 degrees. All surgery was performed by two very experienced consultant orthopedic surgeons using unconstrained mobile bearing low contact stress components. Different bearing devices were utilized: in 40 cases a rotating platform with cruciate substituting function, in two cases posterior cruciate ligament (PCL) retaining anteroposterior glide bearing, and in nine cases PCL retaining meniscal bearings. The postoperative rehabilitation followed a standard protocol similar to that of patients without osteotomy and included criterion-based closed-chain exercises with early weight bearing, except straight leg raise for 8 weeks postoperatively. All patients were assessed both clinically and radiographically after 2, 6, and 12 months.

Surgical Technique

The skin incision is made 5–10 mm more lateral than the standard midline incision, aiming towards Gerdy's tubercle distally, and 1–2 cm lateral to the tib-

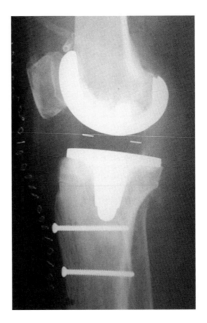

Fig. 4.44. An example of sufficient tibial tubercle osteotomy using two cortical screws only. The surgeon must evaluate both bone quality and stability of the tibial quest

ial tendon insertion. The lateral arthrotomy is begun along the lateral border of the quadriceps tendon. The incision is made approximately 2 cm lateral of the patella and is carried trough to Gerdy's tubercle 7 cm distal to the tibial tendon insertion with preservation of the fat pad. Mobilization of the fat pad and the lateral synovial layer is essential. Lateral releases of various forms include the iliotibial band, the posterolateral corner (arcuate complex), the lateral head of the gastrocnemius or the inner border of the fibula head. The osteotomy is performed using sharp and broad osteotomes rather than an oscillating saw in order to preserve viability. The osteotomy should be at least 7 cm long and 2 cm wide proximally. It is refixed using two or three counter-sunk 3.5 mm lag screws (Fig. 4.44).

Alternatively, wire can be used, but this is not the preferred method in this center. Fixation and patellofemoral tracking is checked in 90 degrees flexion. Expansion of the lateral retinaculum is performed as advocated by Keblish using a coronal Z-plasty (see Sect. 4.4). Fascia and skin are closed in routine fashion with metal clips to skin. In cases with patella baja (infera), the tibial tubercle can be proximalized by up to 1.5 cm, filling the distal gap with autologous bone graft (Figs. 4.45–4.49).

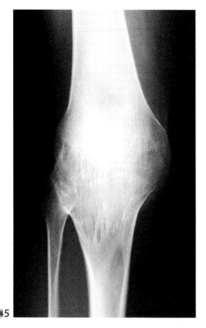

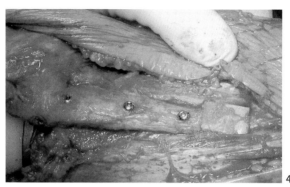

4.48

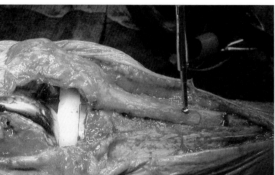

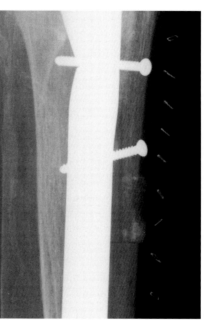

4.49

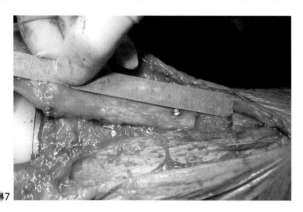

Figs. 4.45–4.49. Lateral tibial tubercle osteotomy was the approach of choice in this arthrodesed knee with severe patella baja. The patella tendon insertion was 2 cm proximalized after take down and the distal bone gap filled with autologous corticocancellous bone graft as shown during surgery and on lateral radiographs

After 12 months the mean score in this group improved significantly from 59.2 to 84.4 points, with 88% of the cases scoring excellent or good results, 8% fair results and 4% poor results. The mean postoperative range of motion was 101 degrees (range 35–130). Radiographic analysis showed primary healing of all osteotomy sites without signs of mal-union or non-union. The mean time for healing of the osteotomy was 2 months in all but one case, which took 4 months for complete union. The average length of the osteotomy was 79 ± 16 mm. No lag screw required removal for anterior knee pain or loosening. After 1 year there was no evidence of patella osteopenia nor avascular necrosis. Complications that occurred included four cases with subcutaneous hematoma, five cases with partial skin demarcation, one compartment syndrome of the anterior tibial compartment and one case with arthrofibrosis. All these complications required a second operation that was successful in all cases without removal of prosthetic components.

Tibial tubercle osteotomy in difficult TKA is a safe, predictable and advantageous procedure that delivers a wide exposure, facilitates soft tissue management, and preserves viability of the extensor mechanism. This technique addresses problematic knee pathologies, which include the valgus knee, stiff knees and any type of patella maltracking or patella baja situation. The clinical results, as shown, are similar or better than those without osteotomy. However, this procedure should be planned preoperatively and is best performed from lateral to medial creating a large tubercle (7×2 cm). The use of cortical lag screws for refixation of the tubercle allows for a postoperative rehabilitation that is similar to conventional TKA except forceful knee extension and straight leg raise in the first 8 weeks. Therefore, TTO has become the method of choice at the Schulthess Clinic in all cases that present with valgus knee deformity, arthrofibrosis, patella maltracking and revision cases.

Acknowledgements. We thank Hubert Burki MD, Zurich, Switzerland for clinical data.

Bibliography

Arredondo J, Worland RL, Jessup DE (1998) Nonunion after a tibial shaft fracture complicating tibial tubercule osteotomy. J Arthroplasty 13:958–960

Barrack RL, Smith P, Munn B, Engh G, Rorabeck C (1998) The Ranawat Award. Comparison of surgical approaches in total knee arthroplasty. Clin Orthop 356:16–21

Buechel FF (1982) A simplified evaluation system for the rating of the knee function. Orthop Rev 11:97–101

Burki H, von Knoch M, Heiss C, Drobny T, Munzinger U (1999) Lateral approach with osteotomy of the tibial tubercle in primary TKA. Clin Orthop 362:156–161

Cosgarea AJ, Freedman JA, McFarland EG (2001) Nonunion of the tibial tubercle shingle following Fulkerson osteotomy. Am J Knee Surg 14:51–54

Davis K, Caldwell P, Wayne J, Jiranek WA (2000) Mechanical comparison of fixation techniques for the tibial tubercle osteotomy. Clin Orthop 380:241–249

Dolin MG (1983) Osteotomy of the tibial tubercle in TKA. J Bone Joint Surg 65A:704–706

Engh GA, Parks NL, Ammeen DJ (1996) Influence of surgical approach on lateral retinacular releases in total knee arthroplasty. Clin Orthop 331:56–63

Insall J, Salvati E (1971) Patella position in the normal knee joint. Radiology 101:101–104

Kanamiya T, Naito M, Ikari N, Hara M (2001) The effect of surgical dissections on blood flow to the tibial tubercle. J Orthop Res 19:113–116

Kayler DE, Lyttle D (1989) Surgical interruption of patellar blood supply by TKA. Clin Orthop 229:221–271

Keblish PA (1991) Lateral approach to the valgus knee. Clin Orthop 271:52–62

Keblish PA (1994) Patellar resurfacing of retention in total knee arthroplasty. J Bone Joint Surg 76B:930–937

Lonner JH, Pedlow FX, Siliski JM (1999) Total knee arthroplasty for post-traumatic arthrosis. J Arthroplasty 14:969–975

Lonner JH, Siliski JM, Lotke PA (2000) Simultaneous femoral osteotomy and total knee arthroplasty for treatment of osteoarthritis associated with severe extra-articular deformity. J Bone Joint Surg Am 82A:1672–1673

Maruyama M (1997) Tibial tubercle osteotomy in revision total knee arthroplasty. Arch Orthop Trauma Surg 116:400–403

Masri BA, Campbell DG, Garbuz DS, Duncan CP (1998) Seven specialized exposures for revision hip and knee replacement. Orthop Clin North Am 29:229–240

Nizard RS, Cardinne L, Bizot P, Witvoet J (1998) Total knee replacement after failed tibial osteotomy: results of a matched-pair study. J Arthroplasty 13:847–853

Ries MD, Richman JA (1996) Extended tibial tubercle osteotomy in total knee arthroplasty. J Arthroplasty 11:964–967

Ritter MA, Herbst SA, Keating EM, Farls PM, Meding JB (1996) Patellofemoral complications following total knee arthroplasty. J Arthroplasty 11:368–372

Scapinelli R (1967) Blood supply of the human patella. J Bone Joint Surg 59B:563–570

Wang CJ (2001) Management of patellofemoral arthrosis in middle-aged patients. Chang Gung Med J 24:672–680

Whiteside LA (1995) Exposure in difficult total knee arthroplasty using tibial tubercle osteotomy. Clin Orthop 3211:32–37

Whiteside LA, Ohl MD (1990) Tibial tubercle osteotomy for exposure of the difficult total knee arthroplasty. Clin Orthop 260:6–9

Wolff AM, Hungerford DS, Krackow KA, Jacobs MA (1989) Osteotomy the tibial tubercle during total knee replacement. J Bone Joint Surg 71:848–852

Younger AS, Duncan CP, Masri BA (1998) Surgical exposures in revision total knee arthroplasty. J Am Acad Orthop Surg 6:55–64

4.6 Soft Tissue Management and Bone Resections

Peter A. Keblish

Options in total knee arthroplasty (TKA) exist from skin incision to final prosthetic implantation. Precise soft tissue balancing and achievement of equal flexion–extension gaps with normal patellofemoral tracking are basic requirements for quality results in primary and revision TKA. Specific factors such as cruciate ligament management and prosthetic design may influence soft tissue approaches (i.e. more stable designs require less precision of soft tissue balance) but basic principles prevail.

Approaches in TKA have evolved into the "soft tissue first" versus "bone first", and "femoral first" versus "tibia first" advocates. Both methods are successful if basic principles are followed. Combinations of all techniques may be required in difficult primary or revision cases. This author favors the "soft tissue–tibia first" approach, which includes pre-cuts and osteophyte removal. Different technique points are addressed in chapters relating to surgical approaches (Sects. 4.2–4.5). This chapter will attempt to relate similarities, differences and advantages of each method, which should be understood by the total knee surgeon, when approaching the varus and valgus knee.

Varus Knee

The varus knee can be approached via the standard medial parapatellar, mid-vastus or sub-vastus routes. The lateral approach has also been used in the varus knee with significant external rotation of the tibia, tight iliotibial band and anticipation of patella maltracking. It has been the standard approach of Prof. W. Muller and associates (Bruderholz Clinic, Basel, Switzerland) for reasons related to neurovascular and soft tissue preservation. Fixed varus with rotational deformities and flexion contractures are common in the osteoarthritic knee (Fig. 4.50).

The soft tissue first approach, including osteophyte and non-essential bone removal to these fixed deformities, has many advantages, which are outlined below.

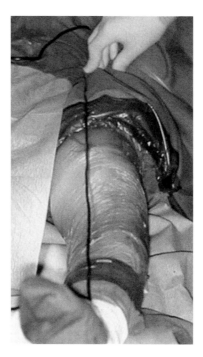

Fig. 4.50. Typical varus knee with tibial rotation. Note deviation from normal axial hip–knee–ankle mechanical line

Enhanced Exposure

Soft tissue releases are case specific and vary from minimal to extreme. A long subperiosteal sleeve elevation of the medial collateral ligament (MCL) to include the pes anserine insertion may be required. The release is begun in extension and completed in flexion as the tibia is externally rotated to expose the posteromedial structures. The meniscal rim is preserved, and the MCL is released from the osteophytic impingement (Fig. 4.51). Osteophytes are removed to the normal tibial contour. The semimembranosus is a major posteromedial stabilizer and should be preserved. If the posterior cruciate ligament is a deforming force and/or is to be sacrificed by the surgeon's choice, it should be released from the femur and tibia at this time. The knee is examined in extension and flexion as the releases progress. Avoid over-releasing and fine tune with trial prostheses.

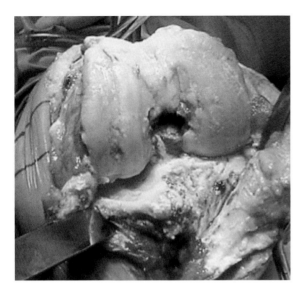

Fig. 4.51. Posteromedial exposure required in fixed varus. Sleeve release technique preserves stability

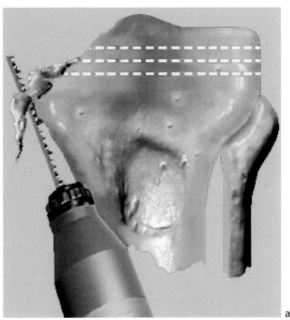

a

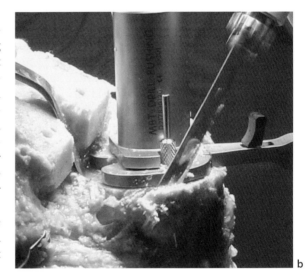

b

Fig. 4.52 a, b. Debulking includes osteophyte removal and downsizing (if necessary) to allow for proper prosthetic sizing and improved soft tissue sleeve closure

Debulking or Downsizing the Remodeled Osteoarthritic Tibial Plateau Debulking or downsizing the remodeled osteoarthritic tibial plateau without bony compromise to the insertion of the semimembranosus is recommended if severe tibial expansion has developed and/or if medial sleeve closure problems are anticipated. Resection of the tibial spine, subchondral bone from the posterior femoral condyles, and peripheral femoral osteophytes, especially under the collateral ligaments, will further enhance exposure and optimize gap balancing. Preliminary distal femoral resections (as discussed in Sect. 4.12) are another option. Fixed flexion deformities require more extensive posterior bone/capsular releases and are best done prospectively, or before the permanent resection (Fig. 4.52).

Assessment of Femorotibial Alignment

Following medial/posterior sleeve release and osteophytic debulking, the knee is examined for axial stability. The medial sleeve is checked for compliance and potential hang-up areas. With the knee held in extension, axial alignment and the medial gap are assessed in preparation for subsequent bone resections.

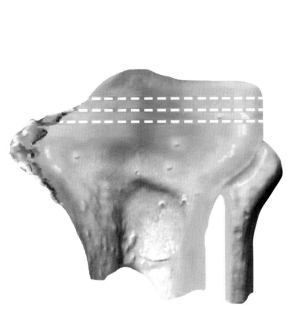

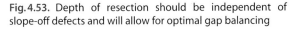

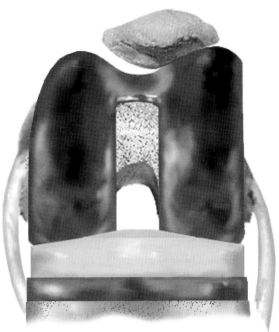

Fig. 4.53. Depth of resection should be independent of slope-off defects and will allow for optimal gap balancing

Fig. 4.54. Prosthetic gap (tibia) is the distance between the lowest articulating interface and the prosthetic undersurface–bone interface. Note common lateral patella subluxation

Tibial Resection

A few points and cautions should be acknowledged regarding the tibial resection. The majority of systems utilize an extramedullary approach. Different landmarks have been recommended and some variations exist within different systems. The goal is to achieve a perpendicular (mediolateral) tibial resection in virtually all systems with varying degrees of posterior slope, ranging from none to the patient's natural slope to an arbitrary 3–10 degrees posterior slope. The most consistent external landmarks are the proximal tibial crest (for rotational alignment) and the tibial anterior tendon distally (axial alignment). The depth of resection should be adequate to allow for prosthetic insertion without elevating the joint line, keeping in mind that posterior cruciate ligament (PCL) resection will increase the flexion gap. Measurement of resection depth can be confusing with different systems. If a stylus is utilized and normal cartilage is present on the lateral side (varus knee), 6 mm from the highest point or 6 mm from a midpoint on the lateral tibial plateau is usually required to allow for an 8 mm polyethylene insert

(Fig. 4.53). Note that the joint line level is a combination of the metallic base plate and the lowest point of the polyethylene articulating surface (Fig. 4.54). Not resecting enough tibia is a common error and results in overstuffing the joint, raising the joint line and limiting extension in this situation; over-resecting of the femur is necessary to achieve full extension. Other situations, such as hyperextension and severe flexion deformity, may also influence depth of resection. Be aware of normal "resection" resections in the loose knee and over-resection in the tight knee. The posterior slope angle is adjusted using an alignment rod and bony landmarks (tibial crest–plateau relationship). Soft tissues and osteophyte first releases will better position the tibia for optimum resections. It needs to be emphasized that a posterior slope must be made with the tibia in a proper neutral rotational alignment. Malrotation will introduce an improperly directed posterior slope, which will negatively affect gap balance and ultimate stability, especially in midflexion. Newer navigation systems will be useful in reducing errors in this most important resection in the tibia first approach.

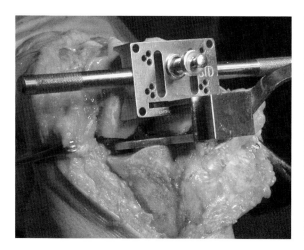

Fig. 4.55. Tibial axis/flexion tension method of determining proper femoral rotation. Note extensive release and medial slope-off deformity

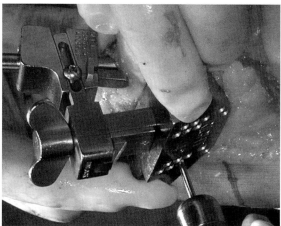

Fig. 4.56. Distal femoral resection angle may vary from 3 to 7 degrees. Fixed varus in short obese patients is best treated with 3–4 degrees varus, while fixed valgus is best treated with a 6–7 degrees valgus resection, maintaining an appreciation for their pre-existing biomechanical alignment

Femoral Rotational Alignment and Anteroposterior Femoral Resection

Flexion gap balance is a major determinant of rotational alignment of the distal femur and correlates with the transepicondylar axis. The longitudinal axis of the tibia, combined with the projected flexion gap and proper ligament tension, therefore, provides for optimal femoral positioning. "Soft tissue first" releases and a perpendicular tibial resection (low contact stress tibial axis approach) allow for precise instrumentation and resection of the distal femur in the correct rotational (coronal) plane. If other landmarks, such as Whiteside's line, arbitrary 3 degrees of external rotation, or transepicondylar axis, are utilized with a femur first approach, the soft tissue releases are still required. Performing the releases before permanent bone cuts better prepares rotational orientation for the subsequent bone resections regardless of instrumentation or technique utilized (Fig. 4.55).

Distal Femoral Resection

The plane and depth of the femoral resection are critical in that they affect soft tissue kinematics, patella positioning, axial and the often-ignored cosmetic/functional aspects of current TKA outcomes. Pre-existing patella baja is not uncommon in the varus knee and is accentuated with an excessive resection and/or too minimal tibial resection (raising the joint line). In the valgus knee patella alta is more common

and the problem less critical, especially in PCL sacrificing/substituting TKA. The MCL–lateral collateral ligament origins should be identified and retained in the most normal relationship to femoral component. The plane of resection may vary depending on pre-existing pathology. The genetically developmental varus knee (especially in short obese females) should be maintained in slight varus to allow for better function (clearing the thighs in gait) and cosmesis (patients do not like the valgus appearance). Therefore, a 3 degrees distal femoral resection is recommended in these cases. The valgus knee, similarly, is accustomed to the "knock knee" attitude and leaving it in slight valgus is more acceptable and technically may allow for an improved lateral extension space and medial stability. Figure 4.56 shows alternative distal femoral resections depending on preoperatively existing severe varus or valgus knee deformities.

Patellofemoral Alignment

Following patella eversion, prospective soft tissue fillet expansion of the vastus lateralis and release of the patellofemoral ligament and the lateral patella rim (when patella tilt exists) improve alignment and enhance overall exposure. The patella eversion is enhanced by the previously described soft tissue pre-cut maneuvers, especially in the tight or more contracted knee. The "soft tissue first" approach, therefore, improves exposure of the extensor mechanism and patella bone management, whether resurfacing

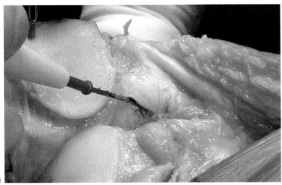
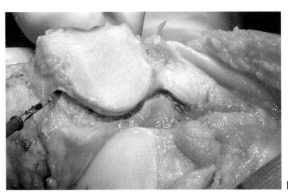

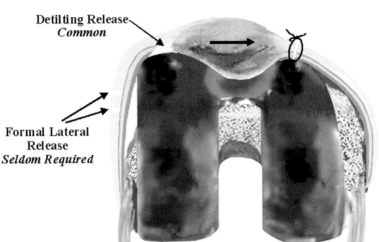

Fig. 4.57 a–c. Vastus lateralis fillet release technique for improving patellofemoral tracking in TKA. a, b Dynamic decompression of the vastus lateralis, which represents the strongest active lateralizing force of the quadriceps mechanism. c Note medialization of the patella with perfect housing within the femoral component trochlea

Detilting Release
Common

Formal Lateral Release
Seldom Required

or non-resurfacing. These methods are more specifically illustrated in Sect. 2.3 on patella management (Fig. 4.57).

Valgus Deformity

The fixed valgus knee presents a different set of challenges because of external tibial contracture, increased Q-angle, and a laterally oriented or subluxed patella. Flexion contractures are common. Lateral structures are contracted, including the iliotibial band, lateral retinaculum, lateral collateral ligament, and popliteus. Sequential releases of these structures, as required, allow for correction of rotational and axial alignment. The "soft tissue first" release via the direct lateral approach results in a sequential correction of the deformity and better preparation for bone resections. The key steps include: (1) proximal release of the iliotibial band; (2) soft tissue relaxation/expansion via a lateral retinacular incision and capsular-retinacular closure (coronal plane Z-plasty); (3) distal osteoperiosteal elevation of the proximal tibia to the posterolateral corner; and (4) distal lateral (concave) side releases, as discussed in

Sect. 4.4. These maneuvers are best performed prior to bone resections.

Tibia First or Femur First?

The issue of tibia first or femur first bone resection raises questions of flexion–extension gap balance problems. Advocates of tibial first resections (low contact stress technique, original Insall technique) note the advantages of this approach, which include: (1) building the reconstruction from "bottom up"; (2) ensuring a properly directed tibial resection in mediolateral and anteroposterior planes; (3) allowing for excellent exposure and a tibial platform to direct proper femoral rotation alignment, arguably the most important factor in patella outcomes in TKA.

Disadvantages of the tibial first approach include: (1) predictability of depth of bone resections; (2) accuracy of the tibial resection as a primary determination of femoral rotation resection; (3) potential for over-resection of the distal femur and subsequent flexion–extension gap imbalances; (4) potential for accentuating a pre-existing patella baja (infera) with under-resection and elevation of the joint line.

Theoretical disadvantages of a femoral first followed by soft tissue approach include: (1) estimation of femoral rotation via methods that rely on approximation of difficult anatomic landmarks such as the transepicondylar axis, Whiteside's line or posterior femoral condyles; (2) estimation of distal femoral resection (depth) – especially if soft tissue releases are not recommended; (3) under-release and/or failure to remove osteophytes or downsize a remodeled tibia to normal anatomy; (4) dictation of tibial resection, perhaps the most important resection.

Soft tissue sleeve stability dictates knee kinematics and quality results in TKA. The "soft tissue first" approach allows ongoing intraoperative assessment of the angular and rotational correction, bone defects and graft needs, as well as bone resection levels. Subsequent instrumentation with flexion–extension gap balancing via bone resection is more accurate and can be titrated at each step. Malresections and/or excess bony resections are minimized, and soft tissue stability is maximized.

Deep approaches in TKA require an understanding of the pre-existing deformity and surgical technique options. The total knee surgeon should have an intrinsic knowledge of all surgical approaches and technique options. The soft tissue, pre-cut, osteophyte removal approach prior to permanent bone resections is recommended to establish a better rotational/axial alignment. This approach will minimize malresections and improve overall prosthetic stability, especially with minimally constrained prostheses. Combinations of soft tissue/bone preparation are often used in order to achieve the final goal, namely a stable implant in all planes.

Bibliography

Attfield SF, Wilton TJ, Pratt DJ, Sambatakakis A (1996) Soft-tissue balance and recovery of proprioception after total knee replacement. J Bone Joint Surg Br 78:540–545

Bizzini M, Boldt J, Munzinger U, Drobny T (2003) Rehabilitation guidelines after total knee arthroplasty. Orthopade 32(6):527–534

Boldt J, Munzinger U, Keblish P (2004) Comparison of isokinetic strength in resurfaced and retained patellae in bilateral TKA. J Arthroplasty 19(2):264

Boldt JG, Munzinger UK, Zanetti M, Hodler J (2004) Arthrofibrosis associated with total knee arthroplasty: gray-scale and power Doppler sonographic findings. AJR Am J Roentgenol 182(2):337–340

Bellemans J, Banks S, Victor J, Vandenneucker H, Moemans A (2002) Fluoroscopic analysis of the kinematics of deep flexion in total knee arthroplasty. Influence of posterior condylar offset. J Bone Joint Surg Br 84:50–53

Clarke HD, Scott WN (2001) Knee: axial instability. Orthop Clin North Am 32:627–637, viii

Emerson RH Jr, Ayers C, Higgins LL (1999) Surgical closing in total knee arthroplasty. A series followup. Clin Orthop 368:176–181

Farrington WJ, Charnley GJ, Harries SR, Fox BM, Sharp R, Hughes PM (1999) The position of the popliteal artery in the arthritic knee. J Arthroplasty 14:800–802

Fishkin Z, Miller D, Ritter C, Ziv I (2002) Changes in human knee ligament stiffness secondary to osteoarthritis. J Orthop Res 20:204–207

Griffin FM, Insall JN, Scuderi GR (2001) Accuracy of soft tissue balancing in total knee arthroplasty. J Arthroplasty 16:545

Hazaki S, Yokoyama Y, Inoue H (2001) A radiographic analysis of anterior-posterior translation in total knee arthroplasty. J Orthop Sci 6:390–396

Johnson R, Barry K, Elloy MA (1994) The collateral ligament flexion-extension test (CLEFT) in total knee replacement. J R Coll Surg Edinb 39:127–130

Keblish PA (1991) The lateral approach to the valgus knee. Surgical technique and analysis of 53 cases with over two-year follow-up evaluation. Clin Orthop 271:52–62

Konig A, Walther M, Kirschner S, Gohlke F (2000) Balance sheets of knee and functional scores 5 years after total knee arthroplasty for osteoarthritis: a source for patient information. J Arthroplasty 15:289–294

Krackow KA, Mihalko WM (1999) The effect of medial release on flexion and extension gaps in cadaveric knees: implications for soft-tissue balancing in total knee arthroplasty. Am J Knee Surg 12:222–228

Luo ZP, Hsu HC, Rand JA, An KN (1996) Importance of soft tissue integrity on biomechanical studies of the patella after TKA. J Biomech Eng 118:130–132

Mahoney OM, McClung CD, dela Rosa MA, Schmalzried TP (2002) The effect of total knee arthroplasty design on extensor mechanism function. J Arthroplasty 17:416–421

Matsuda S, Miura H, Nagamine R, Urabe K, Matsunobu T, Iwamoto Y (1999) Knee stability in posterior cruciate ligament retaining total knee arthroplasty. Clin Orthop 366:169–173

Mihalko WM, Krackow KA (1999) Posterior cruciate ligament effects on the flexion space in total knee arthroplasty. Clin Orthop 360:243–250

Montgomery WH 3rd, Insall JN, Haas SB, Becker MS, Windsor RE (1998) Primary total knee arthroplasty in stiff and ankylosed knees. Am J Knee Surg 11:20–23

Ouellet D, Moffet H (2002) Locomotor deficits before and two months after knee arthroplasty. Arthritis Rheum 47:484–493

Takahashi T, Wada Y, Yamamoto H (1997) Soft-tissue balancing with pressure distribution during total knee arthroplasty. J Bone Joint Surg Br 79:235–239

Tanzer M, Smith K, Burnett S (2002) Posterior-stabilized versus cruciate-retaining total knee arthroplasty: balancing the gap. J Arthroplasty 17:813–819

Whiteside LA, Mihalko WM (2002) Surgical procedure for flexion contracture and recurvatum in total knee arthroplasty. Clin Orthop 404:189–195

Whiteside LA, Saeki K, Mihalko WM (2000) Functional medical ligament balancing in total knee arthroplasty. Clin Orthop 380:45–57

Winemaker MJ (2002) Perfect balance in total knee arthroplasty: the elusive compromise. J Arthroplasty 17:2–10

4.7 Advanced Surgical Technique

David Beverland

Successful outcomes in total knee arthroplasty (TKA) are dependent upon achieving neutral mechanical axes, restored joint lines, as well as equal and balanced flexion and extension gaps. Although these aims apply to all TKAs, both fixed and mobile, in the latter concerns about bearing stability mean that the surgeon has to take more care, particularly with flexion gap stability. Increased awareness is required to achieve flexion gap stability with the mobile bearing knee, which not only provides stability but also encourages the surgeon to adhere to the basic principles as defined by Insall (1984).

Neutral Mechanical Axis

Conceptually the mechanical axis of the lower limb is a line on the frontal plane long leg x-ray running from hip centre to ankle centre, as shown in Fig. 4.58. If the axis is neutral, the line will pass through the centre of the knee. In this situation the mechanical axis of the femur (line from hip centre to knee centre) will be colinear with the mechanical axis of the tibia (line from knee centre to ankle centre). In the normal knee the axis passes just medial to the knee centre and therefore there is a small varus angle between the mechanical axes of the femur and tibia. As can be appreciated from Fig. 4.58, the orientation of the normal joint line is not at right angles to the mechanical axis of the lower limb. Rather it inclines on average by 3 degrees (± 2.5 degrees) such that the distal femoral joint line is in valgus and the proximal tibial joint line is in varus relative to the mechanical axis of the lower limb. With most total knee systems it is customary to cut the proximal tibia and distal femur at right angles to the mechanical axis of each bone. Thus, as can be appreciated from Fig. 4.58, the bone cuts are not parallel to the original joint line and therefore relatively more bone has to be removed from the distal medial femoral condyle than distal lateral and from the proximal lateral tibial condyle than medial. If this is done accurately, postoperatively the mechanical axis will go through the knee centre and the joint line will be at right angles to the mechanical axis. Achieving the above during surgery means having to identify the mechanical axes of the two bones. On the tibia this is more straightforward because during surgery the knee centre and the ankle centre are relatively easy to identify. The femoral side is not as straightfor-

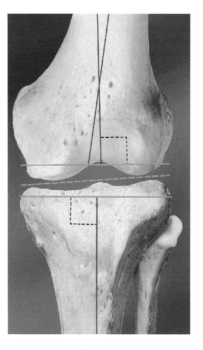

Fig. 4.58. Distal femoral and proximal tibial resections made at right angles to the mechanical axes of their respective bones

ward because location of the femoral head centre is not easy during surgery. Provided that the femur is a normal shape, with care its anatomical axis can be reproduced with the intramedullary (IM) rod. A 5 degrees valgus resection is used routinely in all patients. The concept of using a smaller valgus angle for a patient over 6 feet in height (3 degrees) is not valid. We have shown that there is not a good correlation between patient height or femoral length ($r < 0.45$) and valgus angle; rather femoral head offset is the best predictor ($r > 0.85$).

Although we think of the mechanical axis as a line on the frontal plane long leg x-ray, it is in fact the end-on view of the sagittal plane, as illustrated in Fig. 4.58. This is the plane through which the knee flexes and extends. Anatomically this movement takes place around the transepicondylar axis (TEA). Unlike the orientation of the joint line, the TEA is at right angles to the mechanical axis of the femur (and tibia). Consequently the distal femoral and proximal tibial cuts should be parallel to the TEA. Normally the TEA is thought of as being a flexion gap landmark, but in theory it could be used to check the angle of the distal femoral cut. Unfortunately it is difficult to locate accurately and therefore it is not useful in comparison to the more conventional intramedullary alignment technique for the femur.

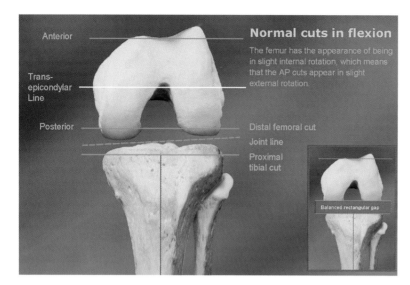

Fig. 4.59. Flexion gap landmarks

The flexion gap landmarks are shown in Fig. 4.59. Compared with Fig. 4.58, the femur is now flexed to 90 degrees but the tibia remains the same. As with the extension gap, the femoral cuts have to be at right angles to the mechanical axis of the femur and will thus be parallel to the proximal tibial cut and also at right angles to the mechanical axis of the tibia. This results in a rectangular flexion gap. As can be seen in Fig. 4.60, the sagittal plane of the mechanical axis still runs through the centre of the femoral head.

Thus the objectives for the plane of orientation of the anteroposterior (AP) femoral cuts in flexion are exactly the same as those used for the distal femoral cut in the extension gap. The difference is that in flexion the femoral landmarks are less easily defined and the potential for error is greater. The AP cuts determine femoral rotation and therefore an error will result in malrotation of the femoral component. In extension, although the femoral head is difficult to locate accurately, the anatomical axis can be defined with the IM rod and from there an estimate of 5 degrees of valgus will rarely err from the femoral head centre by more than 3 degrees.

Figure 4.59 demonstrates landmarks in the flexion gap. Anatomically the mechanical axis of the femur is represented by the patellofemoral groove. This was described by Whiteside as being a useful guide to femoral rotation in flexion and is referred to as Whiteside's line. The TEA or Insall's line is normally just described in the flexion gap. Again, as with Whiteside's line, it does represent a definite anatomical line running between the two epicondyles. With transverse cuts on a computed tomography scan it can be defined precisely, but during surgery both lines are difficult to locate accurately. In the low contact stress

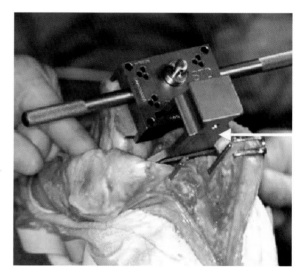

Fig. 4.60. Using the femoral guide positioner to set femoral rotation

(LCS) knee, these landmarks can be used as additional checks, but femoral rotation is set using a unique, simple and very effective method. This is illustrated in Fig. 4.61. Having first performed the proximal tibial cut, a femoral guide positioner is used to separate the femur and tibia. This links the proximal tibial cut to the AP cutting block and ensures that they are parallel to each other. I feel that this is a key step in successful mobile bearing surgery. It provides the most accurate way of first, setting femoral rotation and second, providing a balanced flexion gap. The one important proviso is that the soft tissues must be balanced in flexion before the AP cuts are performed. It

Fig. 4.61 a, b. Restoration of normal extension joint line (*double-ended arrows*)

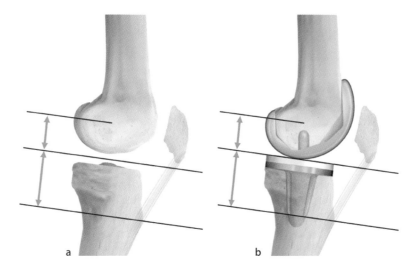

Fig. 4.62 a, b. Restoration of normal flexion joint line (*double-ended arrows*)

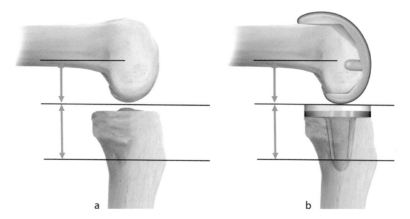

is therefore ideal for knees with mild or passively correctable deformity. The challenge comes in knees with significant fixed deformity.

The Joint Line

It is important to think of the joint line in flexion and not just extension and also in relation to the femur and tibia separately. Figure 4.61 shows the joint line in extension in the normal knee relative to fixed points on the femur and tibia. The surgeon should always try to restore this line and, for example in fixed flexion, the posterior capsule should be released as opposed to resecting more distal femur, as this will raise the joint line relative to the femur.

Figure 4.62 shows the normal joint line in flexion. Again it can be defined relative to the femur and tibia. In theory, on the tibial side, irrespective of how much bone is resected, the joint line can be restored

if an insert of appropriate thickness is used. The exception is when the tibial cut is too conservative and if this is not corrected, even the thinnest insert (10 mm) will still raise the joint line relative to the tibia.

With regard to the femur in flexion, over- or undersizing the femoral component will alter the joint line relative to the femur. Also the placement of the AP cuts relative to the anterior femoral cortex will alter the joint line. The common problems are illustrated in Fig. 4.63.

In the LCS knee, the flexion gap is set first. It can be appreciated from Fig. 4.63 that if the joint line is raised in flexion relative to the femur, this will increase the flexion gap. To compensate for this, a thicker insert is used and therefore the joint line is raised relative to the tibia also. What is perhaps not always appreciated is that raising the joint line in extension by resecting more distal femur is a result of raising the flexion joint line. The two common causes of rais-

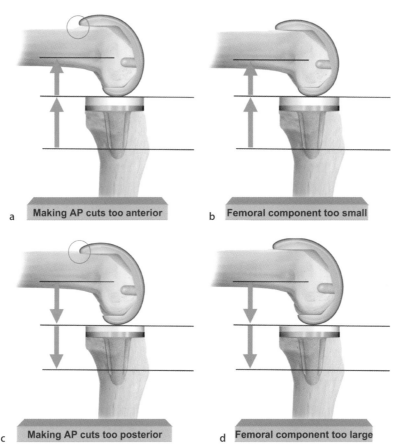

a Making AP cuts too anterior

b Femoral component too small

c Making AP cuts too posterior

d Femoral component too large

Fig. 4.63 a–d. Common causes of raising and lowering the joint line in flexion. All these diagrams assume normal tension in flexion. But other scenarios are possible, for example if the joint line is raised on the femur and left normal on the tibia, the flexion gap will be slack. Conversely if the femoral joint line is lowered in this scenario the flexion gap will be tight. **a** Here the AP cuts have been made too anterior, thus the anterior femoral cut is not flush with the anterior femoral cortex, the flexion gap is increased and the joint line is raised. **b** Here too small a femoral component has been used, which again increases the flexion gap and raises the joint line. **c** Here the AP cuts have been made too posterior, thus the anterior cortex has been notched, which decreases the flexion gap and lowers the joint line. **d** Here the femoral component has been over-sized, which again decreases the flexion gap and lowers the joint line

ing the joint line in flexion are making the AP femoral cuts too anterior (Fig. 4.63a) and choosing too small a femoral component (Fig. 4.63b). Because the joint line is raised relative to the tibia, when it comes to creating an extension gap that is equal to the flexion gap, the surgeon has to remove more bone from the distal femur. It is also interesting to note from Fig. 4.64b that raising the joint line relative to the tibia can create a patella baja. In contrast, if the joint line is restored relative to the tibia but is raised by removing more distal femur, as could happen with fixed flexion, patella baja is not produced because the distance from the tibial tubercle to the joint line is correct, as shown in Fig. 4.64. Therefore if patella baja is created at primary surgery, it is because the joint line has been raised relative to the tibia.

As discussed above, making the proximal tibial cut too conservative can also raise the tibial joint line. If this is not recognised, the surgeon will either raise the flexion joint line relative to the femur or will leave the flexion gap overly tight. The latter will compromise flexion and both will mean either resecting more distal femur or leaving the extension gap tight with resulting fixed flexion.

So, as can be appreciated, even in a knee with minimal deformity, care needs to be taken with the flexion gap. It is not enough to create equal flexion and extension gaps; they also have to be correct relative to the joint line. Clues to these problems arise when the femoral guide positioner is being inserted. The surgeon needs to assess whether insertion is unexpectedly too loose or too tight – see below.

Equal and Balanced Flexion and Extension Gaps

One of the keys to successful mobile bearing surgery is to balance the flexion gap. Therefore, before making the first incision, the surgeon should anticipate potential problems with balancing the flexion gap. As a routine, the surgeon should assess the degree of fixed deformity. Especially in a valgus knee, there can be considerable passive correction, as illustrated in Fig. 4.65. Also ensure that there is normal hip rotation. If the hip is in fixed external rotation, this can distort the flexion gap. I recognise three broad groups of patients: (1) those with mild passively correctable

Fig. 4.64 a, b. The joint line relative to the femur has been raised by an equal amount and the level of proximal tibial resection is also the same. a The joint line relative to the tibia has been restored to normal and there is no patella baja. b The joint line relative to the tibia has been raised by using a thicker insert, thus creating patella baja. This figure illustrates that patella baja is created during surgery primarily by raising the joint line relative to the tibia and not the femur

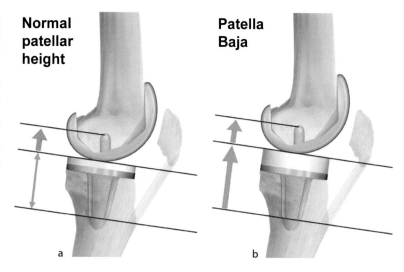

Fig. 4.65. Example of the degree of passive correction that can often be achieved in a valgus knee

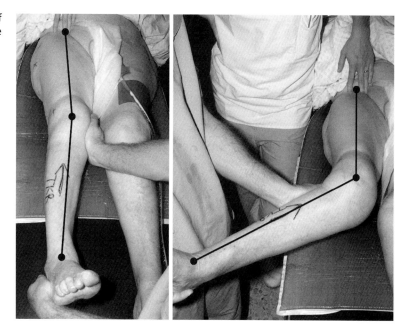

deformity, (2) those with significant varus deformity with or without fixed flexion, and (3) those with valgus deformity.

Patients with Mild or Correctable Deformity

The flexion gap in this group of patients should normally be straightforward in terms of setting femoral rotation. Care needs to be taken to ensure that the proximal tibial cut is neutral relative to the mechanical axis of the tibia. This can be checked using the femoral guide positioner. As an approximate guide,

10 mm of translational error at the ankle represents 1 degree. It is not uncommon to make a 1 degree error into varus (lateral deviation of the rod at the ankle). If this happens I simply use a 6 degree distal femoral cut instead of 5 degrees. In a balanced or neutral knee, when the femoral guide positioner is inserted into the flexion gap, the femur will adopt its correct rotation and the AP block will align itself parallel to the tibial cut, as shown in Fig. 4.61. Although femoral rotation is taken care of, the surgeon still has to give thought to the dimension of the flexion gap. Conceptually this is best considered in relation to the joint line as discussed above.

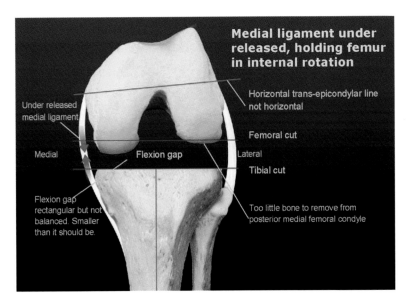

Medial ligament under released, holding femur in internal rotation

Under released medial ligament

Horizontal trans-epicondylar line not horizontal

Femoral cut

Medial   Flexion gap   Lateral

Tibial cut

Flexion gap rectangular but not balanced. Smaller than it should be.

Too little bone to remove from posterior medial femoral condyle

Fig. 4.66. The MCL has been under-released and if the femoral guide positioner is inserted into the flexion gap, the AP cuts will be made in excessive external rotation. At this stage the flexion gap is rectangular but not balanced. If in this same scenario the MCL is later released after the AP cuts have been made, the flexion gap will become both unbalanced and trapezoidal. This can produce flexion instability

Insertion of Femoral Guide Positioner

The femoral guide positioner is easier to insert if the knee is flexed to beyond 100 degrees because the space opens up anteriorly. Once the femoral guide positioner is introduced, the knee is extended to about 100 degrees. This is because at 90 degrees of flexion the proximal tibial cut will not lie in the same transverse plane as the AP guide because of the posterior tibial slope.

Femoral Guide Positioner too Tight

This means that the flexion gap is smaller than expected. There are a number of possible reasons. The posterior medial femoral condyle is blocking entry of the positioning guide or the guide abuts against it. This can usually be prevented by removing a sliver of posterior femoral condyle, as shown in Fig. 4.66. When this happens it usually means that the AP block is positioned too anteriorly. This is a false impression of tightness, as making the AP cuts too anterior actually increases the flexion gap. The medial collateral ligament (MCL) is tight and requires further release, as illustrated in Fig. 4.66. This should not happen in a knee with minimal or correctable deformity. Too large a femoral component has been chosen, which means that the AP resection guide will remove too little bone from the posterior femoral condyles and the flexion gap will be smaller than it should be. In this situation a smaller AP resection guide should be used. The AP cutting block has been

positioned too far posteriorly, as shown in Fig. 4.63c (not common). This means not only that the flexion gap will be too tight, but also that the anterior cut will notch the femur. This is remedied by moving the AP resection guide anteriorly. First of all pin the AP block to set rotation. Use the middle hole of the lower two sets of holes plus the middle of one of the upper sets. These need to be predrilled if not using drill pins. The AP block is then slid off, the IM rod is removed and the AP block is replaced onto the most posterior hole in the three sets of holes. The proximal tibial cut has been too conservative. If all of the above reasons have been excluded, this is the likely explanation. For this reason the fixation pins for the proximal tibial resection guide should not be removed until the flexion gap is satisfactory. The guide is reapplied one set of holes down, allowing a further 2.5 mm of bone to be removed from the proximal tibia. In my experience this happens most commonly with a mild valgus knee.

Femoral Guide Positioner too Slack

The flexion gap is bigger than expected. There are four possible reasons for this. (1) The AP positioning guide has been placed too anteriorly (common). This means that not enough bone is removed anteriorly; too much bone is removed posteriorly and the flexion gap is too large. This is remedied by moving the AP resection guide posteriorly. First of all, pin the AP block to set rotation. Use the middle hole of the lower two sets of holes plus the middle of one of the upper sets. These need to be predrilled if not using drill pins. The AP block is then slid off, the IM rod is removed and the AP block is replaced onto the most anterior hole in the three sets of holes. This moves the block posteriorly by 2.5 mm. If in doubt, perform an initial anterior femoral cut to assess whether it is safe to move the AP guide 2.5 mm posteriorly. (2) Too small a femoral size has been chosen, which again means too much bone will be removed posteriorly and the flexion gap is too large. This is remedied by choosing a larger femoral size with the appropriate AP resection guide. (3) In a varus knee where there has been over-release of the MCL, the flexion gap will also be larger than expected (see below). (4) In a valgus knee where there is an excessive flexion gap laterally following release of soft tissues from the lateral condyle (see below).

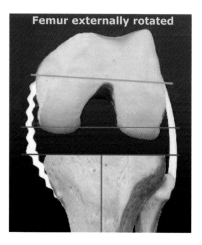

Fig. 4.67. The MCL has been over-released and if the femoral guide positioner is inserted into the flexion gap, the AP cuts will be made in excessive internal rotation. The flexion gap is rectangular but is not balanced, being slacker on the medial side. The flexion gap is also increased, thus raising the joint line

The Flexion Gap in Knees with Significant Deformity

In knees with deformity the surgeon has to pay attention to femoral rotation and flexion gap stability as well as the level of flexion joint line discussed above. The teaching in the LCS knee is that the soft tissues should be balanced prior to making the bone cuts. I find that this is not always easy to achieve in a varus knee and I feel that it is not required in a valgus knee.

Varus Knee

When the femoral guide positioner is inserted in a varus knee that has been correctly released, femoral rotation is automatically set and should be correct. The problem arises particularly with under-release.

Under-release of the Varus Knee

When this happens, the flexion gap will be tighter than expected and the tight MCL will hold the femur down medially. Thus the femur is too internally rotated and the AP resection guide is in excessive external rotation. There are various clues to look for: TEA not parallel to the proposed AP cut (but this line is difficult to define accurately), too little bone to be removed from the posterior lateral femoral condyle and excessive prominence of the lateral supracondylar ridge.

If the AP cuts are made in this situation, any further collateral ligament release performed will result in a flexion gap that is not rectangular and not balanced. When the AP cuts have been done before the MCL was released and the femur is held in too much internal rotation, the AP cuts are in too much external rotation. When the MCL is subsequently released to balance the knee after the distal femoral cut, the flexion gap becomes trapezoidal and is now no longer rectangular or balanced.

As can be appreciated from Fig. 4.67, in flexion the medial gap is increased and the lateral decreased. When the components are inserted and the knee is flexed to 90 degrees with the patella still dislocated, medial lift off may occur. This means that there is a gap between the posterior medial femoral condyle of the component and the insert with the knee flexed to 90 degrees (despite the knee being balanced in extension). Usually with the patella reduced, the gap is decreased or may be obliterated, but this must increase the medial parapatellar tension when the knee is being flexed, which in theory could cause medial parapatellar pain. Other problems are loss of a balanced flexion gap, loss of a rectangular flexion gap (both of these factors combine to produce flexion gap instability with the risk of bearing spinout), external malrotation of the femoral component, or distortion of the axis of rotation in flexion. Consequently every effort must be made to ensure that the knee is balanced before the AP cuts are made.

Over-release of the Varus Knee

When this happens the flexion gap will be larger than expected. The femur appears to be sitting in external rotation. This means that the AP resection guide will be sitting in internal rotation relative to the femur, as illustrated in Fig. 4.67. If this happens the femoral component is either neutral or internally rotated and in flexion the gap is tighter laterally. Recent work, as yet unpublished, from the Schultess Clinic in Zurich, Switzerland has suggested that this is one cause of limited flexion of the knee following surgery and may present as arthrofibrosis.

Excessive external rotation of the femur and therefore internal rotation of the femoral component arises if the femur is in fixed external rotation as a result of hip pathology. The surgeon should be aware of this problem before the operation starts. This is simply done by ensuring that the hip internally rotates on the table with the knee flexed to 90 degrees. If not and there is loss of internal rotation or fixed external rotation, the above problem can be overcome by doing the AP cuts with the lower limb externally rotated.

Fixed Flexion Deformity

In the presence of fixed flexion, achieving equal flexion and extension gaps and avoiding raising the joint line in extension is a challenge. In my experience, when fixed flexion occurs with a varus or valgus deformity, the posterior capsule is usually tight only on the side of the deformity. In other words, with a varus knee the posteromedial capsule is tight and in a valgus knee the posterolateral capsule is tight. For this reason, release of the posterior capsule not only corrects fixed flexion but also contributes to the correction of the varus or valgus deformity but only in extension. The posterior capsule is not tight in flexion.

In a knee with fixed flexion deformity, if prior to performing any bone cuts the varus deformity is fully corrected in extension, the result will be over-release of the MCL in flexion. This increases the flexion gap as well as producing malrotation of the femur. Obviously increasing the flexion gap in fixed flexion exacerbates the problem of achieving an equal extension gap. Later in the operation when the posterior capsule is released, the knee will also be over-released in extension.

Because the posterior capsule is not uniformly tight, I feel it is best released in extension and under direct vision where the tight bands can be cut and released. In a varus knee with significant deformity and

associated fixed flexion, I have modified the LCS technique to allow this to be done before the AP cuts. Having performed the proximal tibial cut, I use the distal femoral resection guide to perform a conservative distal femoral cut before the AP femoral cuts. Instead of removing 10 mm of distal femur, I remove 5 mm. This produces an extension gap, which is correctly aligned relative to the mechanical axis of the lower limb. As a result the extension gap can be balanced and the space created even by the conservative cut usually allows good access to the posterior capsule. I use laminar spreaders to open the extension gap and expose the posterior capsule. The spacer block without the spacer block adapter will usually fit into the gap to provide confirmation of balance. When the fixed flexion is corrected and the extension gap is balanced, the operation proceeds in the usual way with the AP femoral cuts and then the definitive distal femoral cut.

Valgus Knee

I feel that in the majority of valgus knees the lateral side is not tight in flexion even when the knee is approached from the medial side. This means that, prior to doing any releases, the valgus knee is tight laterally in extension but balanced in flexion. In fact, as with the normal knee, the medial side is usually a little tighter than the lateral in flexion. Thus in a valgus knee I am happy to perform the AP cuts before the knee has been balanced in extension. This will usually ensure correct femoral rotation and, if care is taken with the AP positioning of the AP resection guide as discussed above, the flexion joint line will be correct.

The danger for the flexion gap comes when the knee is subsequently released in extension. Table 4.1 shows the various structures that contribute to lateral stability in extension and in flexion. It should not be assumed that because they contribute to stability, they necessarily contribute to contracture and deformity.

Table 4.1. Contribution to lateral stability

	In extension	In flexion
Popliteus	No	Yes
Lateral collateral ligament	Yes	Yes
Lateral head of gastrocnemius	Yes	Yes
Iliotibial tract	Yes	No
Posterolateral capsule	Yes	No

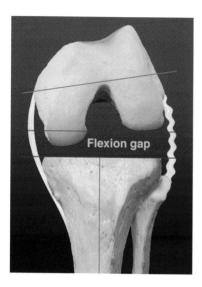

Fig. 4.68. The structures attached to the lateral femoral condyle have been released and if the femoral guide positioner is inserted into the flexion gap, the AP cuts will be made in excessive external rotation. The flexion gap is rectangular but is not balanced, being slacker on the lateral side. The flexion gap is also increased, thus raising the joint line

As can be seen, there are a total of five structures providing stability in either extension or flexion. Only the lateral collateral ligament and the lateral head of gastrocnemius provide stability in flexion and extension and both are attached to the lateral condyle. The popliteus is also attached to the lateral condyle. It has the most distal attachment of the three structures, as shown in Fig. 4.68. As stated above, the valgus knee is not normally tight laterally in flexion and therefore because the popliteus does not contribute to lateral stability in extension it is not rational to release the popliteus in a valgus knee. If any of the three structures attached to the lateral condyle are released, there will be a tendency to create flexion instability. In my experience this is the most common cause of bearing spinout. Thus if flexion stability is to be preserved, ideally only the iliotibial tract and the posterolateral capsule should be released to correct valgus deformity in extension. Fortunately in most valgus knees release of these latter two structures will balance the knee. I feel that the lateral collateral ligament can only be released if the popliteus is intact and functional. Unfortunately in some severe valgus knees the popliteus is not functional.

The standard textbook description of release of a valgus knee does include the release of structures attached to the lateral condyle. This is perhaps satisfac-

tory in a fixed bearing knee but not in a mobile bearing knee. I feel that soft tissue release from the lateral condyle, particularly the popliteus, is contraindicated when using any mobile bearing knee.

If these structures are released from the lateral femoral condyle before the AP cuts are done, there are even more problems. To start with, the AP cutting jig will sit in excessive external rotation because the femur is internally rotated. This then leads to other problems. The flexion gap will be larger than it should be because of the femoral rotation. The gap opens up by hinging on the relatively tight medial structures. Because the AP jig is sitting in excessive external rotation, there will be an excessive amount of bone to remove from the posterior medial femoral condyle and perhaps no bone at all on the lateral side. The error can then be compounded if the AP cutting jig is downsized in order to be able to resect some bone from the posterior lateral femoral condyle. This has the effect of further increasing the flexion gap. Because the flexion gap is artificially increased, the flexion joint line is raised and thus the extension gap becomes tight. In order to achieve full extension, excessive distal femur has to be resected. Because the femur is cut in excessive external rotation, the femoral component goes on to the femur in an abnormal degree of external rotation. Consequently when the knee is extended, the femur rotates the insert externally and because of the posterior slope of the tibia this tends to re-create the preoperative valgus deformity.

As stated above, when using an LCS or any mobile bearing knee, release of the soft tissues from the lateral condyle should be avoided. It should only be considered if the popliteus is intact and well defined and if the amount of release required is small. If the lateral epicondyle is to be released, it needs to be done in a gradual incremental fashion but the popliteus must be left attached. After each incremental release, the extension gap and the flexion gap must be checked. If the flexion gap starts to become slack laterally, the release must stop and if the knee is still tight laterally in extension, an osteotomy of the lateral femoral condyle should be performed, as discussed below.

If the popliteus is inadvertently cut during this procedure or if there is significant lateral instability following this release, the knee should be considered unstable laterally in flexion. If the LCS knee is being used, the knee should be immobilised in plaster with the knee in extension at the end of the operation. The patient should be kept in a plaster cast for 8 weeks.

Osteotomy of the Lateral Femoral Condyle in the Severe Valgus Knee

This technique has been developed by Dr Jean-Louis Briard from Rouen in France. As discussed above, in a fixed valgus knee the major soft tissue problem is shortening or contracture of the soft tissue structures laterally in extension. Flexion balance is not usually a problem unless created by the surgeon. Again as discussed above, the posterolateral capsule and the iliotibial tract can be released without affecting the flexion gap. The problem then is that the only other structures that can be released are attached to the lateral femoral condyle and their release also adversely affects the flexion gap, rendering it potentially unstable. An alternative is to osteotomise the lateral femoral condyle and allow it to move distally. This gains length laterally in extension and if reattached correctly does not alter the flexion gap.

The osteotomy is performed in the sagittal plane. Distally it includes the lateral one third of the femoral condyle and proximally it exits at the proximal limit of the lateral supracondylar ridge. On its lateral aspect from distal to proximal, there is the insertion of the popliteus, the origin of the LCL and the lateral head of gastrocnemius. In order to mobilise the fragment, the latter has to be dissected free, especially at the posterosuperior corner. When the osteotomised fragment moves distally, it is held in place with two 3.5 mm cancellous bone screws.

Another problem in severe valgus knees is that often the MCL is stretched in extension and thus the extension space medially is abnormally large. In this situation it is best to accept some residual medial laxity. This will be stable provided the extension gap is not tight laterally and the flexion gap is balanced. I do not try to advance the MCL. If the extension gap is tight laterally and slack medially, "gapping" is created. This is where in extension a gap appears between the medial femoral and tibial condyles because of excessive lateral tightness. I think this can also lead to instability and the risk of bearing spinout.

Having completed the AP cuts and measured the flexion gap, the distal femur can be cut. As a routine I perform a conservative distal femoral cut. This means that the initial extension gap will be smaller than the flexion gap. This then allows the extension gap to be measured accurately with the spacer blocks. It also allows a final check on balance. Remember any further release of either collateral ligament will alter the flexion gap. When the conservative extension gap has been measured, the femur can then be re-cut, thus making the flexion and extension gaps equal.

Bearing spinout is one of the feared complications in mobile bearing knees. In my personal experience of primary knee surgery, using the rotating platform, I have had 11 spinouts in 2,300 cases, but only one in the last 1,000 of those cases. All were due to one of the surgical errors discussed above and seven of the 11 were in valgus knees. This is despite the fact that only 16% of my knees are valgus. I feel that if the rules above are adhered to, not only will spinout be very rare but also the chances of long-term success will be increased because of restoration of mechanical axis and joint line with balanced and equal flexion and extension gaps.

Bibliography

Arima J, Whiteside LA, McCarthy DS, White SE (1995) Femoral rotational alignment, based on the anteroposterior axis, in total knee arthroplasty in a valgus knee. A technical note. J Bone Joint Surg Am 77:1331–1334

Boldt JG, Hodler J, Zanetti M, Munzinger UK (2003) Is arthrofibrosis associated with femoral component internal malrotation in TKA? AAOS presentation, New Orleans

Chao EYS, Neluheni EVD, Hsu RWW, Paley D (1994) Biomechanics of malalignment. Orthop Clin North Am 25:379–393

Hsu RWW, Himeno S, Coventry MB, Chao EYS (1990) Normal axial alignment of the lower extremity and load-bearing distribution at the knee. Clin Orthop 255:215–227

Insall JN (1984) Surgery of the knee, 2nd edn. Churchill Livingstone, Edinburgh, pp 739–804

Jerosch J (2002) Interindividual reproduceability in intraoperative rotational alignment of femoral components in knee prosthetic surgery using the epicondylar line. AAOS, Dallas, Texas, 13–17 Febr 2002, poster no P105

McAlinden MG, Beverland D (2000) Femoral neck offset predicts distal femoral resection in total knee arthroplasty. J Bone Joint Surg (Orthop Proc Suppl III) 82-B:271

Novotny J, Gonsalez MH, Amirouche FML, Li YC Geometric analysis of potential errors in using femoral intramedullary guides in total knee arthroplasty. J Arthroplasty 16:641–647

Yoshino N, Takai S, Ohtsuki Y, Hirasawa Y (2001) Computed tomography measurement of the surgical and clinical transepicondylar axis of the distal femur in osteoarthritic knees. J Arthroplasty 16:493–497

4.8 Cruciate Ligaments: Retain, Substitute, or Sacrifice?

Jens G. Boldt

Most current knee systems are designed for sacrifice of anterior cruciate ligaments (ACL) with or without retention or substitution of posterior cruciate ligaments (PCL). The function of the PCL certainly deteriorates with an absent or deficient ACL because of its natural four-bar linkage system. Knee designs must, therefore, inhibit increased anteroposterior translation either by sagittal conforming design, providing sufficient space for accommodating the PCL or a cam/post mechanism. Total knee arthroplasty (TKA) requires bone resections as well as careful appreciation of soft tissues, including judgement of both active and passive structures such as extensor, flexor, and rotational muscles, capsule, collateral ligaments and cruciate ligaments. The lateral ligament complexes play a major role in determining a balanced flexion and extension gap throughout the entire range of motion and knee kinematics close to a normal knee joint; however, anteroposterior translation is predominantly controlled by the cruciate ligaments.

Kinematics vary in healthy and arthritic knee joints; however, the durability of any modern prosthetic design (fixed or mobile bearing) decreases with non-physiological motion and lack of stability. Healthy knee joints have six degrees of freedom within a soft tissue envelope, which includes limited physiological translation, rotation, lateral lift off and femoral rollback. These motions are controlled by both active and passive structures as well as proprioception. In general, the collateral ligament complexes control varus–valgus stability, whereas both cruciate ligaments predominantly control anteroposterior and rotational stability of the knee joint. Any total knee system and surgical technique that implements these kinematic issues will increase stability and conformity, ultimately reducing polyethylene wear. One important goal of prosthetic design is to compensate partially for anteroposterior stability, femoral rollback, and lateral lift off without increasing contact stresses above a critical value (usually 5–10 MPa). On the one hand, every TKA will lack stability if the complex soft tissue sleeve of the knee is not individually appreciated throughout the entire range of motion. On the other hand, sacrificing both cruciate ligaments during surgery does not necessarily create generally unstable TKA. Much depends on the premorbid condition, the integrity of the soft tissues, the

components used, and the surgical technique. In summary, there appears to be no general right or wrong with respect to cruciate ligament treatment in TKA.

Normal Function of Healthy Cruciate Ligaments

Both anterior and posterior cruciate ligaments form an inconsistent moving central pivot of the knee joint, which can be described as a four-bar linkage chain. This chain defines the individual rollback gliding pattern of the femoral condyles as well as the anatomic features of both the femoral and the tibial metaphyses. This results in considerable interpersonal variation of anatomic and kinematic features. The physiological central pivot is variable and moves to a certain amount in all three dimensions, allowing anteroposterior and mediolateral translation combined with tibiofemoral rotation and lift off.

The cruciate ligament lever arm is short and therefore has a limited ability to control tibiofemoral rotation. Further rotational and translational stability of the normal knee joint is guided by both menisci and their meniscofemoral ligaments, as well as all collaterals, including the LCM and POL medially and the lateral collateral ligament (LCL), popliteus tendon and iliotibial band laterally.

Ligament Function in TKA

Passive stability such as anatomical shape, menisci, cruciate ligaments and at times collateral ligament function in TKA may be partially compensated by the prosthetic design, particularly with mobile bearings. However, stability is not defined by passive structures alone but by active knee joint muscle forces and proprioception. Rotational and anterior stability of the ACL can be compensated by prosthetic congruency. A healthy PCL controls posterior and mediolateral translation as well as lift off, which may partly be controlled by either design and/or a posterior post and cam mechanism. Because of these concerns, it appears logical that the first prosthetic knee designs were usually overconstrained with at times huge stems, axes, bars and links (Shiers 1954, Walldius 1957, Gunston 1971). The main problem with these designs was increased constraint forces at the implant–bone interface, which ultimately led to early aseptic (mechanical) loosening. The ideal prosthetic design should accommodate all demands in an optimal fashion: minimal contact stress, minimal constraint forces and maximum stability.

Key functions of the PCL in healthy knees include: reduction of posterior tibial translation and lift off, control of mediolateral translation, centralizing of the longitudinal rotational axis, limitation of varus-valgus deviation, and reduction of patellofemoral loads and shear forces.

There is no doubt that osteoarthritic knee joints differ from normal knees in many respects. Soft tissue changes are often underestimated, particularly in degenerative diseases with varus, valgus or fixed deformities. Before retention of the PCL is considered, one must ensure that the PCL is of good quality, since most osteoarthritic knee cases are associated with poor condition of the PCL. A weak and degenerated PCL of poor quality is likely to fail the forces in TKA. Multiple reports in the literature address the insufficient quality and strength of PCL in elderly or arthritic knee joints. Macroscopically abnormal PCL showed more than 50 % degeneration in histology with loss of mechanoreceptors, as demonstrated by Franchi et al (1995). Therefore, PCL with insufficient properties are not recommended for retention, independent of surgeons' preferences and prosthetic design. Perfect tension and positioning of all components is mandatory for acceptable and long-term function of the PCL. Sensitive deviation from perfect positioning and compromise in blood supply will ultimately result in PCL failure.

Surgeons with a preference to retain the PCL must keep the option to sacrifice as a back-up. When retention of the PCL is desired (and possible), the knee design must be selected. Key requirements of such a prosthesis include: anatomical multiradial shape of the femoral component with patellar groove, congruent (mobile bearing) polyethylene bearing with sufficient space posteriorly (impingement), tibial resection with posterior slope, and balanced flexion and extension gaps (nutcracker effect). PCL retention defines the joint line and the tibiofemoral distance, which is less forgiving, since the healing process of TKA offers little biological adaptation (intelligent tissues).

Posterior Cruciate Ligaments and Co-restraints in TKA

1. Retention of PCL requires precise tibial and femoral resections to preserve vascularity.
2. The posterior capsule and the rim of the medial meniscus wall provide further stability.
3. Gaining length in fixed flexion deformity may be achieved by blunt means or posterior capsule pie crusting (transverse/oblique).
4. Posterolateral stability includes preservation of the popliteus tendon, lateral meniscus rim, and Wrisberg–PCL complex, which sends its fibres from the PCL into the posterior rim of both the lateral meniscus and popliteus tendon. This forms a stable posterolateral corner in TKA, improving rotational stability as well as lift off.
5. The PCL and the popliteus tendon are a direct reciprocal system (as are the popliteus tendon and the LCL) with regards to the direction of the forces applied. With voluntary incisions of the fascicles, the extension and flexion gap opens step by step. The lateral rim absorbs the major part (up to 75 %) of the posterior forces from 0 to 30 degrees flexion. The main posterior stabilising force from 30 degrees flexion is the isometric posterior bundle of the PCL followed by the ACL.

Posterior Cruciate Ligaments and Implant Design

Decreased tibial slope and a tight flexion gap in PCL retention increase the risk of a lever effect (nutcracker), which leads to increased contact stresses with polyethylene wear, overstretching of the PCL and lack of flexion. Increased tibial slope and a loose PCL increase anterior tibial subluxation in extension and posterior subluxation in flexion. This will ultimately cause shear forces and increased polyethylene wear. Joint line elevation or lowering has considerable consequences when the PCL is retained, since the biokinematics of the TKA, the PCL tension, and extensor mechanism alter significantly with a difference of as little as 2–4 mm. This can result in reduced extensor mechanism function, as demonstrated in the literature. Independent of PCL preferences, it is essential to preserve a proper joint line in TKA. Two healthy cruciate ligaments provide the best kinematics. That is true for healthy knees, but is different in osteoarthritic knee joints. In most current knee systems, however, the ACL is sacrificed and retention of the PCL alone does not provide the above-mentioned four-bar linkage system. PCL retention or sacrifice will always be a compromise in TKA. There are excellent clinical long-term data with over 13 years track record without PCL retention (Sorrels), as there are excellent results with PCL retention (Hamelynck). The question of PCL management in TKA is certainly multifactorial and may work either way if biomechanical aspects, surgical technique and prosthetic design are well chosen.

Sorger et al. (1997) demonstrated experimentally that the preserved PCL in TKA was able to maintain femoral rollback. When the PCL was cut, significant changes in kinematics were observed. Lewandowski et al. (1997) compared low contact stress (LCS) meniscal bearing (MB) and LCS rotating platform (RP) and found that anterior translation was greater in MB than in RP. The extension gap in MB was 2 mm greater than in the normal knee and in RP it was 4 mm more. The required quadriceps force for full extension was 30% more in MB than in the normal knee and 50% more in RP. This may have an impact on activities such as rising from a chair. Mahoney et al. (1994) looked at three groups of TKA: PCL retaining, PCL excised and posterior stabilized. In PCL retaining, only 37% demonstrated a normal PCL strain, femoral rollback was reduced by an average of 36% and there was 15% loss of extensor efficiency. In PCL sacrificed, rollback was decreased by 70% and there was 19% loss of extensor efficiency. In posterior stabilized, rollback was decreased by 12% and there was 11% loss of extensor efficiency. Montgomery et al. (1993) reported on 2% of late ruptures of the PCL leading to chronic instability and disabling pain in a series of 150 PCL retaining TKA. Yasuda and Sasaki (1986) found that in TKA with PCL retention there were significantly smaller moments and a better and more regular distribution of stresses in the proximal and posterior parts of the tibia than in the posterior stabilized TKA, in which there were large local concentrations of von Mieses stresses in front of the stem under the plateau. They recommended PCL retention whenever possible. Emodi et al. (1999) demonstrated the beneficial effect of the PCL on extensor function. They emphasized how important it is to restore the preoperative joint line and to avoid an overly lax PCL with loss of its function. Waslewski et al. (1998) found early incapacitating instability of PCL retaining TKAs secondary to early PCL deficiency. Typical symptoms and complaints were: persistent swelling, effusions, anterior knee pain and giving way with episodes of instability related to activities of daily living. It is very interesting to note that in the same series of patients, those who did not have PCL deficiency had on average only a 5 mm rise in joint line as compared with the PCL deficient knees, where the average rise was 10.3 mm.

Takatsu et al. (1998) demonstrated that PCL strain and rollback were significantly influenced by the posterior tilt of the tibial component as well as by the external rotation of the femoral component. Ten degrees of tilt as compared to 0 degrees clearly decreased the PCL strain, and rollback was decreased in the medial compartment but increased in the lateral one. Pereira et al. (1998) evaluated the functional outcome of 143 TKAs with the same Kinemax prosthesis implanted between 1988 and 1992. They compared 93 knees with sacrifice and 50 knees with preservation of the PCL and did not find any difference in clinical or early radiological outcome. They recommend that the PCL should be sacrificed in cases where extensive release and complex ligament balance are required. Fluoroscopic kinematic studies by Haas et al. (2002) of the RP with a sacrificed PCL demonstrated similar rollback and lift-off pattern compared with the normal knee joint.

Retaining the PCL seems to be desirable provided the ligament is of a good quality and the surgery is optimally performed. This means placing the tibial component with an anatomical slope and recreating the original joint line. The design of the prosthesis must allow for near-normal kinematics. A good functional PCL may give near-normal kinematics and better gait with more power when climbing stairs. This good functional PCL may be seen in young patients requiring TKA, especially in those patients who also have an intact ACL. In the elderly, most cruciate ligaments are degenerated or weakened by disease. In those patients, cruciate ligament retention should not be considered, as instability may develop in the years after surgery. As fixation of components is no longer a serious problem, it is important during surgery to think not only about the present but also about the future. Fortunately the activity level of elderly patients is usually very different from that of younger and more active patients. So these elderly patients will probably function well with the support of the collateral ligaments only and some more intrinsic constraint of the components, e.g. the RP. When retaining the PCL, the surgeon should think about not only control of anteroposterior translation, but also defining translations, rotations, and condylar lift off. In this respect retention of the PCL may be beneficial for active and younger patients.

The mobile bearing principle with the LCS system offers all possibilities with regards to cruciate ligament management. There is a bicruciate retaining meniscal bearing device, a PCL retaining device with combined rotation and anteroposterior glide bearing, and a bicruciate substituting device (the classic rotating platform used since the late 1970s. The bicruciate retaining meniscal bearing device is a technically demanding prosthesis, which gives good results in the experienced surgeon's hands with the right patient selection. Retention of the PCL may be beneficial in active and younger patients; however, there are no hard data in the current literature to prove this hypothesis. The PCL retaining anteroposterior glide device may cause anterior impingement problems and is, therefore, not generally recommended. The classic rotation platform bicruciate substituting LCS implant is the most frequently used and successful knee prosthesis of all LCS knees. The sagittal design of the conforming femoral component and rotating platform bearing provides sufficient translational stability without both cruciate ligaments. This device has shown excellent long-term results for all types of knee deformities, even in less experienced hands.

Bibliography

Akisue T, Stulberg BN, Bauer TW, McMahon JT, Wilde AH, Kurosaka M (2002) Histologic evaluation of posterior cruciate ligaments from osteoarthritic knees. Clin Orthop 400:165–173

Andriacchi TP, Galante JO, Fermier RW (1982) The influence of total knee replacement design on walking and stair climbing. J Bone Joint Surg Am 64A:1328–1335

Barrett DS, Cobb AG, Bentley G (1991) Joint proprioception in normal, osteoarthritic and replaced knees. J Bone Joint Surg Br 73:53

Buechel FF Sr, Buechel FF Jr, Pappas MJ, Dalessio J (2002) Twenty-year evaluation of the New Jersey LCS rotating platform knee replacement. J Knee Surg 15:84–89

Buechel FF Sr, Buechel FF Jr, Pappas MJ (2003) Ten-year evaluation of cementless Buechel-Pappas meniscal bearing total ankle replacement. Foot Ankle Int 24:462–472

Caton J, Boulahia A, Patricot LM (1999) Natural history of the posterior cruciate ligament in osteoarthritis. ESSKA Nice 1998 and SICOT, Sidney 1999

Chatain F et al Influence du positionnement de l'interligne articulaire sur la cinématique du genou prothèse et sur le comportement des ligaments collatéraux. 9es Journées Lyonnaises de chirurgie du genou La chirurgie prothétique du genou (Chambat, Neyret, Deschamps). Sauramps médical, Montpellier, France

Dennis DA, Komistek RD, Walker SA, Cheal EJ, Stiehl JB (2001) Femoral condylar lift-off in vivo total knee arthroplasty. J Bone Joint Surg 83B:33–39

Draganich LF, Piotrowski GA, Martell J, Pottenger LA (2002) The effects of early rollback in total knee arthroplasty on stair stepping. J Arthroplasty 17:723–730

Emodi GJ, Callaghan JJ, Pedersen DR, Brown TD (1999) Posterior cruciate ligament function following total knee arthroplasty. The effect of joint line elevation. Jowa Orthop J 19:82–92

Franchi A, Maccherotti G, Aglietti P (1995) Neural system of the human PCL in osteoarthritis. J Arthroplasty 10:679–682

Friederich N et al Klinische Anwendung biomechanischer und funktionell anatomischer Daten am Kniegelenk. Orthopäde 21:41–50

Goutallier D, Allain J, Le Monel S, Voisin MC (1998) Evaluation de l'état histologique du ligament croisé postérieur en fonction de l'état macroscopique du ligament croisé antérieur. Intérêt pour l'indication des prothèses conservants le où les ligaments croisés. Communication à la 73me réunion de la SOFCOT, Paris, nov 1998

Gunston FH (1971) Polycentric knee arthroplasty. J Bone Joint Surg 53B:272–277

Haas BD, Komistek RD, Stiehl JB, Anderson DT, Northcut EJ (2002) Kinematic comparison of posterior cruciate sacrifice versus substitution in a mobile bearing total knee arthroplasty. J Arthroplasty 17:685–692

Klein R, Serpe L, Kester MA, Edidin A, Fishkin Z, Mahoney OM, Schmalzried TP (2003) Rotational constraint in posterior-stabilized total knee prostheses. Clin Orthop 410:82–89

Lewandowski PJ, Askew MJ, Lin DF, Hurst FW, Melby A (1997) Kinematics of posterior cruciate ligament retaining and sacrificing mobile bearing total knee arthroplasties. An in vitro comparison of the New Jersey LCS meniscal bearing and rotation platform prothesis. J Arthroplasty 12:777–784

Lombardi AV Jr, Mallory TH, Fada RA, Hartman JF, Capps SG, Kefauver CA, Adams JB (2001) An algorithm for the posterior cruciate ligament in total knee arthroplasty. Clin Orthop 392:75–87

Mahoney OM, Noble PC, Rhoads DD, Alexander JW, Tullos HS (1994) Posterior cruciate function following total knee arthroplasty. A biomechanical study. J Arthroplasty 9:569–578

Montgomery RL, Goodman SB, Csongradi J (1993) Late rupture of posterior cruciate ligament after total knee replacement. Jowa Orthop J 13:167–170

Morberg P, Chapman-Sheath P, Morris P, Cain S, Walsh WR (2002) The function of the posterior cruciate ligament in an anteroposterior-gliding rotating platform total knee arthroplasty. J Arthroplasty 17:484–489

Pereira DS, Jaffe FF, Ortiguera C (1998) Posterior cruciate ligament-sparing versus posterior cruciate ligament-sacrificing arthroplasty. Functional results using the same prosthesis. J Arthroplasty 13:138–144

Race A, Amis AA (1996) Loading of the two bundles of the posterior cruciate ligament: an analysis of bundle function in A-P drawer. J Biomech 297:873–879

Schai PA, Scott RD, Thornhill TS (1999) Total knee arthroplasty with posterior cruciate retention in patients with rheumatoid arthritis. Clin Orthop 367:96–106

Shiers LGP (1954) Excerpta medica. Arthroplasty of the knee. Preliminary report of a new method. J Bone Joint Surg 36B:553

Sorger JI, Federle D, Kirk PG, Grood E, Cochran J, Levy M (1997) The posterior cruciate ligament in total knee arthroplasty. J Arthroplasty 12:869–879

Takatsu J, Itokazu M, Shimizu K, Brown TD (1998) The function of posterior tilt of the tibial component following posterior cruciate ligament retaining total knee arthroplasty. Bull Hosp Jt Dis 57:195–201

Title CI, Rodriguez JA, Ranawat CS (2001) Posterior cruciate-sacrificing versus posterior cruciate-substituting total knee arthroplasty: a study of clinical and functional outcomes in matched patients. JOA 16:409–414

Walldius B (1957) Arthroplasty of the knee using endoprosthesis. Acta Orthop Scand 23 [Suppl]:121

Walker PS, Haider H (2003) Characterizing the motion of total knee replacements in laboratory tests. Clin Orthop 410:54–68

Wasielewski RC (2002) The causes of insert backside wear in total knee arthroplasty. Clin Orthop 404:232–246

Waslewski GL, Marson BM, Benjamin JB (1998) Early, incapacitating instability of posterior cruciate ligament-retaining total knee arthroplasty. J Arthroplasty 13:763–767

Yamakado K, Worland RL, Jessup DE, Diaz-Borjon E, Pinilla R (2003) Tight posterior cruciate ligament in posterior cruciate-retaining total knee arthroplasty: a cause of posteromedial subluxation of the femur. J Arthroplasty 18:570–574

Yasuda K, Sasaki T (1986) Stress analysis after total knee arthroplasty with posterior cruciate ligament resection type and retention type prosthesis with special reference to the significance of retaining the posterior cruciate ligament. Nippon Seigeigrka Gakkai Zasshi 60:547–562

4.9 Femoral Component Rotation

Jens G. Boldt

Femoral rotation positioning is critical for successful total knee arthroplasty (TKA). Three different methods of referencing are generally accepted. These include the transepicondylar axis (TEA), as advocated by Insall, arbitrary external rotation from the posterior condyles, and the so-called Whiteside line. Another less well recognized method, which has been used for over 20 years, is referencing femoral component rotation perpendicular to the tibial shaft axis via a balanced flexion tension gap. Placing the femoral component parallel to the TEA leads to a biomechanically sound knee motion in full flexion and extension. However, this method has potential errors that include any anatomical deviations of the distal femur, which may occur in cases with severe varus or valgus angle deformity, condylar dysplasia, or other rotational pathology of the lower extremity.

Clinical outcomes after TKA are dependent upon multifactorial issues, one of which is femoral component rotational alignment. Prosthetic design and implantation of femorotibial components vary with different total knee systems. The surgeon must evaluate and address variables that include varus-valgus alignment, extra-articular deformities, soft tissue contractions, exaggerated Q-angle, patella position, size, and shape, as well as femorotibial rotation. Intraoperative variables include surgical approach, femorotibial stability, soft tissue management, extensor mechanism and patella treatment, prosthetic selection and positioning. Femoral component rotational alignment has gained more attention in the recent literature, since component malpositioning "negatively" influences knee kinematics, including patellofemoral tracking and range of motion (ROM).

The TEA is the most commonly referenced anatomic landmark for rotational positioning of the femoral component in TKA. It is reported as being more predictable than Whiteside's line or the posterior condyle. However, the TEA depends on estimated landmarks and may be altered in both varus and valgus knees and/or other pathological variations that may change lower limb rotational axes. Tibial rotation position, an important consideration in fixed bearing designs, is also a factor that affects gap balance and the patellofemoral joint. Tibial rotational positioning is of lesser concern in mobile bearing TKA because of the ability (of the bearing) to adapt to tibiofemoral rotation in flexion and extension.

Rotational malpositioning creates a trapezoidal rather than rectangular flexion gap with an altered patellofemoral articulation and unbalanced femorotibial kinematics. Instability in flexion with a tighter medial and more lax lateral compartment occurs when the femoral component is internally malrotated. This is frequently combined with lateral patellofemoral subluxation and instability (lift off) of the lateral compartment in flexion. In most TKA systems, for a given amount of tibial resection, an appropriate amount of posterior condylar resection is required to create a symmetric flexion gap. Different opinions of surgical approach exist regarding soft tissue releases, tibia first or femoral first bone cuts, as well as the femoral rotation resection. The most common method of tibial resection is perpendicular to the mechanical axis with some posterior inclination.

The three established methods of determining femoral rotational positioning in TKA consist of: the TEA, as advocated by Insall (Fig. 4.69), Whiteside's line, or a line perpendicular to the anteroposterior femoral axis (Fig. 4.70), and referencing 3–4 degrees external rotation from the posterior condyles (Fig. 4.71). The posterior condylar reference as described by Hungerford (1995) (Fig. 4.72) is seldom utilized, as it results in consistent femoral internal rotational positioning, often excessive. The low contact stress (LCS) method is based on the tibial shaft axis and balanced flexion gap and has been utilized since 1977 with mobile bearing TKA (Fig. 4.73). Potential advantages and errors of each method will be discussed.

Olcott and Scott (2000) have recently reported that these three widely accepted methods were consistent in yielding a symmetric, balanced flexion gap within 3 degrees. However, significant variables and inconsistencies were noted. The TEA failed to yield flexion gap symmetry in 10% of neutral varus TKA and 14% of valgus TKA, with discrepancies varying

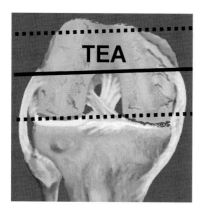

Fig. 4.69. The transepicondylar axis (Insall) is identified after intraoperative identification of both lateral and medial femoral epicondyles. Potential errors are landmark inconsistencies, previous trauma, femoral rotation, and ability to identify digitally both medial and lateral epicondyles

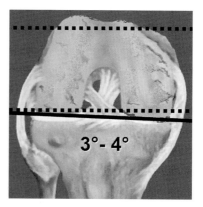

Fig. 4.71. Referencing femoral rotation in 3–4 degrees external rotation to the posterior condylar line leads to a component positioning that approximates to the transepicondylar line, but has a large angular range. This method is arbitrary, based on estimates with variable reference lines in possibly distorted condyles, particularly in valgus or varus deformities

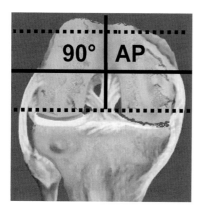

Fig. 4.70. The anteroposterior femoral axis method (Whiteside's line) references femoral rotation perpendicular to that line, which places the component approximately parallel to the transepicondylar line. Potential errors are femoral rotation variables, previous trauma, or patellofemoral diseases that may hinder anatomical identification

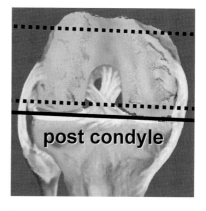

Fig. 4.72. Referencing femoral rotation from the posterior condylar line leads to an internally malrotated component positioning with an average of 4–5 degrees to the transepicondylar axis, which requires varus tibial resection and increased valgus femoral resection to achieve a balanced rectangular flexion tension gap. Internal rotation will also have a negative impact on the patellofemoral articulation

from 9 degrees too little to 6 degrees too much external rotation, which is less than desirable. The authors recommended using a combination of these methods to avoid potential malresections. Clinical studies by Stiehl and Cherveny (1996) compared the tibial shaft axis method with other methods for determining femoral rotation in four different fixed bearing knee systems utilizing a femoral-first approach. With the posterior condylar method, 72% required lateral release with 7% patella fractures reported. When 4–5 degrees of external rotation method was used, 28% lateral releases were reported. When the tibial shaft axis method was utilized, femoral component placement was reported within 1 degree of external rotation compared with the TEA. Fewer lateral releases were required and there were no patella complications. In a cadaver study of eight knees, Katz et al. (2001) (a three-surgeon evaluation) showed that determination of femoral component rotational positioning was more reliable using a balanced flexion gap and the anteroposterior axis. A similar study by Jerosch et al. emphasized that the inaccuracy of anatomically identifying the TEA of the femur by eight surgeons in three knee cadavers was 23 degrees. Intraoperative evaluation of the femoral epicondyles and the TEA is less predictable and accurate than pre-

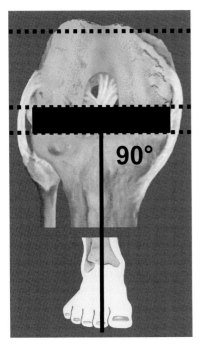

Fig. 4.73. Referencing femoral rotation perpendicular to the tibial shaft axis and a balanced flexion tension gap (LCS method) leads to prospectively predictable alignment parallel to the transepicondylar axis (mean 0.3 degrees)

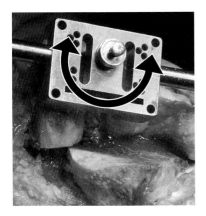

Fig. 4.74. A free moveable femoral resection guide is attached to an intramedullary femoral rod

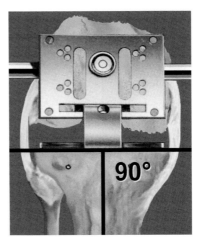

Fig. 4.75. A spacer block (perpendicular to the tibial shaft axis) is attached to the femoral component and sits flat on the tibial resection for flexion balance check and determination of femoral rotational alignment

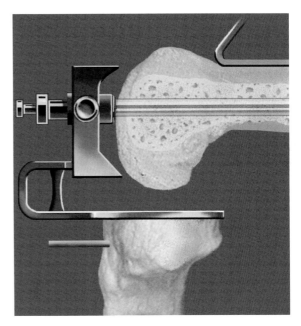

Fig. 4.76. Tibial resection is perpendicular to the tibial shaft axis and femoral resection block is parallel to the tibial resection

viously established methods. The method used to define femoral rotation with the LCS system is referenced on a tibial cut perpendicular to the tibial shaft axis and a symmetrical (rectangular) flexion gap. This method automatically defines the position of the free moveable femoral resection guide (Fig. 4.74), avoiding the need to identify anatomical landmarks. A rectangular spacer block is then applied to the rotationally unconstrained femoral component and sits flat on the tibial resection. The flexion tension is set and checked for proper balance (Figs. 4.75 and 4.76). The extension gap is balanced to the flexion gap with a distal femoral resection, establishing the mechanical axis (Fig. 4.77).

Comparison of this tibial axis method with the TEA methods adds to our understanding of this most important technique step in TKA. Evaluation of computed tomography (CT) scans is the most accurate

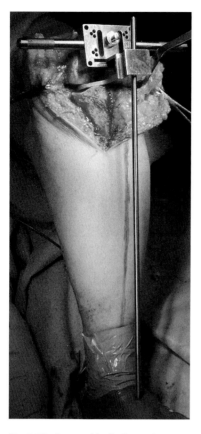

Fig. 4.77. Spacer block determines rotational alignment of the femoral resection block with a balanced rectangular flexion tension gap setting the guide parallel to the tibial shaft axis

method of objectively assessing femoral component rotational placement compared with a known anatomic landmark post-TKA. To investigate clinically the accuracy of the LCS method with regard to femoral component rotational positioning, we performed a study in which helical CT scan investigation was used, referencing the femoral prosthetic placement to the TEA. From a cohort of 3,058 mobile bearing LCS (DePuy Int, Leeds, UK) TKAs, 40 (1.3%) clinically well-functioning knees were randomly selected for evaluation of femoral component rotational alignment. All patients with TKA in this center underwent routine clinical examination and follow-up radiographs at 1 week, 6 weeks, 1 year, 5 years, or when complications occurred. Mean age in this cohort was 67 years (range 54–77). Inclusion criteria for this subset were: ROM over 100 degrees, lack of pre- or postoperative complications, and excellent or good clinical results according to a modified Hospital for Special Surgery 100-point clinical score with a mean of 91.2 points (81–100). One patient had to be excluded

because of inability to identify appropriate anatomical landmarks on CT scans, and another patient refused CT investigation. Of the 38 cases available for this study, the patella was left unresurfaced in 36 (95%) cases, one was previously patellectomized, another patella was resurfaced using a metal-backed rotating patella component.

Follow-ups at regular intervals included a clinical evaluation and x-ray protocol. Radiographic analysis was focused on patella tracking, congruency, and patella tilt with comparable pre- and postoperative skyline radiographs. Patella tracking was based on alignment of the femoral trochlear sulcus and the crown of the patella and measured in millimeters of lateral deviation on comparable pre- and postoperative skyline views.

The ultimate 38 cases were randomly selected from patients who were scheduled by a computerized system for 1-, 5-, or 10-year routine follow-up. These patients were invited to participate in the study until the appropriate number was obtained. Of the two cases eliminated, one patient refused to participate, and another was eliminated for technical reasons, as noted. Of this group, all patients had excellent or good clinical results and no patient refused to participate. The local university ethics committee approved the study.

All cases were investigated by one of two consultant musculoskeletal radiologists with CT experience of more than 15 years. Before the start of the examination, they examined a few patients not included in the investigation in order to use the same criteria, which were identical to those used for everyday examinations. The radiologists were not aware of the patients' knee status (single blinded). They were instructed not to talk with the patients about the status of their knees but only about technical CT aspects. All data for femoral component rotational positioning were analyzed using a helical CT scanner. Femoral component rotational alignment was calculated by referencing the two posterior condyles to the TEA, which was a line drawn between the spike of the lateral epicondyle and the sulcus of the medial epicondyle, as recently recommended by Yoshino et al. (2001) (Fig. 4.78). One case was excluded because of inability to identify the medial sulcus despite 2 mm cuts. Angles were calculated utilizing sophisticated helical CT-implemented software.

An independent statistician analyzed all data. The distribution of angles in each group was analyzed using the one-sample Kolmogorov–Smirnov test, which indicates whether the number of cases is sufficient and a normal "bell-curve" distribution is demon-

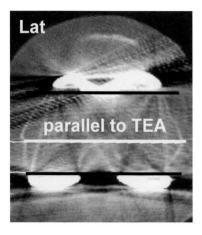

Fig. 4.78. Femoral component alignment parallel to transepicondylar axis ensures optimum patellofemoral tracking

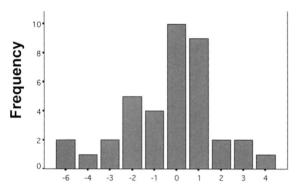

Femoral rotation in degrees

Fig. 4.79. Normal distribution of femoral component rotational alignment in the subset group. Mean rotation of the femoral component was parallel (0.3 degrees) to the transepicondylar axis, ranging from 6 degrees internal to 5 degrees external rotation

strated. A positive Kolmogorov–Smirnov test validates further parametric statistical analyses.

The subset of 38 cases (follow-up 12–120 months) studied in this series had clinical results comparable to a larger cohort group of over 3,000 TKAs. All cases were well-functioning knees with good or excellent clinical results. The mean ROM was 115 degrees (range 100–135). Preoperatively, three of 38 cases had documented patella subluxation and tilt of more than 6 degrees. Postoperatively, all three achieved perfect patellofemoral tracking. Decreased height and sclerosis of the lateral patella facet were seen in two cas-

es without clinical symptoms. There were no fixation failures, no patella failures and no reoperations for any reason in this group.

Mean femoral alignment was near parallel (0.3 degrees internal rotation) to the TEA with a range of 6 degrees internal to 4 degrees external rotation (Fig. 4.79). Standard deviation was 2.2 and standard error 0.4. All angles were normally distributed using the one-sample Kolmogorov–Smirnov test, which validates a statistical mean value and outliers. Four cases fell outside the predicted mean value (more than 3 degrees internal or external rotation). Three had internal rotation and one had external rotation. All four cases with maximum internal and external rotation showed perfect patellofemoral tracking on skyline views (Fig. 4.80). The data from our study emphasize that correct femoral component rotational positioning, utilizing the tibial shaft axis method, results in a high level of consistency for accurate patellofemoral alignment and predictable clinical outcome.

In summary, femoral rotational alignment based on the tibial axis and balanced flexion tension is an instrumented technique that: (1) avoids relationships to arbitrary landmarks; (2) establishes a precise flexion gap, which allows for a stable relationship to the corrected biomechanical axis; (3) is patient-specific regarding bone and soft tissue variations; (4) is reproducible (especially in severe deformities such as the valgus knee); and (5) results in predictable patella outcomes in reported series. Femoral component rotational alignment is technique- and instrument-dependent and influences patella tracking, gap balance, and soft tissue kinematics. Deviation into internal rotation results in less than ideal patellofemoral tracking and clinical outcomes. Potential complications, such as the painful and/or stiff TKA (arthrofibrosis), have been shown to correlate with significant internal rotation of the femoral component. The tibial shaft axis method as used with the LCS system provides perfect rotational alignment without anatomical landmark identification, and is, therefore, felt to be more predictable than all other currently practised methods.

Acknowledgements. I thank C. Varma BS for illustrations (Allentown, PA, USA), J. Hodler MD and M. Zanetti MD for CT data (Zurich, Switzerland), T. Drobny MD for clinical support (Zurich, Switzerland) and P. Keblish MD for manuscript review (Allentown, PA, USA).

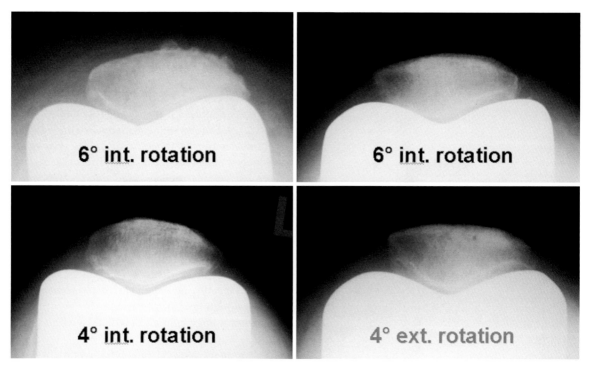

Fig. 4.80. Perfect patellofemoral tracking on skyline views in four cases that fell outside the predicted mean value (more than 3 degrees internal or external rotation)

Bibliography

Akagi M, Matsusue Y, Mata T, Asada Y, Horiguchi M, Iida H, Nakamura T (1999) Effect of rotational alignment on patellar tracking in total knee arthroplasty. Clin Orthop 366:155– 163

Arima J, Whiteside LA, McCarthy DS, White SE (1995) Femoral rotational alignment, based on the anteroposterior axis, in total knee arthroplasty in a valgus knee. A technical note. J Bone Joint Surg Am 77:1331–1334

Berger RA, Rubash HE, Seel MJ, Thompson WH, Crossett LS (1993) Determining the rotational alignment of the femoral component in total knee arthroplasty using the epicondylar axis. Clin Orthop 286:40–47

Berger RA, Crossett LS, Jacobs JJ, Rubash HE (1998) Rotation causing patellofemoral complications after total knee arthroplasty. Clin Orthop 356:144–153

Bizzini M, Boldt J, Munzinger U, Drobny T (2003) Rehabilitation guidelines after total knee arthroplasty. Orthopade 32(6):527–534

Boldt J, Munzinger U, Keblish P (2004) Comparison of isokinetic strength in resurfaced and retained patellae in bilateral TKA. J Arthroplasty 19(2):264

Boldt JG, Munzinger UK, Zanetti M, Hodler J (2004) Arthrofibrosis associated with total knee arthroplasty: gray-scale and power Doppler sonographic findings. AJR Am J Roentgenol 182(2):337–340

Buechel FF (1982) A simplified evaluation system for the rating of the knee function. Orthop Rev 11:97–101

Churchill DL, Incavo SJ, Johnson CC, Beynnon BD (1998) The transepicondylar axis approximates the optimal flexion axis of the knee. Clin Orthop 356:111–118

Dennis DA, Komistek RD, Walker SA, Cheal EJ, Stiehl JB (2001) Femoral condylar lift-off in vivo in total knee arthroplasty. J Bone Joint Surg Br 83:33–39

Eckhoff DG, Piatt BE, Gnadinger CA, Blaschke RC (1995) Assessing rotational alignment in total knee arthroplasty. Clin Orthop 318:176–181

Engh GA (2000) Orienting the femoral component at total knee arthroplasty. Am J Knee Surg 13:162–165

Fehring TK (2000) Rotational malalignment of the femoral component in total knee arthroplasty. Clin Orthop 380: 72–79

Griffin FM, Insall JN, Scuderi GR (1998) The posterior condylar angle in osteoarthritic knees. J Arthroplasty 13:812–815

Griffin FM, Insall JN, Scuderi GR (2000) Accuracy of soft tissue balancing in total knee arthroplasty. J Arthroplasty 15:970– 973

Hungerford DS (1995) Alignment in total knee replacement. Instr Course Lect 44:455–468

Katz MA, Beck TD, Silber JS, Seldes RM, Lotke PA (2001) Determining femoral rotational alignment in total knee arthroplasty: reliability of techniques. J Arthroplasty 16:301–305

Lonner JH, Siliski JM, Scott RD (1999) Prodromes of failure in total knee arthroplasty. J Arthroplasty 14:488–492

Mantas JP, Bloebaum RD, Skedros JG, Hofmann AA (1992) Implications of reference axes used for rotational alignment of the femoral component in primary and revision knee arthroplasty. J Arthroplasty 7:531–535

Nagamine R, Miura H, Inoue Y, Urabe K, Matsuda S, Okamoto Y, Nishizawa M, Iwamoto Y (1998) Reliability of the anteroposterior axis and the posterior condylar axis for determining rotational alignment of the femoral component in total knee arthroplasty. J Orthop Sci 3:194–198

Nagamine R, Miura H, Bravo CV, Urabe K, Matsuda S, Miyanishi K, Hirata G, Iwamoto Y (2000) Anatomic variations should be considered in total knee arthroplasty. J Orthop Sci 5:232–237

Olcott CW, Scott RD (2000) A comparison of 4 intraoperative methods to determine femoral component rotation during total knee arthroplasty. J Arthroplasty 15:22–26

Olcott CW, Scott RD (1999) The Ranawat Award. Femoral component rotation during total knee arthroplasty. Clin Orthop 367:39–42

Poilvache PL, Insall JN, Scuderi GR, Font-Rodriguez DE (1996) Rotational landmarks and sizing of the distal femur in total knee arthroplasty. Clin Orthop 331:35–46

Scuderi GR, Insall JN, Scott NW (1994) Patellofemoral pain after total knee arthroplasty. J Am Acad Orthop Surg 2:239–246

Stiehl JB, Abbott BD (1995) Morphology of the transepicondylar axis and its application in primary and revision total knee arthroplasty. J Arthroplasty 10:785–789

Stiehl JB, Cherveny PM (1996) Femoral rotational alignment using the tibial shaft axis in total knee arthroplasty. Clin Orthop 331:47–55

Stiehl JB, Dennis DA, Komistek RD, Keblish PA (1997) In vivo kinematic analysis of a mobile bearing total knee prosthesis. Clin Orthop 345:60–66

Stiehl JB, Dennis DA, Komistek RD, Crane HS (1999) In vivo determination of condylar lift-off and screw-home in a mobile-bearing total knee. J Arthroplasty 14:293–299

Whiteside LA, Arima J (1995) The anteroposterior axis for femoral rotational alignment in valgus total knee arthroplasty. Clin Orthop 321:168–172

Yamada K, Imaizumi T (2000) Assessment of relative rotational alignment in total knee arthroplasty: usefulness of the modified Eckhoff method. J Orthop Sci 5:100–103

Yoshino N, Takai S, Ohtsuki Y, Hirasawa Y (2001) Computed tomography measurement of the surgical and clinical transepicondylar axis of the distal femur in osteoarthritic knees. J Arthroplasty 16:493–497

4.10 Articular Deformity

Urs K. Munzinger

Articular deformity is a result of a combination of intra- and extra-articular pathology. In a quantitative sense, one can estimate the amount of joint line deformity imparted by a given amount of angular deformity in the femoral shaft. If the angular deformity were centered at the knee joint, the amount of angular bony deformity would contribute to the overall deformity at the knee (Fig. 4.81). At the other extreme, if the shaft angular deformity were closer to the hip or the ankle joint (Fig. 4.82), the impact on overall knee alignment would be minimal. Reconstruction of this very difficult situation would involve several approaches such as corrective osteotomy in two stages or with total knee arthroplasty (TKA) to minimize the articular abnormality. The other option would be placement of the femoral component in proper relationship to the functional mechanical axis of the femur, followed by major adjustments of ligament attachments by release and/or advancement. These options have their limitations and must be pre-planned.

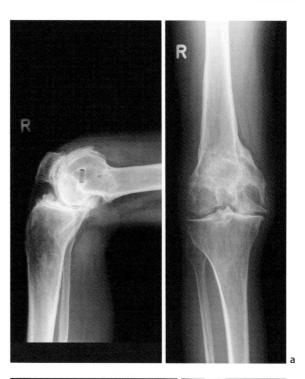
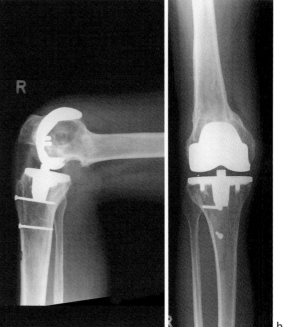

Fig. 4.81. a In a quantitative sense, one can easily estimate the amount of joint line deformity imparted by a given amount of angular deformity in the shaft. b In this patient, deformity is corrected by positioning of the prosthesis components and adequate ligament balancing

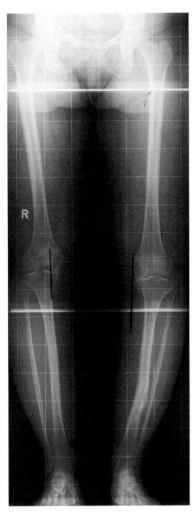

Fig. 4.82. The shaft angular deformity is at the distal third of the tibia; its impact on the overall alignment is minimal

Intra-articular and Extra-articular Deformity

The problems encountered in the management of deformity at TKA are interesting and challenging. Subtleties of deformities may be difficult to appreciate, perhaps because of the complexity of the subject and the wide variability in the relevant pathologic factors relating to intra- and extra-articular (bone and soft tissue) issues discussed in other chapters.

Cases with major deformity (Figs. 4.83, 4.84) present technical challenges for achieving proper alignment and ligament balance. In the extreme, such challenges are essentially eliminated if one resorts to the use of highly constrained or hinged prostheses. Because of the expected and observed problems of loosening and bone loss as a result of higher stress at prosthesis-cement-bone interfaces, most surgeons seek to avoid the highly constrained components.

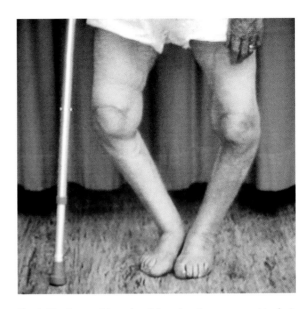

Fig. 4.83. Cases with major deformity always present technical challenges for achieving proper alignment and ligament balance

Many surgeons follow a general principle of trying to minimize prosthetic constraint whenever possible.

The bone cuts and prosthetic joint surface must have the proper angular orientation to the respective femoral and tibial shaft axes for the knee to assume a proper alignment when the prosthesis surfaces are articulated. Although properly oriented cuts – hence properly oriented joint surfaces – imply normal alignment, they do not automatically recreate or maintain normal ligament balance. The goal is for the prosthetic knee to be stable throughout a maximum range of motion. Minor degrees of instability, characterized simply by increased anteroposterior drawer or increased medial or lateral instability are surprisingly well tolerated.

Analysis of Specific Deformities

(Concept by K. A. Krackow)

It is important to understand that this section deals with an analysis of the problems and not specifically with the definitive surgical techniques for managing these problems. Varus and valgus deformities are considered as mirror images of one another. Concave and convex are used to refer to the medial or lateral aspect of the deformed joint with varus or valgus changes. In varus deformity, concave refers to the medial aspect and convex refers to the lateral aspect. In valgus deformity, concave refers to the lateral aspect and concave to the medial aspect.

Fig. 4.84. In the extreme, such challenges are essentially eliminated if one resorts to the use of highly constrained or hinged prostheses. In this patient a condylar prosthesis with reefing of the medial collateral ligament was chosen in the right knee. The left knee was managed with a valgus–varus stabilized prosthesis

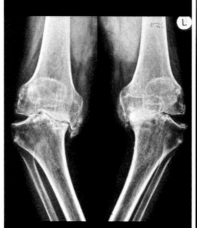
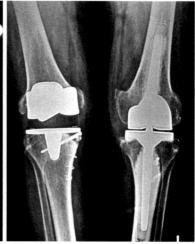

Fig. 4.85. The deformity is evident on weight bearing, and is passively correctable to neutral alignment, i.e. the collateral ligaments are out to normal length when correct alignment is achieved

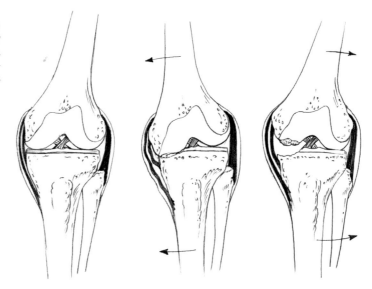

Unicompartmental Bone Loss Without Concave Contracture

To the extent that the loss is present at the tibia, the deformity would be evident in both extension and flexion. On the femoral side, loss distally would appear as deformity in extension, loss from a posterior condyle would appear as subtle deformity in flexion. The deformity would be evident on weight bearing, and it would be passively correctable to neutral alignment (i.e. the collateral ligaments would correct to normal length when alignment is achieved). The deformity is one of bone loss without soft tissue involvement, therefore the deformity will lend itself to replacement or reconstruction of the bone loss.

With the occurrence of abnormal concavity at the side of compression and development of a convexity at the opposite compartment, tension resulting at the periphery of the convex side can lead to alternation of the collateral ligament complex. As this knee is examined, a sense of obvious ligament instability is present on varus–valgus testing. The ligaments on the original concave side may correct to normal length, but the collateral complex at the convex side is lax. The situation could be handled by leaving things as they are, if it is expected that the instability of the convex side is consistent with good function and/or that further minor releasing (fine-tuning) the ligament structures of the concave side will restore normal soft tissue balance between the two sides. This type of defect lends itself to unicompartment replacement if other indications are present to support successful unicompartmental knee arthroplasty (Fig. 4.85).

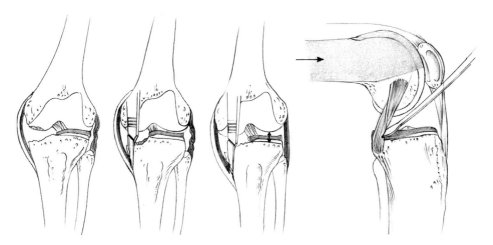

Fig. 4.86. Asymmetrical wear in one compartment and secondary contracture of collateral ligaments. Management is undertaken by concave release, i.e. release that would lead to perfect ligament balance. If not, additional release of the posterior cruciate ligament is necessary

Unicompartmental Bone Loss with Concave Contracture

Asymmetrical wear in one compartment and secondary contracture of collateral, and perhaps, to a lesser degree, contracture of cruciate structures is a common situation in TKA. The deformity is apparent on weight bearing. Ligament testing may reveal normal stability or some laxity on the concave side. Management is undertaken by concave release, the goal being to establish near-normal collateral ligament balance. The tibia is corrected to normal alignment and position with respect to the femur. Not releasing the concave side will lead to a tibial cut that is relatively more distal, creating the problem of asymmetric ligament balance. Depending on the resection level, the concave side may be correct, too loose or tighter than the convex side. Soft tissue release prior to bone resections, therefore, allows for more accurate resection depth and provides more normal kinematic balance. A concave bone loss with a concave contracture will eventually lead to a convex soft tissue stretching, which may be reversible or irreversible. Reconstruction begins with concave release, but it may be difficult to release pathological concave side structures to match the stretched convex side. Limitations of correction and/or pathologic soft tissues will affect prosthetic stability and dictate whether more constrained components are indicated (Fig. 4.86).

Bony Deformity with Concave Contracture

Bony deformities with a severe concave bone loss and a concave tissue contracture are most challenging. With angular deformity of the joint line with respect to the shaft, there is some relative deformity of the epicondylar-epiphyseal-capsular attachment region (Fig. 4.87). This appearance is often seen with a congenitally deformed femur. The distal femoral joint line has a relative varus alignment with respect to the femoral shaft. With time and degenerative process, the wear is proportionately greater at the concave compartment; therefore, relative contracture of the soft tissue develops on the concave side. The knee appears deformed whether the patient is supine or standing. The deformity may be increased with weight bearing depending on the degree of "pseudolaxity", which develops as a result of excessive joint surface wear rather than soft tissue contracture.

Reconstruction involves asymmetric resection from the posteromedial and posterolateral femoral condyles, as well as asymmetric femoral component alignment with respect to the epicondylar axis. The specifics of these resections are discussed in Sect. 4.2.

If concave release is successful in achieving balance at the convex side, satisfactory prosthetic balance can be accomplished. To the degree that correction of the deformity is not achieved in terms of soft tissue release, then femoral and tibial components, properly aligned to the axes, will have some relative laxity on the convex side. One cannot expect to treat this convex laxity simply by putting in thicker components, which will create other problems such as

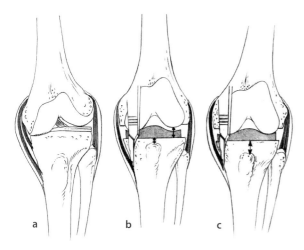

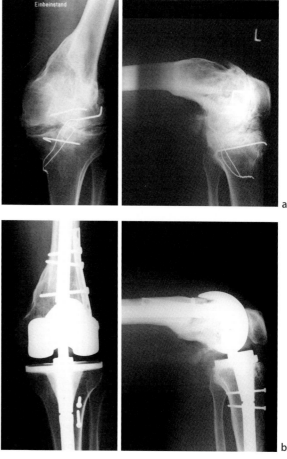

Fig. 4.87. **a** Loss of articular cartilage and bone on concave side of deformity and ligament complex has become contracted. **b** Minimal medial release and sufficient bone resection leads to convex laxity (more distal tibial cut). **c** Adequate medial release and more proximal tibial cut, the convex ligaments are taut, ideal overall correction of deformity

gap imbalance, rotatory instability, etc. The situation of relative laxity on the convex side must either be ignored or dealt with by more effective release on the concave side or by a ligament tightening at the convex aspect (often unsuccessful). If balance cannot be achieved, prostheses with increased constraint must be utilized.

4.11 Varus Knees and Flexion Contracture – Algorithm

Urs K. Munzinger (Concept by K. A. Krackow)

The Problem

Analysis of flexion contracture in total knee arthroplasty requires specific management of soft tissues and posterior capsule. Varus and valgus deformities represent an alignment problem, whereas flexion contracture is a range of motion abnormality with the inability to extend the knee joint fully, a deformity that makes normal walking very difficult and painful. Therefore, soft tissue release and ligament balance maneuvers for flexion contracture require careful planning and an understanding of the pathological and mechanical soft tissue situation in each individual knee joint. With loss of flexion over time, posterior contracture, including (static) capsular ligament as well as hamstring and/or gastrocnemius (dynamic) contracture, will accentuate intra-articular pathology.

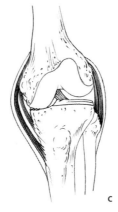

Fig. 4.88. **a,b** Consideration of damage to articular surfaces is important. An acquired molding of the femoral condyles contributes to persistence of flexion contracture. **c** The knee appears deformed whether the patient is supine or standing. The deformity is possibly increased with weight bearing depending on how much "pseudolaxity" develops as a result of excessive joint surface wear

Progression of osteoarthritis produces a variety of significant changes (Fig. 4.88). An acquired molding of the femorotibial articulation contributes to stiffness and flexion contracture. Similarly, although less common, intra-articular adhesions can also block full extension. The complexities of knee kinematics are such that with flexion, collateral ligament relaxation occurs, which permits internal rotation of the tibia. If internal rotation is impeded and the tibia is held initially in neutral rotation as the knee flexes, the collaterals become lax. This relaxed state of the collaterals encourages the development of collateral ligament fibrous and contracture. Clinically (because of pain and effusion) patients often hold the knee in a position of flexion and neutral rotation, encouraging the contractures. Pathological changes occur with time and severity, increasing the difficulty of release techniques and risk of potential instabilities.

Reconstructive Management

Removal of sufficient distal femoral and/or proximal tibial bone can allow passive correction of the deformity. However, it is vital to understand what happens to the soft tissue sleeve and the ligaments with excess resection (Fig. 4.89). A deeper distal femoral cut would serve to lengthen in extension and not in flexion. Deepening the tibial cut, i.e. moving the tibial component distally, will relax the ligaments circumferentially.

Bone removal leads to a collateral laxity, therefore it is important to appreciate the consequences regarding ligament examination. In full extension, tension is created along the posterior capsule and other posterior soft tissue structures. Varus or valgus stressing, therefore, may not produce the sensation of instability. When the taught posterior capsule is lax secondary to flexion contracture correction or bone resection alone, varus/valgus instability in midflexion is a likely consequence.

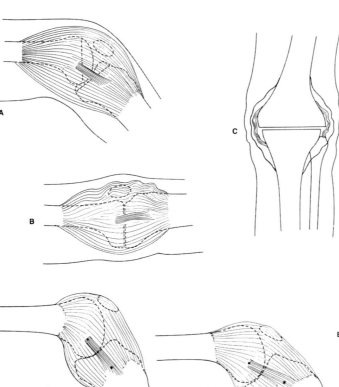

Fig. 4.89. Removal of sufficient distal femoral bone, proximal tibial bone, or some of each can be expected to allow correction of passive deformity. After performing bone resection, the soft tissue sleeve and ligaments may change considerably. Be aware of varus or valgus instability in gentle flexion when tight posterior capsules become lax. (Reprinted with permission of K.A. Krackow)

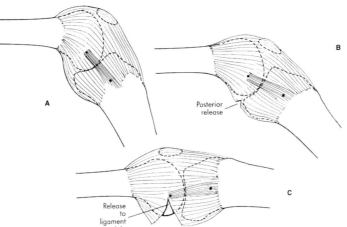

Fig. 4.90. Deformity management via soft tissue releases. Releasing the epicondylar capsule origins may not be sufficient because they are posterior to a mid-anteroposterior femoral plane. Collateral ligament integrity can contribute to a persistence of flexion contracture. (Reprinted with permission of K.A. Krackow)

Soft Tissue Release

Because of the anticipated complexities when bone resection alone is used to correct flexion contracture, one must consider management of the deformity by soft tissue release. Collateral ligament integrity can contribute to the persistence of a flexion contracture. To the extent that the flexion contracture deformity is maintained by relative collateral ligament contracture, lengthening of the collaterals by some technique must be accomplished. Releasing the epicondylar origins may not be sufficient (Fig. 4.90) because the ligament attachments are posterior to a mid-anteroposterior plane on the distal femur. If attempting to preserve anterior and posterior cruciate ligaments (PCL) (uncommon) or PCL (common) retention where firm ligament tension in flexion is desired, deepening the tibial cut may be required. The distal femoral resection must be adequate in order that tension is maintained in flexion. Excessive distal femoral resection produces other problems such as elevation of joint line and patella baja, often consequences of an inadequate depth of tibial resection.

Rotational Deformity

Rotational deformity is present to some degree in most varus or valgus deformed knees. In general, internal rotational deformity occurs in varus cases and external torsion in valgus cases. A large number of patients who have a varus deformity appear to have significant internal torsional deformity such that with the foot held in a normal position, the knee is externally rotated, and with the knee held in neutral, the foot points internally. When the knees are held in a neutral position, internal torsion is very apparent, varus is less obvious, and the knee often appears to demonstrate a flexion contracture. The patient's deformity as viewed from the frontal plane appears to be slightly flexed and internally rotated (Fig. 4.91).

The goal of surgical reconstruction is to re-establish and maintain normal overall rotational alignment. The entire issue of rotation correction, component and prosthesis placement is complex. Addressing rotational deformity with minimally constrained prostheses includes a conservative but adequate release of soft tissue attachments and/or flexion contracture deformity (Fig. 4.92). There is a limitation for soft tissue release to correct rotational deformity. One must appreciate the implications of component position changes on ligament balance and extensor alignment rotationally, as well as its relation to varus–valgus and flexion contracture deformities.

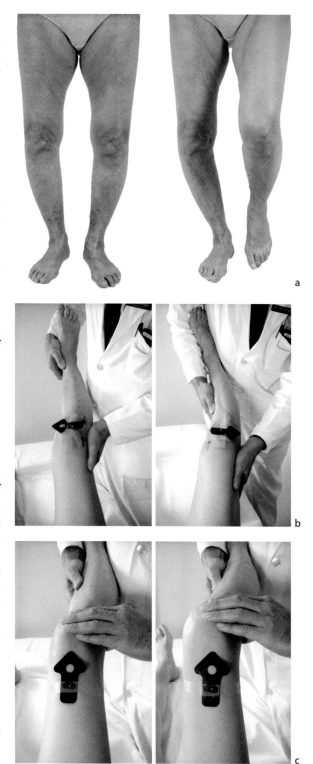

Fig. 4.91 a–c. Rotational deformity. a Flexion contracture deformity and internal torsion combined with varus deformity. b Varus–valgus stress testing reveals laxity due to bone defects and imbalance of collateral ligaments. c Patellofemoral degeneration is palpated during knee motion from extension to flexion

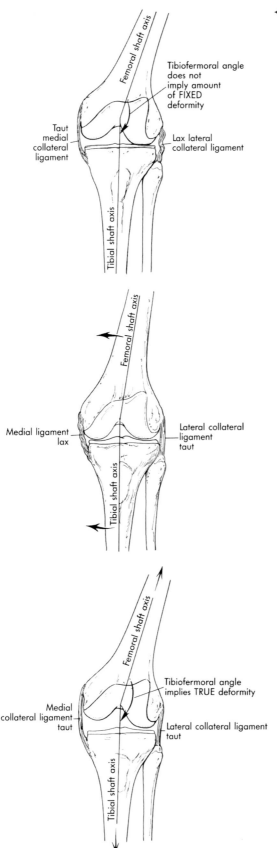

◀ **Fig. 4.92.** Tension stress analysis preoperatively and intra-operatively. Soft tissue ligament balancing is performed by femoral and tibia manipulation. (Reprinted with permission of K. A. Krackow)

Surgical Management

The steps for flexion contracture management at the time of primary arthroplasty are fairly straightforward. Appreciating the potential problems of differential bone resection, it can still be said that the first major technique to employ is additional bone resection, providing that joint elevation or iatrogenic patella baja is avoided. Once access to the posterior aspect of the joint has been developed (following conservative posterior femoral pre-cuts and proximal tibial resection), attention should be addressed to soft tissue attachments of the posterior compartments. Removal of posterior femoral osteophytes and large loose bodies is helpful (Fig. 4.93). At times, division of the posterior capsule and elevation of the gastrocnemius origins may be required. The flexion–extension gap technique directs the surgeon to position the knee at full extension, tense the tibia longitudinally away from the distal femur, and make a distal femoral resection so that an extension gap is created that is equal to or corresponds to the flexion gap. If there is a flexion-contracted knee with extension ex-

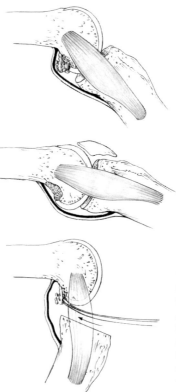

Fig. 4.93.
Removal of posterior femoral osteophytes and large loose bodies is recommended. Posterior capsule release and elevation of gastrocnemius insertion are optional

amination, the separation distance between the femur and the tibia is not determined by the collateral ligament tension, but is secondary to the contracted posterior soft tissues. Therefore, the rationale is to perform the posterior release first, and the distal femoral resection secondary is to reduce potential for midflexion instability. One is advised to pay close attention to the proposed resection level as related to the epicondylar attachments, and the flexion–extension gaps related to the proposed resections. If the surgeon is to manage flexion contracture appropriately, he needs to inspect repeatedly the relative size of the flexion and extension gaps and to determine the relative position of the epicondyles to the femoral joint lines. The maximal distal femoral resection should not infringe on the collateral ligament origins. Epicondylar osteotomy advancement techniques must be considered in extreme cases.

When varus or valgus deformity is present, the posterior aspect of the collateral release for the varus or valgus deformity may be adequate; however, care must be taken in preserving the popliteus and semimembranosus if possible. Intra-articular contracture and the combination of flexion and varus, release of the semimembranosus and the posteromedial capsule may be required. Release of the posterolateral

gastrocnemius and capsule at the femur in cases of severe valgus often aids in correction necessary for coexisting flexion contracture with valgus. Distal lateral collateral ligament release or lateral epicondylotomy (Keblish, Briard) is often required.

Summary of Flexion Contracture Management

(K. A. Krackow)

1. Examine carefully for the amount of flexion contracture and the presence of rotational deformity.
2. Be aware of differences between and pitfalls of the flexion–extension gap and measured resection technique; measured resection may fail to address the flexion contracture abnormality, and the flexion–extension gap technique may lead to instability in midflexion.
3. Expect to position the distal femoral cut, hence the femoral joint line, a bit more proximal than might be anatomic.
4. As early as possible in the procedure, address posterior femoral condylar osteophytes and posterior compartment loose bodies. Be prepared to perform posterior capsular, even gastrocnemius, release for the more severe cases.

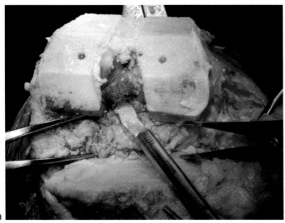

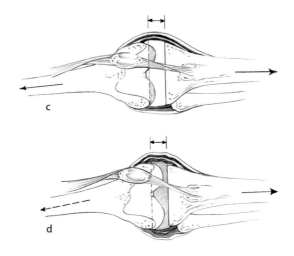

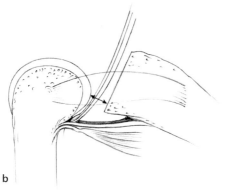

Fig. 4.94. **a** When varus or valgus deformity is combined with flexion contracture, complete release of the capsule from the posterior femur aids in correcting flexion contracture. **b** Because of flexion contracture and tension in posterior aspect of soft tissue sleeve, tibia lies relatively closer to distal surface of femur. Femoral resection line relatively proximal. **c** Posterior release of capsule and – if necessary – gastrocnemius tendons. **d** Release of posterior capsule leads to full length of the collateral ligaments. Femoral resection line relatively distal i. e. less bone resection from distal Femur

5. Assess the collateral ligaments during trial reduction in maximal extension and also in slight flexion. Some of the flexion contracture may be caused by relative collateral contracture. Therefore, consider deepening the tibial cut if the ligaments appear tight and competent.

6. When varus or valgus deformity is combined with flexion contracture, extensive release of the respective posteromedial capsule from the tibia and the posterolateral capsule from the femur aids in creating a significant amount of flexion contracture correction (Fig. 4.94).

Varus Deformity

Handling of varus problems starts with recognition and assessment of the amount of deformity. Careful tension stress examinations with the knee held in neutral rotation is the first stage. The maximum deformity under load and the maximum degree of correction achievable passively may be less important. Attention to proper rotation avoids confusing fixed flexion contracture deformity with varus deformity.

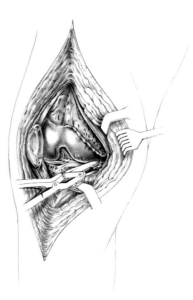

Fig. 4.95. Primary medial release via generous dissection of the deep medial collateral ligament and removal of medial tibial and femoral osteophytes

Osteophyte Removal/Downsizing

Medial osteophytes are commonly present in patients with varus deformity and serve to provoke the deformity as they exert a bowstring effect on the medial capsular ligamentous structures. Removal of the osteophytes is appropriate in virtually all cases of varus deformity and, as an isolated maneuver, can effect a mild amount of correction even before any direct release is undertaken. Access to the posterior capsule is facilitated by the medial sleeve releases and downsizing the "often remodeled" large tibia to normal anatomy (semimembranosus attachment). The large medial femoral condyle and posterior condyle (with osteophytes) are also downsized to allow for the projected prosthetic size. These maneuvers are essential if the optimum exposure and subsequent stable gap balance is to be accomplished.

Any failure to balance the medial and lateral stabilizing structures adequately means that relative instability on one side of the joint persists. Lesser degrees of lateral instability are usually well tolerated, especially in anteroposterior and mediolateral semiconstraint total knee designs.

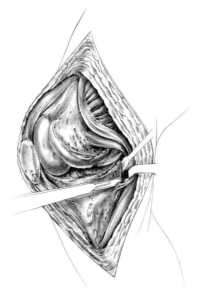

Fig. 4.96. The next stage of medial release includes partial subperiosteal release of the superficial part of the medial collateral ligament

Mild Cases – Primary Medial Release

Almost all varus deformity management involves surgical release of tight soft tissue structures on the medial side of the knee. Generous dissection just below the medial joint line, freeing the deep medial collateral ligament (meniscotibiale ligament), together with removal of medial tibial and femoral osteophytes, may be all that is necessary (Fig. 4.95). This is especially true when leaving some acceptable lateral laxity.

Moderately Severe Cases

The next stage of medial release advocated here is subperiosteal release of the superficial medial collateral ligament from the tibia (Fig. 4.96). Progressive assessment by tension stress maneuver is performed and the dissection proceeds as necessary. It may be necessary to perform some of the major bone cuts prior to a more extensive collateral release, especially when flexion contracture is present; release of the posteromedial capsule is recommended (Fig. 4.97). Removal of osteophytes – downsizing – should be performed at the same time. Preservation of the semimembranosus tendon is recommended (and important for stability) in all but the most severe cases. The joint space and ligaments are repeatedly examined in 0 degrees flexion, with the soft tissue tensed to determine which structures require further release. Occasionally, additional release in the area of the pes tendons and the superficial medial collateral ligament is required. Cruciate limitation to correction in the more severe varus cases is common. Further correction of the varus deformity will not be achieved until the posterior cruciate ligament is removed or released or lengthened.

Severe Cases

Additional release in the area of the pes tendons and the superficial medial collateral ligament is required. Release of the semimembranosus and of the posteromedial capsule is performed (Fig. 4.98). A greater degree of medial release subjects the prosthetic knee to a lateral subluxation. If the tendency of subluxation is found, then the only alternative for the surgeon would be resorting to a prosthesis with more constraint or some form of lateral ligament tightening or stabilizing procedure.

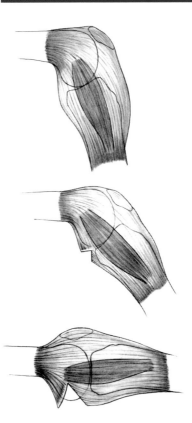

Fig. 4.97. Posteromedial capsule release in flexion contracture

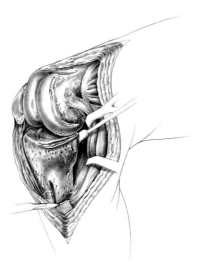

Fig. 4.98. In severe cases only, pes anserinus and if necessary semimembranosus pars directa release may be required

4.12 Severe Valgus: Management of Deep Structures

Peter A. Keblish, Jean-Louis Briard, Jens G. Boldt

The majority of valgus knees can be managed using the methods described in Sect. 4.4. The direct lateral approach provides many advantages, but medial approaches are often used, requiring IB II or more stabilized type prostheses, or posterior stabilized IB III or hinged prostheses, because many surgeons are unfamiliar with the soft tissue stability that can be achieved with the lateral approach. Deep releases will be described in this chapter. A considerable number of situations dictate an understanding of the lateral side if best outcomes are to be accomplished and/or potential catastrophes (wound, extensor tendon necrosis, etc.) avoided. The multiply operated knee with many and/or lateral-based incisions, often with knee contractures that fail to correct with the usual methods, presents a surgical challenge that requires more critical attention. If multiple incisions are present and standard medial approaches require undermining of the skin and rigid soft plane, there is a serious risk of devascularization and the most direct approach to the knee should be used. Observations from the Schulthess Clinic revealed that skin necrosis was always lateral to the skin incision, when the most lateral skin incision was not used.

When severe, fixed valgus deformity is not corrected following usual surgical measures, deep concave side releases are required if reasonably non-constrained total knee arthroplasty (TKA) prostheses are to be used. The problem usually presents as a failure to achieve enough lateral space in extension without excessive bone resection, which leads to predictable flexion gap instability and predictable flexion/extension instability. Deep lateral releases, which preserve posterolateral strength and stability (lateral collateral ligament (LCL), popliteus tendon arcuate complex) are required. Two basic options are available to address this problem: distal or proximal lengthening.

The standard "recommended" release is a pure soft tissue, sleeve, or osteoperiosteal stripping of the lateral femoral condyle. Our experience with this technique, which compromises the strength of the lateral ligament, has shown that posterolateral destabilization may occur, with resultant instability and poor outcomes. The problem has led to the development of two options, which preserve lateral complex strength and stability: deep distal LCL release in continuity via fibular head decompression (enucleation;

Keblish et al. 2002) and proximal lateral sliding condylotomy (Briard). These procedures will be described and illustrated. They are best utilized with a direct lateral approach.

Intra-articular Deep Layer

The popliteus tendon, LCL, fabellofibular ligament, arcuate ligament, and capsule form the posterolateral complex (Fig. 4.99). Anteriorly, the vastus lateralis (VL) inserts at the proximal patellar facet. The tendon of the VL is usually of substantial thickness and joins the lateral aspect of the central quadriceps (rectus tendon). This structure is covered by a capsular and/or synovial layer in the joint. The muscles, by definition, have an extra-articular origin. The LCL differs from the medial collateral ligament (MCL) in that its distal insertion is at the fibular head. The deep anterior and posterior lateral soft tissue layers are usually contracted to different degrees, depending on factors such as the underlying pathology, longevity of the deformity, bony pathology, and others. Management of superficial and deep layer contractures in valgus TKA must be understood, and represents a key to correction of tibial rotation, centralization of the patella, and achieving proper flexion/extension gap balancing. In either case, the direct lateral approach enhances exposure and provides other advantages, which will be discussed in the technique section.

Surgical Technique

When adequate extension space and valgus correction are not achieved after routine exposure with proximal iliotibial band release to the posterolateral corner, options of further soft tissue releases, tibial sleeve releases, or femoral condylotomy must be considered. Three techniques of deep distal and proximal lengthening releases for deep releases (steps 5–7) are suggested:

Step 1. Superficial longitudinal concave release: iliotibial band release/lengthening
Step 2. Lateral arthrotomy: transverse release: coronal plane Z-plasty
Step 3. Tibial sleeve release
Step 4. Patella dislocation: joint exposure (see Sect. 4.4)
Step 5. Deep concave releases
Step 6. Instrumentation/prosthetic insertion
Step 7. Soft tissue closure deep to superficial layer

Fig. 4.99. Deep posterolateral structures are illustrated. Some or all are
contracted or abnormal with fixed valgus deformity

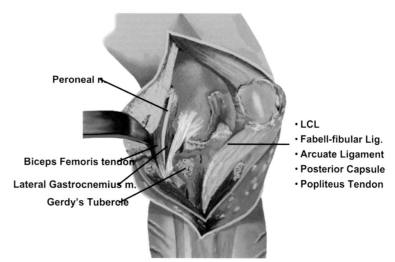

Peroneal n.

Biceps Femoris tendon

Lateral Gastrocnemius m.

Gerdy's Tubercle

- LCL
- Fabell-fibular Lig.
- Arcuate Ligament
- Posterior Capsule
- Popliteus Tendon

Technique Points

In lateral arthrotomy (deep layer), the superficial layer of the retinaculum is separated from the deep layer with a coronal plane Z-plasty, from superficial lateral to deep medial. Proximally, an oblique arthrotomy incision from lateral to medial takes advantage of
the laminated anatomy of the central quadriceps tendon. The VL tendon is non-yielding but substantially
thick and allows for a horizontal (coronal) plane expansion release as well as a longitudinal expansion as
shown. The VL tendon incision begins near the mus-
culotendonous junction and ends distally at the midcoronal plane of the patella insertion. The midportion (lateral retinaculum) separates naturally from the
deep capsule and fat pad. The capsule is incised from
the patella rim. The fat pad incision continues obliquely to the intermeniscal ligament, retaining about
50 % of the fat pad with the patella tendon and 50 %
with the lateral sleeve, which includes the lateral meniscus rim for increased soft tissue stability. The upper tibial sleeve release is considered to be part of the
required releases in virtually all fixed valgus knees,
whether performed from the lateral or medial side.
The technique is more direct with the lateral approach. If, following this release, a tight lateral space
in extension still exists, the distal LCL or femoral
condylotomy is to be considered. When adequate extension space to allow for full extension and valgus
correction is not achieved after routine exposure, including proximal iliotibial band release to the posterolateral corner, options of further bone, tibial sleeve,
or osteotomy or soft tissue releases must be considered. In a technique described by Buechel (1990),
concave side releases in severe valgus deformity include excision of the fibular head.

Type II Valgus with True Laxity or Pseudolaxity

Type II valgus with stretch-out of the medial structures can create instability in the mediolateral and rotational planes. Most pre-existing instabilities represent pseudolaxity and are corrected with the direct
lateral approach (when the medial side is left untouched) and a minimal medial tibial resection. True
medial instabilities due to incompetent soft tissue
structures can be treated with a combination of prosthetic implants such as the posterior stabilized or
varus/valgus constrained and/or proximal MCL advancement.

When using fixed bearing tibial implants, the rotation position of the tibial tray is critical. Rotating
bearings, with or without posterior stabilized or
varus/valgus constrained options, are preferable,
since they self-align to allow for optimum femorotibial interface positioning.

Patella bone bed treatment is important. The lateral facet is often flattened, thin, and/or distorted. If a
severely distorted patella is not seating well but has
adequate bone stalk, resurfacing is favored. However,
if there is any question regarding viability, tracking,
or bone-bed quality, the patella is best left unresurfaced.

Patella alta is more common in congenital/devel-
opmental valgus. Therefore, raising the joint line is
less critical and iatrogenic (problematic) patella baja
is not usually a problem. Autograft enhancement of
lateral defects, when present, is preferred over deeper
resections, which may compromise the flexion/exten-
sion gap stability. Referencing from the medial femoral condyle is recommended. Long-standing posterolateral contractures with severe rotation deformities
require more prospective releases and concern for

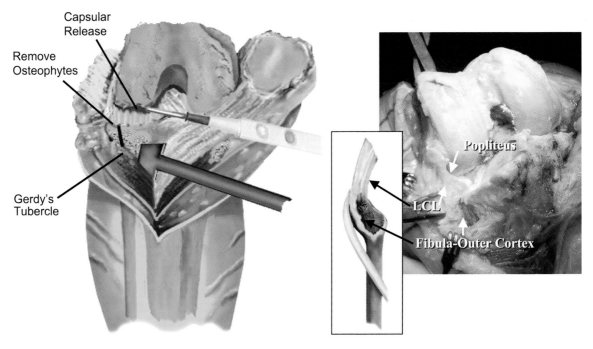

Capsular Release

Remove Osteophytes

Gerdy's Tubercle

Popliteus

LCL

Fibula-Outer Cortex

Fig. 4.100. Instrumentation with flexion/extension gap balancing. The deep distal concave lengthenings can be made prior to this step. However, the more extensive proximal osteotomies should be made following prosthetic insertion

peroneal nerve stretch and/or compression injury. The peroneal nerve can be exposed and decompressed proximally and/or a partial proximal fibulectomy performed as described previously. It is advised to maintain the knee in some flexion postoperatively to avoid tension on the peroneal nerve.

When performing extensive soft tissue dissection in a high-risk rheumatoid type (thin-skinned) patient or after some MCL tightening procedures, splinting for 2–3 days should be considered. In general, the rehabilitation is less intensive in this high-risk group, since achieving good range of motion with the lateral approach is seldom a problem.

In more severe fixed valgus and/or in extra-articular deformity, it may be necessary to lengthen or to slide the deep lateral structures and subsequently the posterior structures. Proximal and/or distal lengthening techniques can be used.

Distal LCL release

When required, direct exposure and removal of the inner proximal fibula (with retention of the outer periosteum and ligament attachments) allows for medial translation and a relative lengthening of the LCL, without the need for fixation. Enough length may be obtained by this maneuver, avoiding the need for femoral side releases. Distal LCL lengthening by this method is illustrated in Fig. 4.100. This is the preferred method to accomplish mild to moderate correction and can be performed before or after bone resections and trial implants.

Buechel (1990) has described a lateral exposure with a three-step release that varies somewhat, but shares the same basic principles.

Instrumentation and Fine-tuning Under Trial Reduction

Instrumentation with a flexion gap and femoral positioner allows for fine-tuning of soft tissue balancing. Flexion and extension gaps are checked with appropriate spacer blocks. The distal femoral resection angle may vary from 4 to 6 degrees and should relate to the hip-knee-ankle axis. Some valgus is tolerable, as patients' soft tissues and cosmetic appearance have adapted to this position over time. If stable gap balancing (in all planes) and/or failure to achieve full extension is not accomplished at this time, the more extensive femoral side releases will be required and are described below.

Femoral sleeve releases are required if severe contractures are present, and large lateral extension space is required. Two techniques are available.

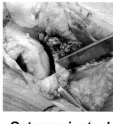
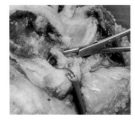
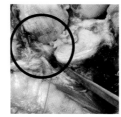
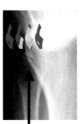

Osteoperiosteal   **Identify LCL**   **Preserve Popliteus**   **Excavate Fibular Head Preserve Outer Cortex**

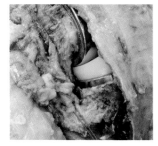
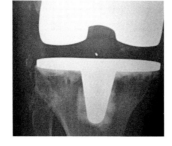
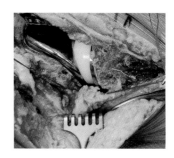

Fig. 4.101. Deep concave side release – distal option. If gap imbalance persists following appropriate level bone cuts, distal LCL lengthening is accomplished by excavating the fibular head and preserving the distal LCL insertion with the periosteum and outer fibular cortex. Note fibular fragmentation and excellent balance on postoperative x-ray

Osteoperiosteal release (limited osteotomy) or soft tissue sleeve release (preferably without the popliteus insertion) extends proximally (Fig. 4.101). The sleeve release is the more commonly recommended method, but it can lead to compromised ligament attachment and resultant instability. A proximal periosteal sleeve or limited osteotomy may not be very strong because of the absence of continuous soft tissue attachments.

The sliding lateral condyle osteotomy has been described by Briard to overcome the potential for lateral instability. The osteotomy allows for a strong and stable retention of femoral soft tissue (LCL and popliteus) attachments with correction of soft tissue contractures and achievement of an adequate extension gap. The osteotomy steps are outlined in Fig. 4.102. The initial cut is performed in the sagittal plane (just outside the anchoring hole that preserves a large bone segment (with ligament attachments), which can be inset into the lateral condyle of the femoral implant and fixed securely. Extension of the knee allows the osteotomy fragment to migrate distally to the appropriate position, achieving correction of the coronal deformity. Resection and contouring of the distal bony fragment (preserving the ligament attachments of the popliteus and LCL) allows the large bony fragment to self-adjust (at the proper tension). The fragment is then inset and fixed with one or two screws inside the housing of the lateral condyle of the prosthesis, which ensures stability.

Trial component insertion is recommended in order to check position, stability, and mobility prior to permanent prosthetic insertion. Soft tissue sleeve closure is accomplished in flexion. The expanded soft tissue closure is completed using sutures of choice proximally. The distal (bony) portion of the iliotibial band is re-attached with trans-osseous sutures. Prosthetic joint seal can be accomplished in all cases. Use of the fat pad may be required, especially in soft-tissue-deficient rheumatoid knees.

Clinical Case Example

Severe valgus correction in a 63-year-old white female resulted in excellent patellofemoral tracking and femorotibial stability at 3 years. The patella was left unresurfaced. If satisfactory correction is accomplished following the tibial sleeve, capsular/posterior cruciate ligament releases, and downsizing maneuvers, proceed with bony resections and fine-tune the ligament releases at the time of trial reduction. If the lateral structures remain tight and do not allow for satisfactory varus/valgus balance, proceed with distal LCL lengthening (fibula or proximal lengthening femoral side).

Osteoperiosteal ⬅ OPTIONS ➡ Epicondylectomy

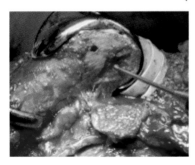

**Sleeve Advancement
Fix to Bone**

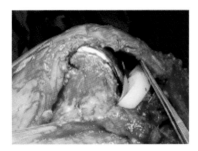

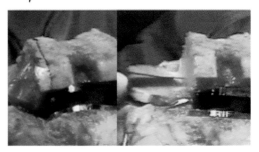

Trim Bone Distal to LCL

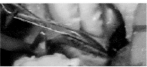

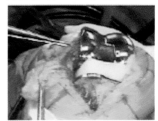

ADVANCE - INSET - FIX

Fig. 4.102. Deep concave side release – proximal options. If the knee cannot be fully extended because of severe lateral contractures, proximal femoral release options include: (1) the more commonly performed soft tissue or small osteoperiosteal sleeve release with/without reattachment (especially with the medial approach); or (2) sliding lateral condyle osteotomy that preserves soft tissue attachments and allows for extensive correction without loss of stability. X-ray example of severe valgus correction with lateral and tibial tubercle osteotomy

When concave side releases of the LCL, popliteus, and secondary structures are required, they can be performed prior to or following trial reduction. Keep in mind that the LCL affects both the flexion and extension gap stability, while the popliteus tendon affects flexion and rotation stability. The more commonly recommended technique (with the medial approach) is a soft tissue release of the iliotibial band and posterolateral complex from the femur. The sliding lateral condyle osteotomy with a more extensive bone segment is a newer concept that has the advantage of maintaining a strong proximal soft tissue ligament attachment. When correcting a valgus deformity, distal femoral resection of 6–7 degrees is often acceptable because it allows for improvement of extension gap balancing and tensioning of intact medial structures. Slight residual valgus is cosmetically acceptable in the patient with long-standing valgus deformity.

Long-standing posterolateral contractures with severe rotation deformities require more prospective releases and concern for peroneal nerve stretch and/or compression injury. The peroneal nerve can be exposed and decompressed proximally and/or a partial proximal fibulectomy can be performed as described previously. It is advisable to maintain the knee in some flexion postoperatively to avoid tension on the peroneal nerve. When performing extensive soft tissue dissection in a high-risk rheumatoid (thin-skinned) patient or after some MCL tightening procedures, splinting for 2–3 days should be considered. In general, the rehabilitation is less intensive in this high-risk group, since achieving good range of motion with the lateral approach is seldom a problem.

Fixed valgus deformity presents a major challenge in TKA. The literature suggests that correction of fixed valgus deformities via the standard medial parapatella approach leads to higher failure rates, primarily at the patellofemoral joint. A common factor in all reports is the medial surgical approach. Therefore, the surgeon should be familiar with and consider the direct lateral approach in challenging total knee replacements that include: (1) fixed valgus deformity with patella subluxation; (2) partially correctable valgus with lateral orientation and/or patella subluxation; (3) varus knee with severe tibial rotation, increased Q-angle, tight retinaculum, and iliotibial band with patella tilt and/or subluxation; (4) grossly unstable knee in a rheumatoid patient with expanded suprapatellar pouch; (5) previous lateral incisions in a multiply operated knee when skin is at risk (with undermining); (6) lateral unicompartmental replacement; and (7) high tibial osteotomy conversion to TKA, especially if there is a lateral incision and/or retained metal.

Bibliography

Arnold MP, Friederich NF, Widmer H, Muller W (1998) Patellar substitution in total knee prosthesis – is it important? Orthopade 27:637–641

Buechel FF (1990) A sequential three-step lateral release for correcting fixed valgus knee deformities during total knee arthroplasty. Clin Orthop 260:170–175

Burki H, von Knoch M, Heiss C, Drobny T, Munzinger U (1999) Lateral approach with osteotomy of the tibial tubercle in primary total knee arthroplasty. Clin Orthop 362:156–161

Fiddian NJ, Blakeway C, Kumar A (1998) Replacement arthroplasty of the valgus knee. A modified lateral capsular approach with repositioning of vastus lateralis. JBJS [Br] 80: 859–861

Insall JN, Scott WN, Keblish PA et al (1994) Total knee arthroplasty exposures and soft tissue balancing. In: Insall JN, Scott WN (eds) Videobook of knee surgery. Lippincott, Philadelphia

Keblish PA (1985) Valgus deformity in TKR: the lateral retinacular approach. Orthop Trans 9:28

Keblish PA (1991) The lateral approach to the valgus knee: surgical technique and analysis of 53 cases with over two-year follow-up evaluation. Clin Orthop 271:52–62

Keblish PA, Boldt JG, Varma C, Briard JL (2002) Soft-tissue balancing in fixed valgus TKA: methods of achieving concave side releases. Presented at AAOS 2002 scientific exhibit, Dallas, Texas

Krackow KA, Jones MM, Teeny SM et al (1991) Primary total knee arthroplasty in patients with fixed valgus deformity. Clin Orthop 273:9–18

Lootvoet L, Blouard E, Himmer O, Ghosez JP (1997) Complete knee prosthesis in severe genu valgum. Retrospective review of 90 knees surgically treated through the anterio-external approach. Acta Orthop Belg 63:278–286

Merkow RL, Soudry M, Insall JN (1985) Patellar dislocation following total knee replacement. J Bone Joint Surg Am 67: 1321–1327

Ranawat CS (1988) Total-condylar knee arthroplasty for valgus and combined valgus-flexion deformity of the knee. Tech Orthop 3:67–76

Scapinelli R (1967) Blood supply of the human patella. J Bone Joint Surg 49B:563

Tsai CL, Chen CH, Liu TK (2001) Lateral approach without ligament release in total knee arthroplasty; new concepts in the surgical technique. Artif Org 25:638–643

Whiteside LA (1993) Correction of ligament and bone defects in total arthroplasty of the severely valgus knee. Clin Orthop 288:234–245

Wolff AM, Hungerford DS, Krackow KA et al (1989) Osteotomy of the tibial tubercle during total knee replacement. J Bone Joint Surg Am 71:848–852

4.13 Bone Defect Management

Urs K. Munzinger, Peter A. Keblish, Jens G. Boldt

Bone defects in the proximal tibia and distal femur are common and may present as obvious or more subtle, intra- or extra-articular and may or may not be structurally significant. When superimposed on osteopenic bone structure, these defects and their management may determine the success or failure of a given case. The evaluation and decision of how to manage these defects becomes an intraoperative decision in both primary and revision total knee arthroplasty (TKA). This chapter addresses the index or primary operation, with emphasis on the use of readily available autograft material (Fig. 4.103). Revision situations require more extensive approaches with use of stemmed, shimmed, and specialized devices, allografts, or a combination of structural grafts, reinforced cement utilizing re-bar screws, etc. Basic principles and goals prevail with primary and revision TKA, namely to achieve a strong biomechanical bony structure on which to anchor the prosthetic device.

The evolution of TKA principles was greatly enhanced by the development of biological fixation, which dictated an improvement in technique to provide optimal implant stability. A better understanding of bone biology and need for structural integrity has stimulated the use of bone graft enhancement, which is required in potentially and/or obviously weakened areas of the distal femur and proximal tibia.

Principles of Utilizing Autograft

Contained isolated defects with stable cortices are best treated with cancellous autograft material that can be milled or rongeured into aggregate material, which is compliant and compacts easily (Fig. 4.104).

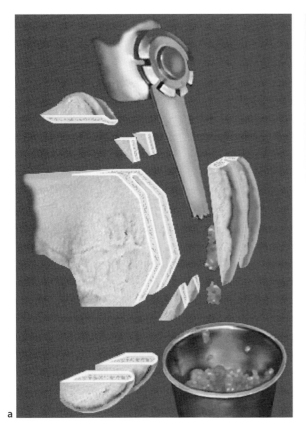

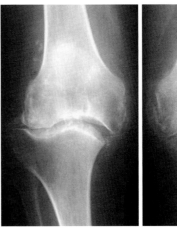

Fig. 4.104. Bilateral varus knee deformities with typical erosive medial tibial slope-off defects, usually combined with soft lateral compartment bone and competent mediocollateral ligaments

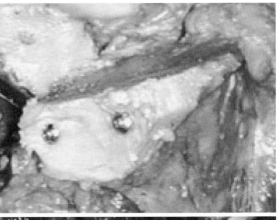

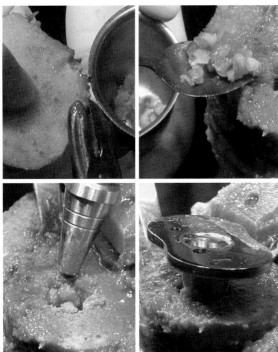

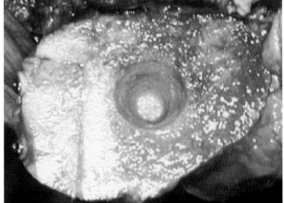

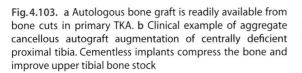

Fig. 4.103. a Autologous bone graft is readily available from bone cuts in primary TKA. **b** Clinical example of aggregate cancellous autograft augmentation of centrally deficient proximal tibia. Cementless implants compress the bone and improve upper tibial bone stock

Fig. 4.105. Medial slope-off deformity of less than 15 degrees treated with a wedge autograft that is fixed with two horizontally placed cortical screws

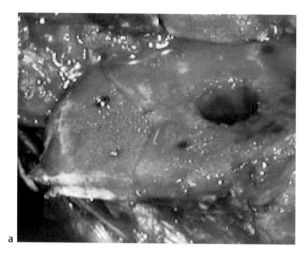

a

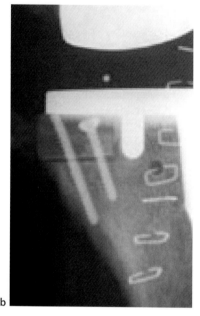

b

Fig. 4.106. a Autograft inset with key-in technique for slope-off non-contained defect. **b** Postoperative radiograph demonstrating block autograft technique

Contained defects with marginal cortical support can be supported with corticocancellous struts removed or preserved from the bone resections (distal femur best).

Non-contained defects are most common with severe varus knees on the tibial side in primary TKA. Options of treatment include corticocancellous strut grafting (Fig. 4.105), inset "key-in" with screw fixation (Fig. 4.106), cement fill with or without buttress (rebar) screw augmentation. The issue of graft fixation depends on factors of size, location, and possibly whether or not cement is being used. Screw fixation techniques work well when applied to larger fragments. Smaller, contained grafts need no internal fix-

ation. Alternative methods include use of prosthetic shims or augments to filling uncontained defects, and newer bone graft substitutes for contained defects. These methods are more costly, as they require use of additional implant material.

Femoral Bone Loss

Femoral bone loss is less common in primary TKA, but extreme cases may present primarily in post-traumatic osteonecrosis and long-standing severe valgus. These non-contained defects are managed using the methods illustrated. The majority of difficult primary knees with good bone stock can be managed without long-stemmed prostheses and/or augments. However, this remains a surgeon's choice. Autograft is readily available, therefore economical, cost-effective, and has the advantages noted; primarily improving "biological" structural support. The surgeon must weigh the cost, practicality, and time requirement in the choice of surgical options in bone defect management.

The management choices include cement filling, bone grafting, use of a more built-up or shimmed prosthesis, and stemmed partially constrained or constrained implant if the combination of soft tissue and bone correction is adequate. In cases with a severely worn condyle, the cuts are normal on the opposite side with little to no bone resection from the hypoplastic condyle (intraop. 21056). Cemented and cementless femoral components can be utilized to stabilize distal grafts, bone grafts with cement fill or buttress screws with cement. Cases with major femoral bone loss are analogous to many revision cases. Basic principles should be honored, even in very large defects when prosthetic augmentation is required; available autograft material should be utilized in the methods described, as biologically proven autograft material improves the underlying bone deficiency. The combination of impaction grafting (auto- or allograft) has a proven track record in total hip arthroplasty and TKA.

Tibial Defects

The pathology–anatomy of most tibial defects includes peripheral depression or slope deformities secondary to wear and possibly avascular necrosis, contained midplateau wear areas, and isolated cystic defects. The issue of resection level with regard to planning and instrumentation is discussed in

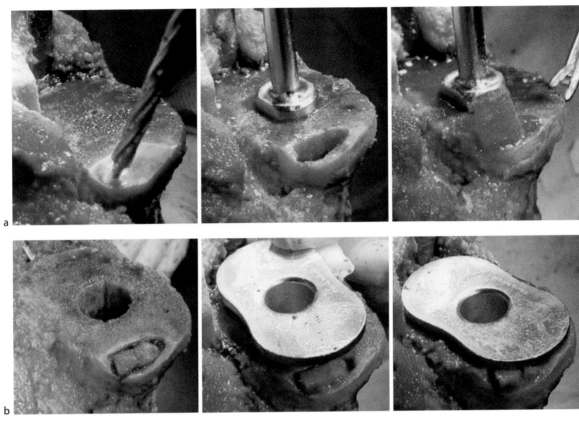

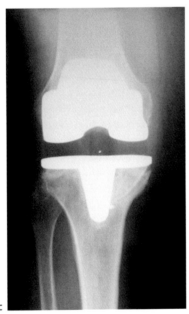

Fig. 4.107. a Technique of corticocancellous strut autografting of partially constrained posteromedial tibial defect, b which is impacted utilizing the final component. c Immediate postoperative x-ray of corticocancellous strut grafting supporting incompletely contained medial wall plus central impaction graft without requiring screw fixation

Sect. 4.1. The best approach is a normal conservative resection (Fig. 4.107) while addressing the resulting area of depression with either grafting, prosthetic filling, or some combination as described. Bone grafting in combination with a normal level tibial resection, rather than a lower resection (cemented or uncemented) is our preference. Postoperative x-ray films confirm an improved biological appearance and interface fixation in grafted cases compared with cemented cases in terms of lucent line formation and bone quality. Metallic wedge substitution may be easier and may prove to be as durable in slope deformities, but long-term results are not available.

The management of contained defects on the tibia is more straightforward. The rounded hole is converted to a circular shaped depression with a flat base and vertical walls. Technically, this is most easily done using a cylindrically shaped high-speed burr. Drilling and curetting of base exposes the vascularized substrate for graft impaction. Internal fixation is seldom necessary, as the contained grafts are mechanically stable.

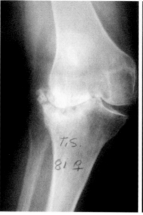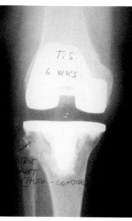

Fig. 4.108. Valgus knee deformity with collapse of lateral tibial plateau treated utilizing supportive corticocancellous strut grafting in combination with cement. Radiographic result 8 years postoperatively

Angular Deformity

The problems encountered in the management of structural deformity in TKA are interesting and challenging. Cases with major deformity frequently present technical challenges for achieving proper alignment and ligament balance (Fig. 4.108). In the extreme, such challenges are essentially eliminated if one resorts to the use of highly constrained or hinged prostheses. Because of the expected and observed problems of loosening and bone loss as a result of higher stress (GSB-Wechsel) at prosthesis-cement-bone interfaces, most surgeons seek to avoid the highly constrained components. Current teaching encourages surgeons to follow a general principle of minimizing prosthetic constraint whenever possible.

Bone cuts and prosthetic joint surfaces must have the proper angular orientation (respective femoral and tibial shaft axes) for the knee to assume a proper alignment. Properly oriented joint surfaces may imply normal alignment, but they do not automatically recreate or maintain proper ligament balance. The goal is for the prosthetic knee to remain stable throughout a maximum range of motion, therefore requiring precise soft tissue balancing. Minor degrees of instability (increased anteroposterior drawer or increased medial or lateral instability) may be well tolerated for the short term, but progressive ligament instability is becoming recognized as a long-

term problem, and is related to many factors including bone defect management and prevention of loosening or subsidence.

Unicompartmental Bone Loss without Contracture

To the extent that the loss is present at the tibia, the deformity would be evident in both extension and flexion. On the femoral side, loss distally would appear as deformity in extension; loss from a posterior condyle would appear as subtle deformity in flexion. The deformity would be evident on weight bearing, and it would be passively correctable to neutral alignment (i.e. the collateral ligaments would be out to normal length when correct alignment is achieved). The deformity is one of bone loss and not soft tissue involvement, and it will automatically yield to replacement or reconstruction of the bone loss. This deformity is amenable to unicompartmental replacement or medial open wedge osteotomy, especially in a very young patient.

With the occurrence of abnormal concavity at the side of compression and development of a convexity at the opposite compartment, tension resulting at the periphery of the convex side can lead to alternation of the collateral ligament complex. As this knee is examined, a sense of obvious ligament instability is present on varus-valgus testing and lateral tibial subluxation may be present. The ligaments on the originally concave side are out to normal length, but the collateral complex at the convex side is lax and slight lateral tibial translation is commonly seen. At this point, unicompartmental knee arthroplasty is probably ill advised and TKA the treatment of choice. Instability of the convex side is correctable with TKA and consistent with good function by releasing the ligament structures of the concave side until there is soft tissue balance between the two sides.

Unicompartmental Bone Loss with Contracture

Asymmetrical wear in one compartment and secondary contracture of collateral, and perhaps to a lesser degree, contracture of cruciate structures results in a fixed contracture. The deformity is apparent on weight bearing. Ligament testing may reveal normal stability or some laxity on the concave side, but there is incomplete correction.

Management is undertaken by concave release, i.e. release that would lead to perfect collateral ligament balance, bringing the tibia back out to normal length and position with respect to the femur. Not releasing the concave side first may lead to a tibial cut that is relatively more distal, resulting in an (iatrogenic) asymmetric ligament imbalance. The concave side remains tighter than the convex side, creating high contact stress and potential for instability and early wear or failure. A concave bone loss with a concave contracture may eventually lead to a convex soft tissue stretching. Reconstruction with concave release will usually balance the opposite pseudolaxity or reversible ligament instability commonly seen in the type II valgus medial side. Cruciate contracture may limit correction and will need to be released in these fixed contracture type cases. These topics are covered in more detail in chapters dealing with the valgus knee and varus with severe flexion contracture.

Bony Deformity with Concave Contracture

The general bony deformity (metaphyseal widening) with a concave bone loss and a concave tissue contracture is the most common deformity seen in the typical fixed varus osteoarthritic knee. In addition to the angular deformity of the joint line with respect to the shaft, there is a relative deformity of the epicondylar–ligament–capsular origin. This appearance is most commonly seen in congenitally varus deformed femura, where the distal femoral joint line has a relative varus alignment with respect to the femoral shaft and the tibial plateau is neutral to slight valgus. With time and progression of the degenerative process, the wear is proportionately greater at the concave side, and progressive contracture of the soft tissue on the concave side develops.

The knee appears deformed whether the patient is supine or standing. The deformity is increased with weight bearing and is dependent on the amount of "pseudolaxity" that develops as a result of excessive joint surface wear rather than soft tissue contracture.

Reconstruction involves asymmetric resection of the medial and lateral femoral condyles and it also necessitates asymmetric component placement with respect to the epicondylar axis. This placement is more valgus and the epicondyle of the concave side remains in the proper relationship, whereas the convex side is slightly closer (more valgus) to the prosthetic surface, as more bone is resected. Conversely, the convex epicondyle is in the proper relationship, but the epicondyle (ligament origin) of the concave side is further from the prosthetic joint line when more medial bone is resected (valgus knee). Therefore, subtle changes in the rotational axes occur with required resections in most deformities.

To the degree that concave releases may sufficiently achieve balance at the convex aspect, prosthetic components would be expected to correct convex ligament instability. If correction of the deformity is not achieved via soft tissue release, relative laxity on the convex side will be a potential consequence. Relative laxity on the convex side may be ignored, or may be treated by more significant release on the concave side or by a ligament tightening on the convex side. It may be necessary to consider using a prosthesis with increased constraint (such as posterior stabilized or varus/valgus constrained) in these types of deformity. Mobile bearing knee prostheses with excellent congruity are most beneficial in addressing these subtle alterations in TKA.

Bone defects occur more commonly at the tibia than the femur in advanced degenerative arthritis of the knee joint. Whereas small defects may be sufficiently and safely addressed with slight increase of resection levels, larger defects require other methods such as prosthetic augments and/or bone autografting, with or without cement. Autograft is recommended as the method of choice, as it is a proven biologic and cost-effective technique.

There are three basic types of bone deficiencies: contained, uncontained and structural defects. Most defects are contained defects that are easily treated with readily available autograft. Larger, uncontained defects are preferably addressed with stemmed components and corticocancellous (strut) autograft augments (Fig. 4.109), or buttress screws with cement

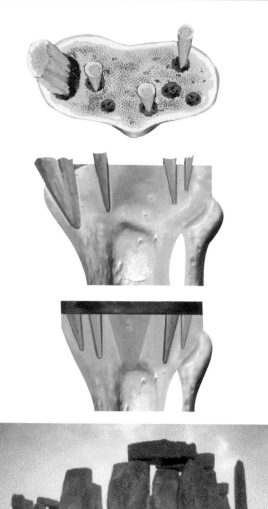

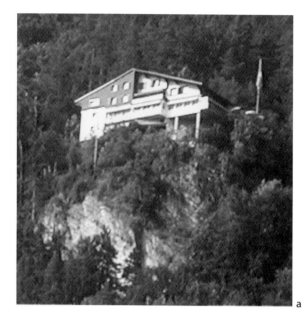

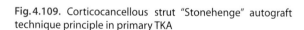

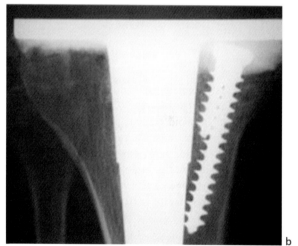

Fig. 4.109. Corticocancellous strut "Stonehenge" autograft technique principle in primary TKA

Fig. 4.110. a Constructional example of supporting (buttress) house pillars used in the Swiss mountains. b Radiographic example of buttress screw supports in a bone-deficient primary tibia

(Fig. 4.110) and revision stems. Bone defects that include epicondyles, collateral ligaments, tendon insertions, or the diaphysis, as often found in revision situations, require composite allografts and stemmed prostheses with or without shims.

Midsize defects may also be treated with metal or acrylic augments (Fig. 4.111) and assisted soft tissue balancing. Augments do not restore lost bone and do not depend on vascularized host bone as much as bone graft. Block and wedge augments may be superior to autografts in cases with osteopenic bone quality, but have their limitations. Wedge augments work well up to 10–15 degrees of slope, but should be re-

placed by block augments or block inset autografts with or without screw fixation and stemmed components if the slope exceeds 15 degrees.

Autologous bone graft is an attractive and recommended alternative to metal or acrylic augments and has the potential to restore bone stock. Incorporation and remodeling depend on healthy and vascularized "host" bone. The shape and size of autologous bone grafts follow basic mechanical principles and require stable fixation. The tibial surface should be prepared in a fashion that allows access of viable cancellous bone to the bone graft for incorporation. Wedge or block autografts are best secured with screws, while

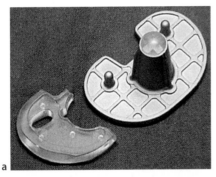
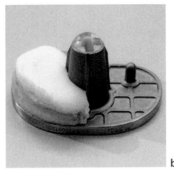
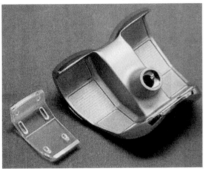
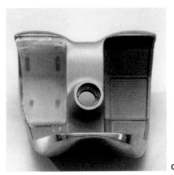

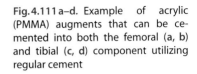

Fig. 4.111 a–d. Example of acrylic (PMMA) augments that can be cemented into both the femoral (a, b) and tibial (c, d) component utilizing regular cement

corticocancellous strut grafts do not require fixation, which is a distinct advantage. When cement is used, it is important to avoid cement entering the interface between host bone and autograft. Sclerotic bone surfaces do not provide sufficient potential for bone ingrowth and should, therefore, be drilled and/or removed to encourage cancellous bone access. Poor supporting bone quality in osteopenic cases may require general bone-enhancing techniques independent of type of augments. Cement fillings alone can be used successfully in small central defects, but are mechanically inferior to other options and, therefore not recommended in larger defects unless buttress (re-bar) type screws and stemmed prosthetic devices are utilized.

Ligament-stable knees, which have sufficient host bone–prosthetic contact areas available for prosthetic seating, may well suffice with primary implants. However, uncontained defects may require stemmed components or more constraint type devices (posterior stabilized, varus/valgus constrained). In destructive situations with ligament incompetence, semiconstrained to constrained components (central stems) are recommended as devices of choice. In cases with massive bone destruction, structural allografts (composites) should be utilized, even in primary TKA. The goal of bone defect management in TKA is to achieve "lifetime" structural support for the prosthetic implant.

Bibliography

Aglietti P, Buzzi R, Scrobe F (1991) Autologous bone grafting for medial tibial defects in total knee arthroplasty. J Arthroplasty 6:287–294

Altchek D, Sculco TP, Rawlins B (1989) Autogenous bone grafting for severe angular deformity in total knee arthroplasty. Arthroplasty 4:151–155

Boldt J, Munzinger U, Keblish P (2002) Biological fixation in cementless TKA. Results of 255 cases after 2 to 15 year follow-up. AAOS, abstract P254

Brand MG, Daley RJ, Ewald FC, Scott RD (1989) Tibial tray augmentation with modular metal wedges for tibial bone stock deficiency. Clin Orthop 248:71–9

Cameron HU, Turner DG, Cameron GM (1988) Results of bone grafting of tibial defects in uncemented total knee replacements. Can J Surg 31:30–32

Dennis DA (1998) Repairing minor bone defects: augmentation and autograft. Orthopedics 21:1036–1038

Dorr LD, Ranawat CS, Sculco TA, McKaskill B, Orisek BS (1986) Bone graft for tibial defects in total knee arthroplasty. Clin Orthop 205:153–165

Franceschina MJ, Swienckowski JJ (1999) Correction of varus deformity with tibial flip autograft technique in total knee arthroplasty. J Arthroplasty 14:172–174

Gorlich Y, Lebek S, Reichel H (1999) Substitution of tibial bony defects with allogeneic and autogeneic cancellous bone: encouraging preliminary results in 18 knee replacements. Arch Orthop Trauma Surg 119:220–222

Hernigou P, Ma W (2001) Open wedge tibial osteotomy with acrylic bone cement as bone substitute. Knee 8:103–110

Laskin RS (1989) Total knee arthroplasty in the presence of large bony defects of the tibia and marked knee instability. Clin Orthop 248:66–70

Lindstrand A, Hansson U, Toksvig-Larsen S, Ryd L (1999) Major bone transplantation in total knee arthroplasty: a 2- to 9-year radiostereometric analysis of tibial implant stability. J Arthroplasty 14:144–148

Loon CJ, de Waal Malefijt MC, Verdonschot N, Buma P, van der Aa AJ, Huiskes R (1999) Morsellized bone grafting compensates for femoral bone loss in revision total knee arthroplasty. An experimental study. Biomaterials 20:85–89

Loon CJ, Wijers MM, de Waal Malefijt MC, Buma P, Veth RP (1999) Femoral bone grafting in primary and revision total knee arthroplasty. Acta Orthop Belg 65:357–363

Loon CJ, de Waal Malefijt MC, Buma P, Stolk T, Verdonschot N, Tromp AM, Huiskes R, Barneveld A (2000) Autologous morsellised bone grafting restores uncontained femoral bone defects in knee arthroplasty. An in vivo study in horses. J Bone Joint Surg Br 82:436–444

Parks NL, Engh GA (1997) The Ranawat Award. Histology of nine structural bone grafts used in total knee arthroplasty. Cin Orthop 345:17–23

Ries MD (1996) Impacted cancellous autograft for contained bone defects in total knee arthroplasty. Am J Knee Surg 9: 51–54

Ritter MA (1986) Screw and cement fixation of large defects in total knee arthroplasty. J Arthroplasty 1:125–129

Rosenberg AG (1997) The use of bone graft for managing bone defects in complex total knee arthroplasty (review). Am J Knee Surg 10:42–48

Sayampanathan SR, Ali MA (1997) Reconstruction of a medial tibial plateau defect using a "pillar" bone graft – a report of two knee reconstructions. Singapore Med J 38:295–296

Smith S, Naima VS, Freeman MA (1999) The natural history of tibial radiolucent lines in a proximally cemented stemmed total knee arthroplasty. J Arthroplasty 14:3–8

Stuchin SA, Ruoff M, Matarese W (1991) Cementless total knee arthroplasty in patients with inflammatory arthritis and compromised bone. Clin Orthop 273:42–51

Stuchin SA (1993) Allografting in total knee replacement arthroplasty (review). Semin Arthroplasty 4:117–122

Watanabe W, Sato K, Itoi E (2001) Autologous bone grafting without screw fixation for tibial defects in total knee arthroplasty. J Orthop Sci 6:481–486

Whiteside LA (1989) Cementless reconstruction of massive tibial bone loss in revision total knee arthroplasty. Clin Orthop 248:80–86

Windsor RE, Insall JN, Sculco TP (1986) Bone grafting of tibial defects in primary and revision total knee arthroplasty. Clin Orthop 205:132–137

4.14 Conversion of Knee Fusion to Total Knee Arthroplasty

Jens G. Boldt, Thomas Henkel

Takedown of any arthrodesed knee to total joint replacement is a challenging and technically demanding procedure with a reported high failure rate. However, some patients wish to have a moveable knee joint despite in-depth counselling about being much worse off after surgery. It is recommend that, if considered, a conversion of fused knees to total knee arthroplasty (TKA) should be performed only in carefully selected cases and in highly motivated patients, who comprehend the procedure and have realistic expectations.

Renewed mobility of a fused knee joint correlates with increased pain on walking. Postoperative problems include skin necrosis, extensor mechanism contracture, insufficient collateral ligaments and arthrofibrosis. Few reports are available in the literature and clinical outcomes are rarely successful. The best results, reported by Cameron (1996), revealed a success rate of ten out of 17 patients, with a postoperative complication rate of 53%. Another study reported just two patients with excellent results without postoperative complications. Mahomed et al. (1994) described a technique of preoperative soft tissue expansion with good results in two patients. We evaluate the clinical and radiographic midterm results of all consecutive patients who had undergone conversion of knee joint arthrodesis to TKA in a large joint replacement center.

Between 1984 and 1998, seven TKAs in seven patients with previously fused knee joints were performed by two senior surgeons. Demographics included six women and one man with a mean age of 58 years (range 40–72) at time of surgery. The mean time since fusion was 28 years (range 4–47) and the time since fusion varied from 4 to 47 years. The reason for the initial fusion was infection in five cases (two tuberculosis, three staphylococci) and posttraumatic arthritis in a further two cases. Previous fusion was performed with one or two plates in three patients (Fig. 4.112) and screws or pins in four patients. One patient had a previous patellectomy. Patients' dissatisfaction with their ability to perform activities of daily living was the predominant reason for "takedown" of the fused knee joint. Patients with neuromuscular disease, poor general health conditions, persistent local infection and non-realistic expectations were advised against a takedown procedure.

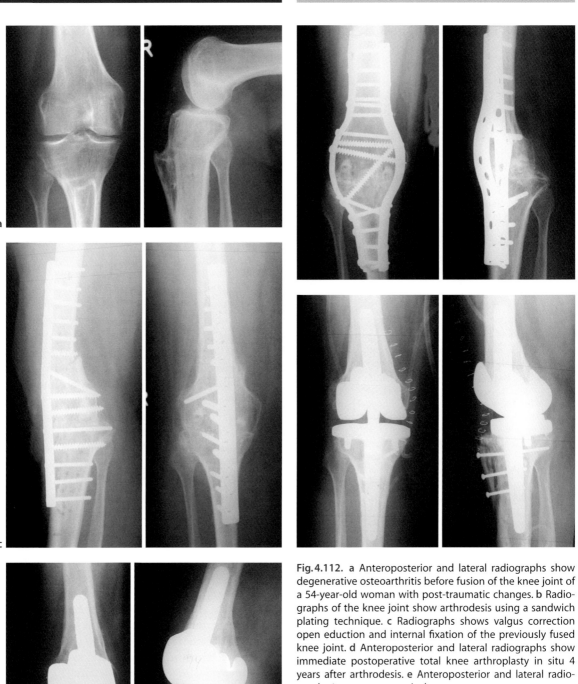

Fig. 4.112. a Anteroposterior and lateral radiographs show degenerative osteoarthritis before fusion of the knee joint of a 54-year-old woman with post-traumatic changes. b Radiographs of the knee joint show arthrodesis using a sandwich plating technique. c Radiographs shows valgus correction open eduction and internal fixation of the previously fused knee joint. d Anteroposterior and lateral radiographs show immediate postoperative total knee arthroplasty in situ 4 years after arthrodesis. e Anteroposterior and lateral radiographs 1 year postoperatively

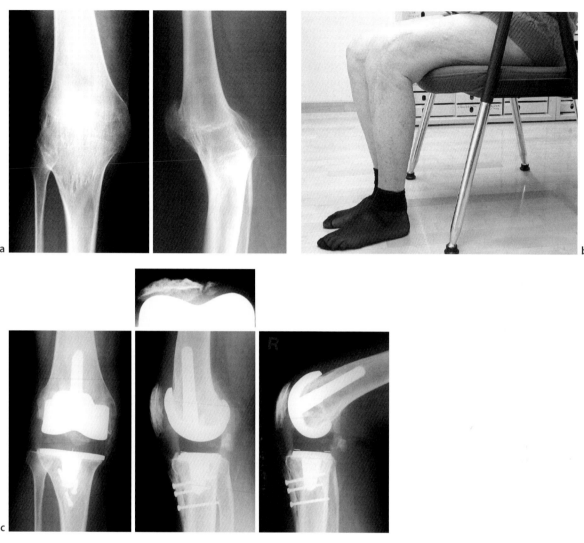

Fig. 4.113. a Anteroposterior and lateral radiographs show post-tuberculosis arthritis 44 years after knee joint fusion in a 26-year-old woman. **b** Radiographs 2 years postoperatively with good clinical result. **c** Excellent clinical result with 90° active ROM, walking distance more than 2 km, and satisfactory ability to perform activities of daily living

Operative Technique

A tibial tubercle osteotomy, as described in Sect. 4.5, was performed in all patients and was reattached with two or three cortical screws. Four patients had a bony fusion between the patella and the femur and two patients had a fibrous ankylosis of the patella, which required . The fusion site between the femur and tibia was identified by comparing intraoperative bony landmarks with radiographs and takedown of the fusion was carried out with an oscillating saw. The prosthesis was unconstrained (Fig. 4.113) in four patients (LCS, De Puy, Warsaw, USA) and constrained (AGC Dual Articular, Biomet, Warsaw, USA) in three patients. The tibial component was cemented in four patients (in all unconstrained prostheses) and the femoral component in three patients. The patella was resurfaced in two cases. In one patient the medial collateral ligament complex was absent and was reconstructed with a synthetic band. One thin patellar tendon was reinforced by an artificial ligament.

Continuous passive motion of the knee from 0 to 90 degrees was employed on the first postoperative day, followed by intensive physiotherapy. Preventive measures against thromboembolism were commenced 1 day preoperatively with low molecular weight heparin followed by cumarine on the 4th postoperative day until full weight bearing was permitted. Partial weight bearing was allowed in the first 8 weeks postoperatively. Progression to full weight bearing was permitted when the tibial tubercle osteotomy showed signs of bony healing on plain radiographs.

The average length of follow-up was 56 months (range 12–161). No patient was lost to follow-up. The modified Hospital for Special Surgery (HSS) score was used for clinical evaluation (maximum score 100 points; pain 30 points). The patient subjective assessment was graded as excellent, satisfied, non-committal or disappointed. Radiographs (anteroposterior, lateral and axial views) were reviewed for component positioning, joint axes and radiolucent lines.

The mean modified HSS score improved from 54 before TKA surgery to 68 points at the latest follow-up. The mean pain score decreased from 22.5 to 19 points. On walking, two patients had slight pain and three patients had moderate pain. Mean range of motion (ROM) at follow-up was 74 degrees (range 55–90). The patients' subjective ratings were "excellent" in two cases, "satisfied" in three cases, and "disappointed" in two cases. The latter underwent refusion. No progressive radiographic lucent lines were observed in any of the cases.

Complications

Of the seven knee joints, six underwent further surgery. Three patients with arthrofibrosis were treated with open arthrolysis (one patient with an additional VY quadriceps plasty). All patients had at least two operations prior to conversion. Two cases with lateral skin necrosis required a lateral gastrocnemius flap. Two of the three patients who were fused with one or two metal plates developed skin necrosis after TKA and required a lateral gastrocnemius flap. In one patient the skin coverage was performed with a gastrocnemius flap 3 months postoperatively, which developed chronic deep infection despite longstanding antibiotic treatment. This case ultimately required refusion 1 year later. Another case with a lateral gastrocnemius flap had gained 65 degrees ROM by 55 months follow-up.

All tibial osteotomies healed without complication. The patella was present in all but one case. One patient with an absent patella lever-arm mechanism reached 55 degrees of ROM at follow-up and was able actively to elevate the knee in extension. One patient with a very thin patellar tendon underwent reinforcement with an artificial ligament. At follow-up she had 85 degrees of flexion and full extension. A magnetic resonance imaging (MRI) investigation was carried out in the last two cases prior to conversion surgery

and was considered to improve preoperative evaluation and understanding of the integrity of extensor mechanism and both collateral ligaments.

Two TKAs underwent refusion, one after 12 months because of chronic bacteriological infection after delayed soft tissue healing and gastrocnemius flap revision and the second after 2.5 years because of persistent and painful collateral ligament instability in a mobile bearing knee prosthesis. One patient underwent neurolysis of the fibular nerve for painful paresis, which occurred postoperatively. At the time of revision (3.5 years postoperatively), the nerve was found to be entrapped in fibrotic scar tissue at the level of the fibular head and was exposed with limited success.

Conversion of formal knee joint fusion to TKA is a challenging procedure and is seldom reported in the literature. The main complaints of patients with fused knee joints appear to be the inability to sit properly, the utilization of public transport and, in particular, managing stairs. Another issue in arthrodesis of knee joints seems to be the inability to get used to the situation, even after decades. Therefore, indications for takedown of fused knee joints are complex and require consideration of the patients' motivation, the presence of sufficient musculoskeletal and neurovascular anatomical structures, and extensive experience in TKA surgery.

The largest series was analyzed by Cameron (1996), who reported 17 patients with a postoperative complication rate of 53% including myositis ossificans, early tibial component loosening, ligamentous laxity and quadriceps tendon rupture with further complication and subsequent refusion. Of the 17 patients, one developed postoperative wound breakdown requiring a medial gastrocnemius flap, leading to a restricted ROM of 35 degrees. Five out of nine complications were resolved successfully with further surgery. Two patients underwent refusion for infection. General recommendations remain unresolved. In two independent studies, both Mahomed et al. (1994) and Holden and Jackson (1988) reported two patients with good results without postoperative complications or reoperations. Mahomed recommended soft tissue expansion prior to TKA surgery in two patients with fused knee joints. This technique involves placement of a subcutaneous soft tissue expander between the femur and the quadriceps tendon in order to gain length of the extensor mechanism. Active ROM of 80–85 degrees flexion was obtained in both patients without any postoperative complications. Legaye et al. (1994) reported one patient with 90 degrees of flexion 1 year postoperatively.

The overall complication rate and reoperation rate in this study was 86 % and all complications were related to soft tissue problems. Four types of problems were noted and included skin necrosis, extensor mechanism contracture, insufficient collateral ligaments and adhesion/arthrofibrosis.

Skin Problems

The status of the skin around the knee joint is crucial for conversion to knee arthroplasty. All patients had at least two operations prior to conversion. Two of the three patients that were fused with one or two metal plates developed skin necrosis after TKA. In one patient the skin coverage was performed with a gastrocnemius flap 3 months postoperatively, which developed chronic deep infection despite longstanding antibiotic treatment. This case ultimately required refusion 1 year later. Another case with a lateral gastrocnemius flap had gained 65 degrees ROM at 55 months follow-up. Cases that developed postoperative skin demarcation were likely to develop infection, and intervention by a vascularized flap should be considered at an early stage. Utilizing subcutaneous inflatable cushions is another reported method to enlarge the skin successfully prior to TKA.

Extensor Mechanism

Tibial tubercle osteotomy (Sect. 4.5) provides adequate exposure and has become the routine management for revision TKA and valgus knee deformities in this hospital. All tibial osteotomies healed without complication. Knee joint fusions are associated with contracture of the extensor mechanism and tibial osteotomy provides proximalization of the tubercle of up to 2 cm. The patella was present in all but one case. The patient with no patella lever-arm mechanism reached 55 degrees of ROM at follow-up and was able to elevate the knee actively in extension. One patient with a very thin patellar tendon underwent reinforcement with an artificial ligament. At follow-up she had 85 degrees of flexion and full extension. An MRI investigation was carried out in the last two cases prior to conversion surgery and was considered to improve preoperative evaluation and understanding of the integrity of the extensor mechanism and both collateral ligaments. In addition, MRI investigation provides detailed information about the quality and quantity of both muscle fibers and the extent of fibrosis of the quadriceps muscle group (Fig. 4.114). A contracted and overloaded extensor mechanism might be responsible for the restricted mobility and pain on walking postoperatively. Nerve conduction studies are also strongly recommended to ensure nerve function.

Collateral Ligaments

Special consideration should be given to potentially inadequate or non-functioning collateral ligaments. At the time of surgery, collateral stability was considered to be sufficient to implant an unconstrained prosthesis in four patients. One of these patients developed painful lateral instability and had to undergo reconstruction of the lateral ligament, which failed 1.5 years after TKA. The patient was recommended to undergo revision using a more constrained arthroplasty but in preference opted for a refusion 2.5 years later. In our experience, collateral ligament insufficiency is better treated with a condylar semiconstrained knee prosthesis (LCCK, NexGen, Zimmer, Warsaw, USA) or hinged components in severe laxity.

Arthrofibrosis with severe painful limitation of ROM was the most frequent complication in this series. Three patients underwent open arthrolysis, which included partial resection of the entire knee joint capsule and mobilization of the extensor mechanism. One patient had a VY quadriceps plasty and one a proximal detachment of the femoral rectus and sartorius muscle. Two patients gained 30 degrees of motion. One patient had to be refused for chronic collateral ligament instability.

This study shows that a takedown of arthrodesed or fused knee joints to TKA has a high complication rate. Therefore, the indication for takedown must be carefully evaluated and the unfavorable risk/gain ratio fully explained to the patient. According to the results of the present study, desarthrodesis of fused knee joints to TKA should be performed only in well-equipped centers, by experienced surgeons and in highly motivated patients with realistic expectations who are able and willing to face a procedure that does not guarantee success.

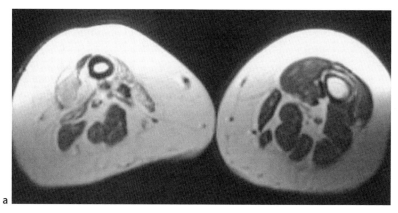

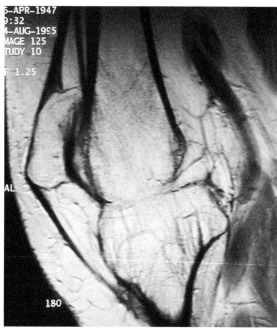

Fig. 4.114. a Preoperative MRI scan with considerable atrophy of quadriceps femoris muscles on the right side excluding the rectus femoris muscle compared with the opposite side. **b** Lateral MRI section shows intact extensor mechanism. Nerve conduction studies are also strongly recommended to ensure nerve function

Bibliography

Buechel FF (1982) A simplified evaluation system for rating of the knee function. Orthop Rev 11:9

Burki H, von Knoch M, Heiss C, Drobny T, Munzinger U (1999) Lateral approach with osteotomy of the tibial tubercle in primary total knee arthroplasty. Clin Orthop 362:156

Cameron HU, Hu C (1996) Results of total knee arthroplasty following takedown of formal knee fusion. J Arthroplasty 6: 732

Holden DL, Jackson DW (1988) Considerations in total knee arthroplasty following previous knee fusion. Clin Orthop 227:223

Legaye J, Emery R, Lokietek W (1994) Desarthodèse de genou par prothèse total. A propos d'un cas. Acta Orthop Belg 60: 26

Lindenfeld TN, Wojtys EM, Husain A (1999) Operative treatment of arthrofibrosis of the knee. J Bone Joint Surg 81A:12

Mahomed N, McKee N, Salomon P, Lahoda L, Gross A (1994) J Bone Joint Surg 76B:88

Naranja J, Lotke P, Pagnano M, Hanssen A (1996) Total knee arthroplasty in a previously ankylosed or arthrodesed knee. Clin Orthop 331:231

CHAPTER 5

Jens G. Boldt · Yaw Jakobi · Thomas Guggi

Computer Assisted Surgery and Minimal Invasive Surgery

5.1 Computer Assisted Surgery, Robotics, and Minimal Invasive Surgery in Knee Arthroplasty

Jens G. Boldt

Computer assisted surgery (CAS) and robotics have gained increased popularity in the planning and execution of orthopaedic surgery, particularly in Europe. They have become valuable and reliable tools for many specific procedures, including pedicle screw insertion, cruciate ligament reconstruction, as well as knee and hip arthroplasty. Complex primary and difficult revision cases appear to benefit the most from CAS guidance.

This chapter will not cover all orthopaedic applications available today, nor will it contribute new data from personal studies. However, close observation, personal communication, practical experiences, and intense literature research have revealed information regarding this new technology that is worth sharing. The principle of computer navigation is based on either matching preoperative digital imaging (fluoroscopy, computed tomography-CT, magnetic resonance imaging-(MRI) with available intraoperative landmarks, which then directs optically guided surgical tools into best anatomical (or desired) position, or intraoperative navigation. The disadvantages of CT scan guided systems are additional radiation, time, and costs, which is why more modern CAS systems offer intraoperative and CT-less "online" navigation. MRI guided systems are favoured in neurosurgery and maxillofacial operations, but less so in orthopaedic applications. The advantages of CAS include preoperative planning, virtual simulation, and online guided surgical execution. Digital landmark registration pre- and intraoperatively may enhance surgical accuracy, which, in some cases, may lead to improved fine-tuning via mental registration of stored patient parameters. Newer systems and technology.

The three aspects of CAS are: (1) registration of anatomy and pathological morphology, (2) instrument calibration, and (3) monitored three-dimensional tool navigation and surgical execution, including visual feedback. There is a difference between data guided navigation and anatomical landmark navigation, which is defined by the surgeon intraoperatively. This procedure is referred to as "virtual reality" and requires attachment of optical LED or (now seldom used) magnetic markers to hooks, probes, resection blocks, and other equipment. Infrared cameras are preferred for various reasons and have become the leading technology because of their accuracy and practicability (Figs. 5.1–5.3).

Robotic surgery has come full circle from early skepticism to enthusiastic fascination (from surgeons and patients) to recent drawbacks in less than a decade of its use. Although bone resections were remarkably precise, soft tissue damage led to increased concerns. The intensity of wound damage in orthopaedic applications was at times significant and evolved to a major medicolegal lawsuit in middle Europe. Therefore, the number of centres withdrawing from this technology increased, but it will remain an interesting field worth observing in the future.

Total knee arthroplasty (TKA) requires attention to the entire knee joint mechanics, active muscle forces and passive ligament structures. Prosthetic component design must accommodate the patient's knee anatomy, biomechanical stability, function, and mobility. It is generally accepted that the longevity of any knee prosthesis is patient specific and depends upon proper component design and alignment, implant fixation, soft tissue balancing and physiological mechanical axes. Minimal malpositioning of any component may lead to considerable postoperative problems, including increased wear, early loosening, pain, stiffness, and other functional impairments. Thus reconstruction of the correct mechanical lower extremity axis as well as soft tissue balancing is vital for good outcome. Survivorship of TKA should be in the region of 80–90 % after 20 years. Even slight malposition of any prosthetic component may potentially cause inferior results.

As far as knee surgery is concerned, unicondylar and TKA, as well as both anterior and posterior cru-

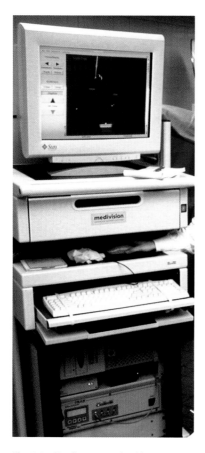

Fig. 5.1. Hardware required for computer assisted navigation, including a monitor, PC, software, and LED camera

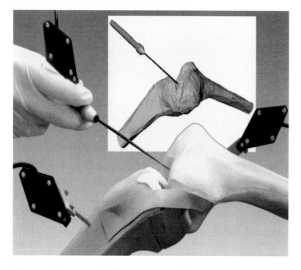

Fig. 5.2. Knee model demonstrating femoral and tibial reference markers as well as LED probe

ciate ligament (ACL/PCL) reconstruction surgery, have become established to a point of routine use in most clinics. Numerous studies and literature reports have evolved since the introduction of this technology. The thrust of most publications includes the following messages with regards to CAS in TKA: computer navigation and assisted surgery show significantly increased three-dimensional accuracy of bone resections, and resulting mechanical axes; however, ultimate functional long-term outcomes are expected, but have yet to be confirmed in long-term studies.

Advantages in ACL and PCL surgery include optimal and accurate transplant placement, minimally invasive surgical techniques, and perioperative virtual testing for tunnel placement, impingement and elongation of the ligament during full range of motion prior to implantation (Fig. 5.4). Recent clinical prospective, randomized, comparative outcome studies have uniformly demonstrated significantly improved results, both morphologically and clinically. Again, long-term clinical outcomes are expected, but have to be confirmed.

Computer navigation in knee arthroplasty holds multiple challenges, particularly due to the fact that TKA requires both accurate bone resections and proper soft tissue balancing. It is generally accepted that the survival of each individual knee prosthesis (unicompartmental knee arthroplasty and TKA) depends significantly on the accuracy of bone resection, appreciation of joint anatomy and biomechanics, and optimal ligament tensioning. Component orientation is dealt with (nearly) perfectly when navigation technology is utilized, as has been reported in many excellent studies. Bone resection accuracy has now reached 0.5 degrees positioning. However, as soft tissue balancing and fine-tuning play a major part in the long-term success of knee arthroplasty, further appreciation of ligament tension, joint stability, and near to normal biomechanics cannot be emphasized enough and should be included in future navigation tools. Development of tools (Komistek) that become capable of measuring interface and bearing pressures will certainly enhance the possibilities of guided soft tissue (or bone) releases and fine-tuning in order to optimize knee function and long-term outcome.

The vast majority of large knee prosthesis manufacturers offer their own navigation system, as do independent navigation tool companies. Problems may exist when tools require the specific use of an unfamiliar knee system or even new evolved knee implants without a proven track record with conventional methods. Today, all major navigation manufac-

Fig. 5.3 a, b. Typical setup and TKA navigation tools, including LED probes, touch pad, and reference markers

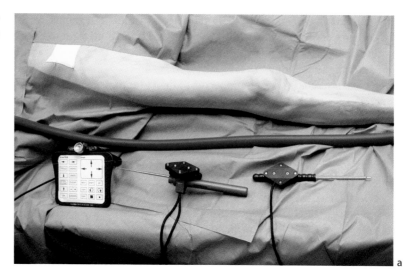

a

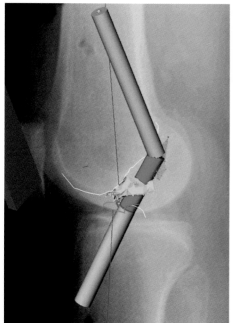

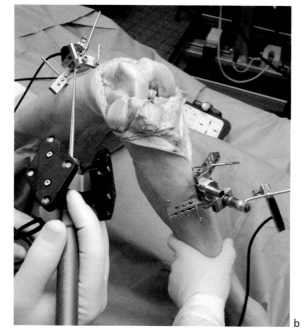

b

Fig. 5.4. Virtual ACL radiographic overlay animation prior to implantation, allowing for testing best graft position, thickness, elongation, and potential impingement

turing companies have agreed to an international consensus for component interchangeability, keeping the choice of desired implants open.

Since reconstructive knee arthroplasty surgery does not depend on accurate bone resections alone, long-term success is equally if not more dependent on individual proper soft tissue balancing and ligament stability. Therefore, computer navigation in TKA should be considered as an additional tool, which adds accuracy to conventional alignment guides. However, navigation should not lead to a

blind trust in modern technology. Neither should it replace the experienced surgeon's eye or his or her dexterity for proper biomechanical alignment and soft tissue balancing. Utilizing CAS may, however, distract attention from a critical view of the experienced (and successful) conventional surgeon and unappreciated trust of the less experienced orthopaedic resident. In addition, navigation should not be considered as a warrant to improving surgical skills in the less experienced surgeon. Further disadvantages include a learning curve (cadaver studies are strongly recommended), additional costs and surgery time (15–30 minutes), as well as additional skin and bone injuries. The immense positive public relation effect of computer technology in various hospitals and regions has attracted a large number of patients (and customers) with the economical pressure of prosthetic centres in offering similar services.

Future success will determine the "clinical utility" of CAS. This term was introduced in the USA by the Clinton administration, and is now part of the Food and Drugs Administration mandate for new devices. In essence, clinical utility is "true marketability." To have a place in today's medicine product range, a new device must answer the following questions:

1. Does it solve a real problem in clinical medicine?
2. Does it improve the clinical outcome?
3. Is it safe for the patient without compromising health?
4. Does it result in economic savings without lowering quality?

Currently, these questions cannot all be answered in the affirmative; therefore, more studies, clinical data, and outcome results are required.

In summary, one can state that knowledge of conventional surgical skills and techniques in knee arthroplasty remains the golden standard, with excellent long-term outcomes when utilizing proven prosthetic designs and appreciation of soft tissue balancing. Computer navigation should be handled as a helpful tool for improvement of bone resection and (hopefully in the future) soft tissue balancing. Critical and careful double checking throughout all surgical steps remains an absolute necessity, as knee arthroplasty represents a highly complex, individual, and challenging procedure in orthopaedic surgery today.

Minimal Invasive Surgery (MIS) in Knee Arthroplasty has gained immense popularity and has become a major marketing tool in the last years. There is now doubt that minimizing soft tissues and musscle trauma will lead to better function of the operated site, but the real value of these goals should not compromise on important surgical steps, namely, posterior capsular releases, ligament releases, tendon reslease, osteophyte removal, parapatellar denervating techniques that are required to maintain the golden standard of obliterate total knee arthroplasty with excellent clinical and functional outcomes since 30 years. There is no hard evidence today that a long skin and capsular incision in TKA has significant dis-

advantages with regards to propioception, postoperative pain, knee function, or longevity.

As far as total knee arthroplasty is concerned MIS may work well in the mild arthritic knee, with little or no patello-femoral problems, no osteophytes, no major valgus-varus deformity, no bone defect, and no extension lack, because in all other cases capsular and soft tissue releases as well as denervating techniques can not be addressed sufficiantly. When MIS knee arthroplasty is performed, the patella is usually not everted 180 degrees, therefore the full patelloplasty procedure including denervation, cheilectomy, and improvement of tracking cannot be carried out. This is likely cause increased patello-femoral problems both represented in less than optimal tracking and anterior knee pain. In comparison to hip arthroplasty where most of the surgical approach affects muscle tissue, knee arthrotomy during knee arthroplasty had not been an issue of concern in TKA.

There is no evidence of decreased function and mobility of the TKA when a conventionally long skin cut and arthrotomy is used. If, however, outcome and function relevant surgical soft tissue manoeuvers are neglected because of minimal invasive techniques, MIS in TKA has a considerable chance leading to inferior results and should, therefore, be critically observed.

Bibliography

Babisch J, Layher F, Ritter B, Venbrocks R (2001) Computergestützte biomechanisch fundierte zweidimensionale Operationsplanung hüftchirurgischer Eingriffe. Orthop Prax 37: 29–38

Bargren JH, Blaha JD, Freeman MAR (1983) Alignment in total knee arthroplasty. Clin Orthop 173:178–183

Bernsmann K, Rosenthal A, Sati M, Stäubli H.U, Cassens J, Menestrey J, Wiese M (2001) Multicentererfahrungen mit einem System zur computerassistierten vorderen Kreuzbandrekonstruktion. Orthop Prax 37:1–5

Davies BL, Harris SJ, Lin WJ, Hibberd RD, Cobb JC (1997) Active compliance in robotic surgery. The use of force control as a dynamic constraint. J Eng Med Proc H IMechE 211:H4

Delp SL, Stulberg SD, Davies B et al (1998) Computer assisted knee replacement. Clin Orthop 354:49–56

Delp SL, Stulberg SD, Davies BL, Picard F, Leitner F (1998) Computer assisted knee replacement. Clin Orthop 354:49–56

Dessenne V, Lavallee S, Julliard R, Orti R, Martelli S, Cinquin P (1995) Computer-assisted knee anterior ligament reconstruction: first clinical tests. J Image Guid Surg 1:59–64

DiGioia AM (1998) What is computer assisted orthopaedic surgery? Clin Orthop Relat Res 354:2–4

DiGioia AM, Jaramaz B, Colgan B (1998) Computer assisted orthopaedic surgery: image guided and robotic assistive technologies. Clin Orthop Relat Res 354:8–16

DiGioia AM, Jaramaz B, Blackwell M, Simon DA, Morgan F, Moody JE, Nikou C, Colgan BD, Aston CA, Labarca RS, Kischell E, Kanade T (1998) Image guided navigation system to measure intraoperatively acetabular implant alignment. Clin Orthop Relat Res 355:8–22

Dorr LD, Conaty JP, Schreffler R, Mehne DK, Hull D (1985) Technical factors that influence mechanical loosening of total knee arthroplasty. In: Dorr LD (ed) The knee. University Park Press, Baltimore, pp 121–135

Jenny JY, Boeri C (2001) Computer-assisted implantation of total knee prostheses: a case control comparative study with classical instrumentation. Comput Aided Surg 6:217–220

Julliard R, Lavallee S, Dessenne V (1998) Computer assisted reconstruction of the anterior cruciate ligament. Clin Orthop 354:57–64

Khadem R, Yeh CC, Sadeghi-Tehrani M et al (2000) Comparative tracking error analysis of five different optical tracking systems. Comput Aided Surg 5:98–107

Klos TVS, Habets RJE, Banks AZ, Banks SA, Devilee RJJ, Cook F (1998) Computer assistance in arthroscopic anterior cruciate ligament reconstruction. Clin Orthop 354:65–69

Krackow KA, Bayers-Thering M, Phillips MJ, Mihalko WM (1999) A new technique for determining proper mechanical axis alignment during total knee arthroplasty: progress toward computer-assisted TKA. Orthopedics 22:698–702

Leitner F, Picard F, Minfelde R et al (1997) Computer assisted knee surgical total replacement. Proceedings of the first joint conference on computer vision, virtual reality and robotics in medicine and medical robotics and computer assisted surgery. Grenoble, France. Springer, Berlin Heidelberg New York, pp 630–638

Mai S, Lörke C, Siebert W (2000) Implantation von Knieendoprothesen mit dem neuen Operationsroboter-System CASPAR. Orthop Prax 36:792–800

Petermann H, Kober, R. Heinze P (2000) Computer assisted planning and robot-assisted surgery in anterior cruciate ligament reconstruction. Operat Tech Orthoped 10:50

Picard F, Leitner F, Raoult O, Saragaglia D Computer assisted total knee arthroplasty. In: Rechnergestützte Verfahren in Orthopädie und Unfallchirurgie. Steinkopff, Darmstadt, pp 461–471

Simon D, Hebert M, Kanade T (1995) Techniques for fast and accurate intrasurgical registration. J Image Guided Surg 1:17–29

Stulberg SD, Picard F, Saragaglia D (2000) Computer-assisted total knee replacement arthroplasty. Oper Techn Orthop 10:25–39

Taylor RH, Mittelstadt BD, Paul HA, Hanson W, Kazanzides P, Zuhars JF, Williamson B, Musits BL, Glassman E, Bargar WL (1994) An image-directed robotic system for precise orthopaedic surgery. IEEE Trans Robot Automat 10:261–273

Wiesel U, Boerner M (2001) First experiences using a surgical robot for total knee replacement. Proc CAOS/USA, Pittsburgh, USA, 6–8 July 2001, pp 143–146

Yanof J, Haaga J, Klahr P, Bauer C, Nakamoto D, Chaturvedi A, Bruce R (2001) CT integrated robot for interventional procedures: preliminary experiment and computer-human interfaces. Comput Aid Surg 6:352–359

5.2 Outcome Measures and Quality Control

Yaw Jakobi, Thomas Guggi

Outcomes are important and are the basis of continuous improvement of joint replacement. To find the best treatment and solutions for cost-effectiveness, evidence needs to be developed as a guide for the decision-making process. Policy-makers and purchasers are interested in identifying sources of cost without benefit. Physicians need to select effective treatments and patients want to make informed treatment choices. All require accurate information on the likely benefits of alternative procedures, in order to make an informed choice.

Codman is considered to be one of the pioneers of evaluation and documentation of results after orthopaedic interventions. In 1934, he introduced the concept of understanding the effect of medical and operative treatment on patient function, as well as the meaning of patient satisfaction, quality of life (QOL), and registering these details using standardized documentation. Since the 1990s, there has been increased interest in outcome measures in orthopaedic studies. The 1990s were, therefore, dedicated as the decade of outcomes. Data gained through outcome measures help to evaluate the effectiveness of treatment in terms of patient outcome as well as patient satisfaction with the outcome. A number of different scoring systems have been developed to rate the results after knee arthroplasty. Factors measured in the assessments include pain, function limitations, deformity and QOL. Results from different knee scoring systems vary because of different weightings of the score components. Despite efforts to standardize clinical scoring systems for knees and other joints, an ideal system is not currently available. The most commonly utilized scoring system is the HSS knee score, introduced more than 20 years ago by John Insall at the Hospital for Special Surgery in New York. It consists of two ratings with a maximum of 100 points and includes the measurement of function, pain, mobility, deformity, stability and strength. A separate radiographic score, the Knee Society Roentgenographic Evaluation and Scoring System (KSRESS) requires a clinician for x-ray judgement. Not all systems are suitable to allow for comparison of outcomes within individual units and between orthopaedic units worldwide. Traditional methods of reporting clinical outcomes include data on complications, revisions, mortality rates (survival analysis), and clinical rating scores.

Each scoring system demands particular properties. First, it should assess what is important in successful knee surgery outcomes: reduction of pain and improvement of function. Furthermore, it should be reliable and reproducible. This will ensure that the change in clinical score reflects the same change in knee joint status. This so-called "psychometrics" includes further sensitivity or responsiveness to changes in clinical status. Psychologists specializing in psychometry spend much of their time studying the application of questionnaires and examinations.

Patient self-administered questionnaires capture data on the patient's experience of pain, functional disability, and general health status. This subjective collection of data by the patient reduces the possibility of observer bias. These questionnaires are considered as additional information completing both subjective and objective data. Different patient-based outcome measures include: (1) general health status instruments such as the Medical Outcomes Study short forms (MOS SF-36, SF-12), (2) the Nottingham Health Profile (NHP), and (3) the World Health Organization Quality of Life (WHOQOL). These are intended to address a wide range of health problems, and include disease-specific and condition-specific health status instruments focusing on patients' perceptions in relation to a single condition. Examples for the latter are the Western Ontario and McMaster Universities Osteoarthritis Index (WOMAC) and the Oxford-12 knee score.

Advantages and disadvantages are associated with both generic and disease-specific measures. Disease-specific measures are more relevant to patients and physicians than generic instruments. They are preferred for detecting the effects of treatment because of their sensitivity to specific problems. Generic measures have a higher discrimination than condition-specific measures between subjects with different levels of self-reported general health status and comorbidities. Patients who have reached a ceiling on disease-specific measurements continue to experience pain and physical disabilities as a result of comorbidity, which is expressed by lower general scores. Generic instruments also allow the impact of treatment to be compared across various medical conditions (a highly relevant feature for policy makers). Literature reports support inclusion of both general and condition-specific health-related QOL measures in cross-sectional studies.

Patient satisfaction is another measure often asked in addition to standardized outcome measures. Surgeons frequently ask their patients whether they are satisfied with the operated knee replacement. Patient satisfaction is a subjective description that is based on a variety of factors. However, when a validated self-administered form is used to ask patients about satisfaction with the operated knee directly after the operation, they relate their perceived surgical result to that expected of the operation, even though the knee function is not necessarily comparable to that of a healthy subject. In a validated survey comparing patient satisfaction (4-point scale) with the MOS SF-36 and the WOMAC score, patient satisfaction correlates significantly with general health and disease-specific outcome measures, with the highest correlation to domains that relate to pain and function. In conclusion, patients who undergo knee arthroplasty usually state in self-administered surveys that they are satisfied with their knee, when they have gained good pain relief and improved function.

Standardized documentation is a central point of evidenced-based medicine. To analyze the outcome in long-term prospective studies, large databases are needed for documentation of all core data in addition to mentioned outcome measures: clinical data of the hospital course and medical record (demography, diagnosis, admission, therapy, discharge, co-morbidity, early complications, and re-hospitalization) and follow-up, including late complications.

With the help of new technologies, electronic databases have been and continue to be developed: registries, documentation instruments, electronic medical records, etc.

Registries such as the Swedish knee arthroplasty registry have contributed considerably to improvements in regional and worldwide standards of practice. Other registries, such as the Canadian joint replacement registry and the New Zealand joint registry were started. So far, registries have provided survival analysis with, for example, revision as an endpoint, aiming for integration of patient-derived outcome assessments.

The first standardized documentation of patient history was performed by M.E. Mueller in Switzerland, based on structure and consensus about terminology for reporting results of total hip arthroplasty (THA) by the Hip Society, the American Academy of Orthopedic Surgeons (AAOS) and the Société Internationale de Chirurgie Orthopédique et de Traumatologie (SICOT). This is the International Documentation and Evaluation System (IDES), which includes clinical and radiological data of hospital course and later follow-up.

Another example is the Musculoskeletal Outcomes Data Evaluation and Management System (MODEMS), utilized by the AAOS from 1997 to 2000 to improve quality and value of musculoskeletal care by providing physicians with tools and methods to collect, organize and analyze information about the outcome of the health care. The main goals of the MODEMS project were to develop a national database on the outcomes of musculoskeletal procedures and to provide a method by which physicians can assess the results of musculoskeletal care in an outpatient setting and compare those outcomes with a national norm (benchmarking).

Modules for standardized documentation in four areas of orthopaedics (upper limb, lower limb, pediatrics, and spine) are offered by the AAOS. New technologies such as handheld computers, workpads, or barcode readers can further improve the method of documentation. In a pilot project for the Canadian joint registry, data were collected electronically at the point of care (operating room) through handheld computers and on paper. A validation process compared the paper and electronic records, with the electronic data proving to be superior. "Electronic data collection is not only futuristic, but an assessment tool whose time has come. Electronic data are more accurate than paper collection and provide timely, immediate data and add several benefits including real-time feedback" (Bourne 1999).

Clinical Outcome Assessments

The American Knee Society (AKS) score was developed by consensus and is today the most commonly used and cited objective clinical assessment of total knee arthroplasty (TKA). It includes two parts, the knee score and the functional score. Separation in a dual rating system influences factors linked to the patient's general health and condition. The function score allocates points for walking distance, and stair-climbing ability, and deducts points for the use of walking aids. A maximum of 100 points represents unlimited walking distance and normal stair-climbing without the use of an aid. The knee score considers pain, the clinical assessment of stability and range of motion as the main parameters, with deductions for flexion contraction, extension lag and malalignment. Fifty of 100 points in the knee score reflect pain assessment (a score of 50 points represents no pain). The pain component of the knee score requires the evaluator to rate the patient's knee pain with one question, which combines frequency and severity of pain on a 7-point scale. The other 50 points reflect the clinical assessment of range of motion, stability and alignment (50 points represent at least 0–125 degrees

of knee flexion with no active lag, no instability, and normal alignment).

A patient categorization system is included in the AKS to identify patients whose function may be undermined by factors other than the knee. Patients without substantial disease in the contralateral knee (a) are categorized differently from those with substantial osteoarthritis (b), or those with multiple joint problems and/or generalized debility (c). In order to validate the AKS, Lingard et al. (2001) confirmed that the system has a poor correlation among items, but that it has adequate convergent construct validity. The AKS knee score was a responsive instrument for assessing the outcomes of TKA, but the function score was not.

Condition-Specific and Disease-Specific Health-Related Quality of Life

The Oxford-12 knee score is a validated and reliable self-administered questionnaire specifically designed for patients with TKA. Twelve questions with a 5-point scale (Likert 1932) require some 9 minutes on average. A single score ranks from 12 to 60, with 12 indicating the best possible health state. Balancing among patients' burden, feasibility, content validity and reliability, the Oxford-12 knee score appears to be the best TKA-specific questionnaire for use with large databases in a cross-sectional population. Dunbar et al. (2001) proved this in his research with the Swedish knee arthroplasty registry, adding the MOS SF-12 to the Oxford-12.

Western Ontario and McMaster Universities Osteoarthritis Index

The WOMAC index represents a disease-specific health questionnaire and was developed in patients with osteoarthritis of the hip and knee, including the following parameters: pain, stiffness, activity, and limitation. In order to scale 24 items, there are two versions of the WOMAC: (1) a 5-point Likert (1932) scale (answers for pain can range from none to extreme), and (2) a 10 cm visual analogue scale. The self-administered WOMAC takes approximately 11 minutes to complete. The reliability, internal consistency, and validity have been tested in the context of knee and hip replacement studies, as well as in clinical trials of anti-inflammatory drugs. Today it is considered the most commonly used questionnaire for patients with osteoarthritis.

Knee Injury and Osteoarthritis Outcome Score

The KOOS assesses knee injuries and knee osteoarthritis and is based on the WOMAC. This validated and responsiveness questionnaire consists of the following parameters: pain, stiffness, swelling, activities of daily living, sports and recreational activities, and knee-related QOL. To answer the 42 questions of this self-assessment takes approximately 10 minutes. Standardized answer options are given (5-point scale) and each question gets a score from 0 to 4. The optimal score is 100 points with no symptoms and the worst score is 0 points with severe symptoms.

Medical Outcomes Study Short Forms

The SF-36 or SF-12 outcomes studies assess general QOL with either 36 or 12 questions. Both are most commonly utilized for international general health questionnaires.

Their reliability has been documented in general and chronic disease populations, validity in relation to clinical indicators in the presence or absence of a disease, severity within disease category, and changes in disease-related symptoms over time. The SF-36 short form is a 36-item questionnaire that includes eight areas of QOL considering health status in the last 7 or 30 days, physical function, physical pain, bodily pain, general health, vitality, social function, emotional status, and mental health.

Physical function is defined in health-limiting physical activities, whereas physical health is defined in interference with work or other daily activities. Bodily pain is the intensity of pain and effect of pain on normal work, both inside and outside the home. General health is the personal evaluation of health including current health, health outlook and resistance to illness. Vitality is feeling energetic and full of pep. Social functioning is the extent to which physical health or emotional problems interfere with normal social activities. Emotional and mental health is the extent to which emotional problems interfere with work or other daily activities. The SF-36 generates scores for each of the eight domains and for two summary scales, physical (PCS) and mental component summary (MCS). An estimated 14 minutes is required for completion of this form.

The SF-12 uses 12 items from the SF-36 and generates directly the PCS and MCS. It takes about 7 minutes for the documentation. The SF-12 is meant to be used in studies with large sample sizes (over 500), having severe constraints on questionnaire length, and in studies focusing on patient-based assessment of physical and mental health.

Nottingham Health Profile

The NHP is commonly used for validation in different languages and for patients with rheumatic arthritis or osteoarthritis. It includes 38 items with six parameters: physical mobility, pain, social isolation, emotional reactions, energy, and sleep. Scores from 0 to100 are calculated for each dimension and for an overall score. The higher the score, the greater the health problem. It takes about 11 minutes to complete the dichotomous (yes/no) structured questions.

World Health Organization Quality of Life

In 1991, the WHO initiated a project to develop a QOL instrument simultaneously in 15 countries: WHO-QOL. This was intended as a generic tool for use with patients across varying disease types, severities of illness, and cultural subgroups. The definition of QOL was described as: "an individual's perception of his/her position in life in the context of the culture and value systems in which he/she lives, and in relation to his/her goals, expectations, standards and concerns."

The WHOQOL is available in over 20 languages. Currently there are two versions: the complete WHO-QOL-100 with 100 items and WHOQOL-bref with 26 items. The latter is a short form, which is appropriate for clinical research. The answers are given on a 5-point scale. The WHOQOL-bref is selfadministered and has a form for interviewer-assisted or interview-administered assessment. The WHOQOL-100 produces scores relating to particular facets of QOL, positive feelings, social support, financial resources, physical health, psychological health, level of independence, social relationships, environment, spiritual domain, and a score relating to overall QOL and general health. The WHOQOL-bref produces the above domain scores, and general scores, but no individual facet scores.

Fig. 5.5. The IDES system is structured as three forms: primary operation, revision operation and follow-up. The forms collect a set of core information analogue to the patient medical record, including demographic, clinical, radiological evaluation, and details about the operation technique and type of prosthesis

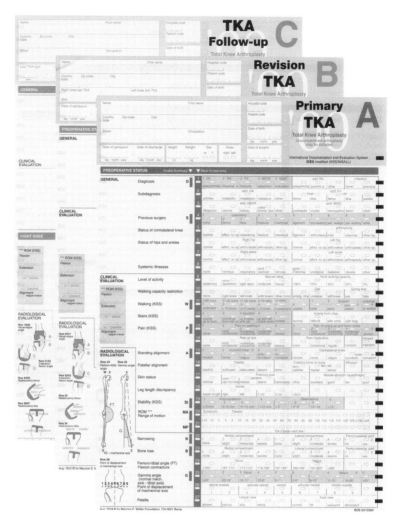

International Documentation and Evaluation System

The IDES allows standardized documentation of clinical and radiological information. The database system using standardized terminology for research and evaluation includes forms for hip and knee replacements. The IDES system database is supported by the Maurice E. Mueller foundation, Bern, Switzerland. The system is structured in three forms: (a) primary operation, (b) revision operation and (c) follow-up (Fig. 5.5). The forms collect a set of core information analogue to the patient medical record. This core set includes demographic, clinical, and radiological evaluation, and details about the operation technique and type of prosthesis. Forms a and b contain information concerning medical history, diagnosis, treatment, operation, postoperative course, recovery and discharge. Form c for the follow-up provides information on physical and radiological examination,

pain, mobility, walking ability and evaluation of the results by the surgeon as well as the patient.

The comprehensive one-page code sheets are economically reported during normal clinical assessment or after the operation. With the help of optical marks, the sheets are easily entered into a database. A customization module allows existing questions and answers to be changed or completely new questions

The development of the IDES was supported and utilized in 1977 by the executive committee of SICOT as a basis for the development of a uniform method of reporting and evaluating results in orthopaedic surgery after the world congress in Munich. A SICOT commission on documentation and evaluation formed the first version of the hip IDES. It was further developed by the American Hip Society, AAOS and SICOT. A subcommittee of SICOT was formed to address similar problems in knee surgery related to the treatment of arthritis and knee replacement arthroplasty. Today, three forms for hip and knee arthroplasty are internationally accepted and more than 66,000 THAs and more than 3,000 TKAs have been documented with these standardized forms.

American Academy of Orthopedic Surgeons Outcomes Questionnaires

The AAOS has developed outcome questionnaires to assess musculoskeletal results of most patient populations and conditions. During this process, the AAOS has been supported since 1990 by the musculoskeletal specialty societies, the council of spine societies, and approximately 23 specialty societies. There are four orthopaedics subspecialties: upper limb, lower limb, paediatrics, and spine, all of which require similar information: diagnosis, history, general health status, co-morbidities, expectations, social status. This information is supplemented by questions that gather information about the specific condition. Each form takes about 15 minutes to complete.

The lower limb outcomes instrument includes four specific modules: knee osteoarthritis, foot and ankle, sports medicine, and general musculoskeletal condition questionnaires. THA and TKA modules include six forms: baseline questionnaire, follow-up, physical examination, operations, discharge, and complications (www.aaos.org/wordhtml/research/outcomes/question.htm).

Outcome assessments and questionnaires are summarized in Table 5.1.

Table 5.1. Summary of outcome assessments and questionnaires

Name	Dimensions	Number of questions/ items	Time (min)
Clinical assessment			
American Knee Society (AKS) score	Functional (walking distance, stair climbing, walking aid)	10 –	
	Knee (pain, stability, range of motion, deformities)		
Condition-, disease-specific quality of life			
Oxford-12 knee	Total knee arthroplasty score	12	9
Western Ontario and McMaster Universities Osteoarthritis Index (WOMAC)	Osteoarthritis of knee and hip	24	11
	Pain, stiffness, activity limitation	24	11
Knee injury and Osteoarthritis Outcome Score (KOOS)	Knee injury and knee osteoarthritis:	42	10
	pain, other symptoms, activities of daily living, sport and recreation, knee-related quality of life		
General quality of life			
Medical Outcome Study short form 36 (MOS SF-36)	Physical health, mental health, physical function, role-physical, body pain, general health, vitality, social functioning, role-emotional, mental health	36	14
Medical Outcome Study short form 12 (MOS SF-12)	Physical health, mental component health	12	7
Nottingham Health Profile (NHP)	Physical mobility, pain, social isolation, emotional reactions, energy, sleep	38	11
World Health Organization Quality of Life (WHOQOL-bref)	Physical, psychological, independence, social relationships, environment, spiritual	26	10
Documentation instruments			
International Documentation and Evaluation System (IDES)	Hip and knee arthroplasty		
AAOS outcome questionnaires	Upper limb, lower limb, paediatrics, and spine		

Bibliography

Aichroth PM (1993) The evaluation of results of knee replacement arthroplasty. Internal, unpublished paper

Amadio PC et al (1993) Outcome measurements. J Bone Joint Surg Am 75A:1583–1584

Arslanian C, Malcolm B (1999) Computer assisted outcomes research in orthopedics: total joint replacement. J Med Syst 23:239–247

Bach CM, Steingruber IE, Peer S, Nogler M, Wimmer C, Ogon M (2001) Radiographic assessment in total knee arthroplasty. Clin Orthop 385:144–150

Barck AL (1997) Agreement among clinical assessment scales for knee replacement surgery. Knee 4:155–158

Bellamy N, Buchanan WW, Goldsmith CH et al (1988) Validation study of WOMAC: a health status instrument for measuring clinically-important patient relevant outcomes following total hip or knee arthroplasty in osteoarthritis. J Orthop Rheum 1:95

Bellamy, Buchanan WW, Goldsmith CH et al (1988) Validation study of WOMAC: a health status instrument for measuring clinically important patient relevant outcomes to antirheumatic drug therapy in patients with osteoarthritis of the hip or knee. J Rheumatol 15:1833

Bourne RB (1999) The planning and implementation of the Canadian Joint Replacement Registry. Bull Hosp Jt Dis 58:128–132

Bourne RB (2000) Outcome measurements in total knee arthroplasty: in search. Orthopedics 23:995–996

Clancy CM (1998) Outcomes research: measuring the end results of health care. Science 282:245

Codman EA (1914) The product of a hospital. Surg Gynecol Obstet 18:491

Dawson J (1998) Questionnaire on the perceptions of patients about total knee replacement. J Bone Joint Surg Br 80:63–69

Dolley RL, Engel C, Müller ME (1992) Automated scanning and digitising of roentgenographs for documentation and research. Clin Orthop 274:113–119

Drake BG, Callahan CM, Dittus RS, Wright JG (1994) Global rating systems used in assessing knee arthroplasty outcomes. J Arthroplasty 9:409–417

Dunbar MJ, Robertsson O, Ryd L, Lidgren L (2001) Appropriate questionnaires for knee arthroplasty: results of a survey of 3600 patients from the Swedish Knee Arthroplasty. J Bone Joint Surg Br 83B:339–344

Ewald CF et al (1989) The Knee Society total knee arthroplasty roentgenographic evaluation and scoring system. Clin Orthop 248:9–12

Guyatt GH, Deyo RA, Charlson M, Levine MN, Mitchell A (1989) Responsiveness and validity in health status measurement: a clarification. J Clin Epidemiol 42:403–408

Gyatt GH, Feeny DH, Patrick DL (1993) Measuring health-related quality of life. Ann Intern Med 118:622

Harcourt WGV, White SH, Jones P (2001) Specificity of the Oxford knee status questionnaire. J Bone Joint Surg Br 83B:345

Huskisson EC (1982) Measurement of pain [VAS]. J Rheumatol 9:768–769

Insall NJ (1989) Rational of The Knee Society clinical rating system. Clin Orthop Relat Res 248:13–14

Johnston RC, Fitzgerald RH, Harris WH, Poss R, Müller ME, Sledge CB (1990) Clinical and radiographic evaluation of total hip replacement, a standard system of terminology for reporting results. J Bone Joint Surg 72A:161–168

Keller RB, Rudicel SA, Liang MH (1993) Outcomes research in orthopedics. J Bone Joint Surg Am 74A:1562–1574

König A, Scheidler M, Rader C, Euler J (1997) The need for a dual rating system in total knee arthroplasty. Clin Orthop 345:161–167

König A et al (1998) Ist die Verwendung des Knee Society Roentgenographic Evaluation and Scoring System zur radiologischen Kontrolle von Knieendoprothesen sinnvoll? Z Orthop Ihre Grenzgeb 136:70–76

Lieberman JR, Dorey F, Shekelle P et al (1996) Differences between patients' and physicians' evaluations of outcome after total hip arthroplasty. J Bone Joint Surg Am 78A:835–838

Likert T (1932) A technique for measurement of attitudes. Arch Psychol 140:44–60

Lingare E, Hahimoto H, Sledge H (2000) Development of outcome research for total joint arthroplasty. J Orthop Sci 5:175–177

Lingard EA, Katz JN, Wright RJ et al (2001) Validity and responsiveness of the knee society clinical rating system in comparison with the SF-36 and WOMAC. J Bone Joint Surg Am 83A:1856–1864

Medical Outcomes Trust (1993) How to score the SF-36 health survey

Müller ME Lessons of 30 years of total hip arthroplasty. Clin Orthop 274:12–21

Patrick DL, Deyo RA (1989) Generic and disease-specific measures in assessing health status and quality of life. Med Care 27:217

Ranawat CS, Insall JN, Shine JJ (1976) Duo-condylar knee arthroplasty: hospital for special surgery design. Clin Orthop 120:76–82

Ritter MA, Albohm MJ (1997) Overview: maintaining outcomes for total hip arthroplasty. Clin Orthop 344:81

Robertsson O, Dunbar MJ, Pehrsson T, Knutson K, Lidgren L (2000) Patient satisfaction after knee arthroplasty. A report on 27,372 knees operated on between 1981 and 1995 in Sweden. Acta Orthop Scand 71:262–267

Roos EM et al (1998) Knee injury and Osteoarthritis Outcome Score (KOOS): development of a self-administered outcome measure. J Orthop Sports Phys Ther 78:88–96

Rothwell AG (1999) Development of the New Zealand Joint Register. Bull Hosp Joint Dis 58:146–160

World Health Organization (1994) Protocol for new centres. WHO (MNF/PSF/94.4), Geneva, p 43

Wright JG, Rudicel S, Feinstein AR (1994) Ask patients what they want: evaluation of individual complaints before total hip replacement. J Bone Joint Surg Br 76B:229–234

CHAPTER 6

Mario Bizzini · Jens G. Boldt

Rehabilitation Before and After Total Knee Arthroplasty

Rehabilitation programs are as important in the overall success of total knee arthroplasty (TKA) as surgical technique and implant design. However, most rehabilitation protocols are based on empirical guidelines rather than on scientific facts and are seldom supervised by the surgeon. As a result, the variety of recommended programs is large and confusing in content, ranging from unsupervised walking to complete instruction in functional activities and specific exercises. Popular programs include active and passive range of motion (ROM) exercises, continuous passive motion (CPM) and isometric quadriceps strengthening.

A panel of American physical therapists agreed that basic categories of TKA rehabilitation programs should include treatment frequency, transfer training, gait training, exercises and discharge criteria. ROM is considered to be the primary indicator of successful TKA outcomes because restricted knee mobility affects functional activities the most. Campbell's Operative Orthopaedics (Canal 1998) states that "postoperative physical therapy and rehabilitation greatly influence the outcome of total knee arthroplasty". Further studies have been devoted to CPM and ROM exercises, but have failed to provide evidence. Results of large clinical trials are contradictory: whereas some show improvement of early postoperative ROM with additional CPM, others demonstrate no difference at all.

Profound analysis of current literature reports showed that the majority lack in study design quality and methodological set-up. Beaupre et al. (2001) compared three different TKA rehabilitation protocols in a randomized controlled trial: standardized exercises and CPM; standardized exercises and a slider board; and standardized exercises only. Postoperative early mobilization of the patient appeared sufficient and no additional benefit was encountered with CPM or slider board. There were no differences between groups in self-reported pain, function, and overall quality of life 3–6 months after surgery. Other studies indicated significant improvement of ROM after CPM treatment in the first week after surgery.

Reported benefits of CPM in the acute postoperative phase include decreased rate of knee manipulation, increased ROM, decreased swelling, less postoperative pain, and possibly reduction in pain relief medication and deep vein thrombosis. Yashar et al. (1997) conducted a prospective randomized study in 210 TKAs. They showed that CPM with an accelerated protocol of 70–100 degrees flexion in the recovery room allowed safer early discharge compared with CPM of 0–30 degrees flexion 1 day postoperatively. However, no overall difference was noted in ROM at 4 weeks or 1 year postoperatively. These results could not be duplicated when MacDonald et al. (2000) repeated the study. Worland et al. (1998) found that CPM is an adequate and more economical rehabilitation alternative after hospital discharge. In summary, CPM after TKA remains controversial.

Rehabilitation of TKA patients is not about ROM alone. Modern protocols are more specific and scientific and include important factors such as neuromuscular joint stabilization, propioception, and joint motion coordination movements. What use is a knee that flexes 110 degrees but is unstable while managing stairs or walking (jogging) on uneven ground? Today, patients with TKA have tremendously increased expectations and daily living activities. Sports and recreational activities are performed by more than 75%, and in extreme situations TKA patients desire to perform contact sports such as football, squash or alpine skiing. Sapega (1990) addressed this lack of goals in knee exercise programs.

Improvements in TKA design, surgical technique and data collection support the concept of accelerated and early rehabilitation after TKA. CPM treatment and the use of crutches are often determined by the surgeon, based upon his or her experience alone. There are no established peer-reviewed guidelines for decision making in rehabilitation programs available today.

Rehabilitation Programs

Local musculoskeletal surgery leads to several impairments for the entire system, as shown in Fig. 6.1 (Nagi 1991). After TKA, neuromuscular stabilization is lacking at the operated knee, leading to functional limitations (managing stairs) and problems returning to work or sports activities. Rehabilitation should focus on physical and functional limitations. Physiotherapists must choose the most appropriate intervention with the aim of optimizing the patient's individual functional outcome, keeping in mind that physiotherapy is only one part of the equation.

Surgery and rehabilitation may be regarded as external factors, motivation and lifestyle as internal factors. Further individual characteristics include general health, age, gender, diagnosis, healing potential, and specific risk factors, most of which are often neglected in rehabilitation protocols. There has certainly been a trend towards increased activity in the past three decades. The time interval of crutches is seldom included, as are weight-bearing characteristics. This chapter emphasizes the fact that modern TKA rehabilitation protocols should be more individualized and criterion-based rather than based on fixed time frames

Time-based rehabilitation programs are restrictive and focus on surgical procedure and expected healing time, in which all patients receive identical (imperceptive) interventions, neglecting individual progress and abilities.

Criterion-based rehabilitation programs are adapted to individual progression and are dictated by the achievement of specific criteria (functional goals). Furthermore the level of therapy is based on the patient's response to treatment, and therapeutic goals are the result of patient and physiotherapy teamwork. Criterion-based rehabilitation programs are based on six basic principles:

1. Healing tissue should never be overstressed
2. Immobilization must be prevented
3. Patient criteria determine progression to the next stage
4. Rehabilitation must be based on current scientific research
5. Rehabilitation programs are not a cookbook
6. Surgeon, patient, and physiotherapist must communicate in a team.

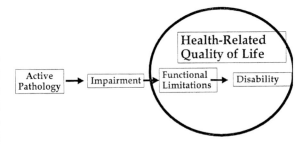

Fig. 6.1. The Nagi scheme of disablement

The ultimate goal of TKA rehabilitation is the clinical outcome, a process that requires close communication between the surgeon and the physiotherapist, as well as regular follow-ups and monitoring. Intense and understandable preoperative information about TKA is crucial to guide the patients' expectations. There have been numerous improvements in the knowledge of normal and prosthetic knee biomechanics and kinematics. However, this information is seldom transferred into rehabilitation programs. Adequate knee motion is only one of multiple important factors in rehabilitation outcomes. Practice and improvement of overall muscle function, loading tolerance, sensor–motor control, and functional activity level are superior determinants of TKA function and are discussed below.

Phase I

Neuromuscular knee and lower limb stabilization is crucial for optimal activities of daily living. Muscle groups are trained in partial or full weight bearing according to the loading responses: pain, swelling, or muscle activity. Accurate monitoring and observation allows safe functional progression, taking subjective parameters of the patient into consideration. Successful activities of daily living include: sitting, rising from chair, standing, walking, managing stairs, and kneeling.

Phase II

Rehabilitation is focused on the patient's own goals, including his or her desire to participate in previous professions, recreational activities and sports. Safety and a realistic approach must have the highest priority to achieve these goals. Neuromuscular stabilization, sensorimotor coordination, motor control, strength and endurance of the operated knee are a necessity and only obtainable after intense, specific, and controlled training.

The following points must be considered in the management of TKA patients:

1. Criterion-based rehabilitation program
2. Interventions, education, and documentation of progress and complications
3. Intensity of rehabilitation based on patient's response to treatment
4. Improvement of function until maximum is obtained
5. Communication between patient, surgeon, and physiotherapist.

Biomechanics of Exercises

Primary concerns in postoperative TKA rehabilitation are soft tissue healing, implant osseointegration and minimizing complications. Long-term follow-up studies demonstrated excellent or good outcome results in 98 % after 20 years with both cemented and cementless mobile bearing TKA (Buechel et al. 2001). Personal experiences showed that early CPM contributes to improved soft tissue healing with considerable differences in individual wound healing. Muscles and tendons require an average of 3 weeks for the fibroblastic phase, a time in which potentially stressful exercises should be avoided.

Tibiofemoral and patellofemoral biomechanics in TKA have shown peak loads at level walking of 2 times body weight and 3.1 times while descending stairs. Justification for early full weight bearing is more based on successful clinical experience rather than kinematic studies. Resulting forces and pressures in TKA components and soft tissues are highly complex and difficult to calculate in vivo. The following degrees of flexion and extension are considered to be safe:

1. Isolated knee flexion throughout full ROM
2. Isolated knee extension from 90 to 40 degrees
3. Squat from 0 to 40 degrees
4. Leg press machine from 0 to 60 degrees.

Isolated knee motions represent open chain exercises without floor contact of the involved leg and are considered disadvantageous in comparison to closed chain exercises such as squats and leg presses. Closed chain exercises should be preferred in knee and TKA rehabilitation because of the more natural leg function, increased muscle coordination, joint surface compression, facilitation of muscular activation, and enhanced joint stability. For optimal neuromuscular control, both open chain and closed chain exercises should be integrated in rehabilitation programs.

Research has demonstrated that lateral step-ups is a task predominantly affecting the quadriceps, retrograde stair climbing is a more hamstring-loading task, and lateral lunges with knees at 30 flexion a more co-activation task. A ventrally inclined trunk reduces quadriceps work by increasing dorsal musculature activity and is a commonly observed compensatory protecting mechanism when rising from a chair. Because of extensive soft tissue trauma in TKA, functional weight bearing is more protective than isolated knee flexion and extension exercises during the first 2–3 months. Repetitive knee open chain extension exercises, especially between 40 and 0 degrees of flexion, as well as deep knee closed chain exercises over 40 degrees of flexion, should be avoided. These situations can potentially exacerbate soft tissue inflammation and extensor mechanism healing. Further exercises to avoid in TKA rehabilitation include leg press machines over 90 degrees flexion because of extremely high compressive loads in all three joint compartments and high quadriceps tension, and significantly increased patellofemoral contact stresses after patella resurfacing in TKA.

Sport Activities after TKA

Cycling is considered the best and safest exercise for TKA because of minimal loads and maximal isokinetic/isometric forces and desired vascularity. Highest loads were recorded during downhill walking and jogging. Healy et al. (2000) listed recommended activities after TKA including low-impact aerobics, stationary bicycling, dancing, golfing, and swimming. For patients with previous experience, road cycling, hiking, skiing, tennis, and weight machines are also allowed. Activities such as high-impact aerobics and contact sports in general are not recommended. TKA patients should be encouraged to participate in low-impact and low-demand sports and to return to previous activities.

Sensorimotor System

Gait analyses, electromyographic activity, proprioception, and balance investigations provide unique information and have the potential to improve treatment planning. Gait analyses allow for objective assessment of function, performance and understanding of gait physiology after TKA. Andriacchi et al.

(1982) reported that TKA design influenced stair climbing (more normal in less-constrained cruciate retaining designs), but not level walking. TKA patients typically have a reduced gait velocity, shortened stride length, decreased duration of single-limb stance, and leaning of the trunk over the weight-bearing leg in order to reduce the moment arm. Kramers et al. (1997) found that gait pattern seen in five subjects (bilateral TKA with two different systems within each subject) lacked several of the principal elements described by Inman et al. (1984). Others have compared posterior stabilized versus posterior cruciate ligament retaining TKA and reported no significant differences with regard to gait parameters, knee ROM, isokinetic testing and electromyographic waveforms during level walking and stair climbing. Most results indicate that the gait pattern observed before TKA continues (prolongation of stance time, reduced gait velocity, reduction of vertical component of the floor reaction force), although pain during walking is reduced or absent and the passive ROM of the knee is sufficient for gait after TKA.

Compensatory mechanisms accommodate decreased knee ROM, velocity, and muscle performance by substituting other methods of advancing and lifting the lower limbs. Altered upper-body motions can also bring the body anteroposterior center of mass position closer to the knee joint center, thus decreasing the net knee flexion moment that must be resisted by the extensor. Jevsevar et al. (1993) found that locomotor activities of daily living (ADL) demand relatively slow loaded angular velocities and low knee torques, and that this factor should be considered in TKA exercise prescription. Patients with TKA were less able to perform effective knee deceleration during stair descent, which suggests that rehabilitation programs should be more tailored to knee demands during gait and ADL.

Berman et al. (1991) presented an evaluation of 68 TKA patients using isokinetic testing and found marked muscular deficits in flexion and extension preoperatively in the involved knee. Postoperatively, hamstring peak-torque values were able to attain strength levels of the uninvolved knee within 7–12 months after surgery, whereas quadriceps muscles maintained a residual deficit at 2 years follow-up. Huang et al. (1996) reported long-term results of muscle strength in 50 TKA patients compared with 16 matched healthy subjects, showing that the hamstring to quadriceps ratios after successful TKA were not the same even after 6–13 years. Lorentzen et al. (1999) stated that knee pain during measurements decreased significantly from the preoperative level

within 3 months after TKA. The isokinetic tests showed a pronounced increase in flexor muscle strength and a slight decrease of extensor muscle strength in the involved knee. Isometric flexor strength decreased and isometric extensor strength returned to the preoperative level only at 6 months in the TKA knee. Walsh et al. (1998) compared 29 TKA patients with 40 age/gender-matched control subjects and found decreased strength in walking (13–18%), stair climbing (43–51%), and knee extension (28–39%), as well as reduced walking speed.

Weakness of both quadriceps and hamstrings compared with the contralateral limb is commonly observed in patients with osteoarthritis (OA) and quadriceps atrophy, and has been shown histologically. An age-related decline in overall muscle strength also begins in adulthood, with a significant increase in the rate of strength loss beyond the age of 50. Proprioception measurements in OA and TKA are diminished with age, joint laxity, surgery, and inflammation. Weiler et al. (2000) reported an adverse effect of joint receptors and proprioceptive performance in OA. Comparing posterior cruciate ligament retaining with substituting TKA designs, Simmons et al. (1996) and Lattanzio et al. (1998) found no difference in proprioceptive values. Comparing TKA patients with healthy subjects, Fuchs et al. (1997) concluded that TKA conducts to loss of proprioception in the operated and healthy leg in TKA. Swanik et al. (2001) reported that TKA patients exhibit mild improvements in proprioception and balance with modified quadriceps activation patterns. No significant differences were found between the two TKA designs.

Sensorimotor systems represent composites of physiological systems with complex neurosensory and neuromuscular mechanisms. They are often simplified and inappropriately described as proprioception. The sensorimotor system also describes mechanisms involved in the acquisition of sensory stimuli to a neural signal, along with signal transmission via afferent pathways to the central nervous system (CNS). This signal is processed and integrated by the various centers of the CNS and central command generators, as well as the motor responses, resulting in muscle activation from locomotion and the performance of functional tasks and joint stabilization (Fig. 6.2)

Lephart et al. (2001) defines the sensorimotor system as "the system of sensory, motor and central integration and processing components involved with maintaining joint homeostasis during functional activity". Peripheral afferents originate from sensory receptors located in the joint (capsuloligamentous

Fig. 6.2. Sensorimotor system and neuromuscular control pathways

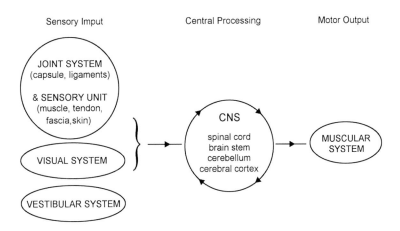

structures), muscle (muscle spindle, golgi tendon organ), myofascial and cutaneous tissue. Afferents also include inputs from the visual and vestibular systems. The respective contribution of all these peripheral afferents in regulation of the neuromuscular control (necessary for joint stability) is still controversial, but all information appears to contribute in the motor control mechanisms. The process by which afferent peripheral signals are utilized for motor control can be categorized into either feedback or feedforward mechanisms. Feedback is characterized by a reactive reflex to imposed forces to the joint, and the feedback neuromuscular control mechanisms are involved in maintaining posture and regulating slow movements.

For example, a TKA patient exercises neuromuscular stabilization during descending a step. The muscle activations are continually mediated by all available sensory information (modulated by the CNS). With several repetitions of the same task, the patient will acquire motor strategies.

Feedforward is characterized by preactivated muscle control in anticipation of loads or subsequent events, and feedforward mechanisms are used to evaluate results and help preprogram future muscle activation strategies. The idea is that preactivated (stiff) muscles recognize unexpected (destabilizing) joint loads quicker and can also facilitate feedback neuromuscular control. The same TKA patient is now, for example, exercising neuromuscular stabilization of the operated knee on different surfaces, while descending a step. In these new situations, the muscle activations have to occur in an anticipatory manner.

Recent investigations show that numerous free nerve endings are located at the interfaces of different tissues in surrounding structures of a peripheral joint. These free nerve endings can adapt and modify their receptive functions depending on the nature of the structure that contains them, so that differentiation between receptors may be difficult. Sensory receptors in the joint, muscle, tendon, fascia, and skin present a functional unit, which sends afferent inputs (information about joint position, motion, and tension) depending on the load and deformation experienced by this functional unit. Sensory functional units are important in understanding the efficacy of sensorimotor rehabilitation after TKA. As 90 % of the OA synovial tissue is removed, motor control would depend upon joint receptors only, jeopardizing all neuromuscular stabilization of the knee. However, no significant functional differences between the two TKA designs were reported, indicating that TKA patients can utilize the peripheral inputs to develop the motor strategies necessary to control the "new" knee joint.

Different theories of motor learning and motor control exist. Schmidt and Lee (1999) define motor learning as a series of internal processes, which, combined with training and experience, lead to long-term adaptations or changes in the motor skills. Three main stages of motor learning have been proposed. During the (verbal) cognitive phase, the patient learns the goals and the appropriate responses. In the motor (or intermediate) phase, the patient focuses more on the effective strategies to respond. In the last (autonomous) phase, the patient's responses are automatic and executed on a subconscious level.

Cognitive, perceptual and motor mechanisms are not independent elements, but are inseparable parts of the motor behavior. A large amount of rehabilitation can be seen as a learning process, during which the patient must master new skills. Physiotherapists may actually inhibit this learning process. Different activities involving motion are seen as motion strategies to solve specific tasks. Essential requirements include availability of adequate verbal feedback of results, variability of practice, and adequate design of the learning situation. No physiotherapist should teach the patient how to walk, but should rather give guidelines on how optimally to regain walking patterns. Lower extremity rehabilitation should include body weight bearing against gravity, as in real-life situations, to allow the patient to develop his own motor strategies. Based on this knowledge, one can appreciate abnormal patterns and deficits in gait analyses, muscle strength and proprioception measurements in knee OA and TKA.

Rehabilitation Guidelines

The first week after surgery represents the basis for successful TKA rehabilitation outcomes. Further goals have to be achieved for functional weight-bearing progress:

1. Adequate knee joint mobility of at least 90 degrees flexion and full extension. We recommend immediate CPM with accelerated flexion combined with ROM exercises, including heel on a pillow and dangling leg exercises. Manual mobilizations of the patellofemoral joint are performed by the physiotherapist followed by sitting from day two.
2. Sufficient quadriceps activation. The patient should be able to contract the quadriceps actively while performing isometric contractions in the knee extension position. Knee extensor lag is the term used for cases of weak quadriceps muscles.
3. Low muscular tightness and tension. To prevent and treat muscular problems, gentle massage and soft gastrocnemii and hamstring stretching are important interventions.
4. Pain and swelling may inhibit quadriceps function and motion, consequently slowing down rehabilitation. A combination of the above interventions plus pain management help to improve pain and swelling.
5. Progressive weight bearing from day one postoperative and encouragement of walking on crutches with 50% body weight is considered a golden rule. Walking distance is progressively increased daily, aiming to walk 100 meters and to manage stairs with proper crutches technique by days 4–5.

After the first postoperative week, TKA patients enter phase I of rehabilitation with recovery of global body functions and continuation of the exercise program. Daily home exercises and discipline are crucial for successful rehabilitation. After wound healing, hydrotherapy is useful, as water exercises improve knee ROM and walking patterns. Weight-bearing allowance with crutches is progressively increased according to knee status and neuromuscular stabilization skills. A cane can be utilized in the transition period, usually 6–8 weeks postoperatively. Flexion is expected to increase gradually to 110 degrees after 6 weeks and 120 degrees after 2–3 months. Any loss of motion or complication should be reported to the surgeon, in order to ensure rapid intervention.

Phase I is characterized by criterion-based rehabilitation:

1. Respect of knee pain and swelling
2. Respect of safe ROM during exercises
3. Qualitative coordinated motion and stabilization strategies only.

Phase II of rehabilitation intensifies individual progression of phase I:

1. Functional progression after correlation with criterion-based program plus gradual progression, such as: from double- to single-leg body positions, from static to dynamic low-reactive motor tasks, and from low-speed to high-speed motor tasks
2. Learning of individual motor tasks under different conditions in random practice for long-term skill acquisition, variable practice under varying degrees of difficulty, speed and environmental conditions, and finally verbal feedback
3. Training devices for functional progression to enhance neuromuscular stabilization, by increasing the muscular activation and proprioception on balance devices, external resistance devices, visual devices, and the patient's own devices.

Milestones in the sensorimotor training progression include: controlled loading of the operated knee (Figs. 6.3–6.5), rising from a chair (Figs. 6.6–6.8), level walking (Figs. 6.9–6.11), ascending/descending stairs (Figs. 6.12–6.14), and low-reactive activities (Figs. 6.15–6.17).

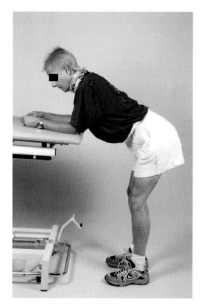
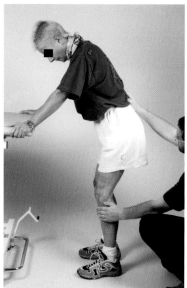
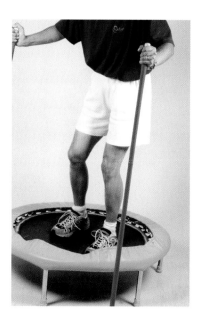

Figs. 6.3–6.5. Controlled loading of the operated knee

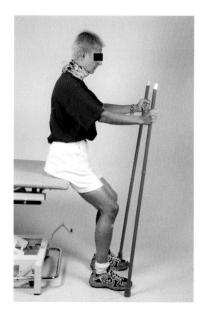
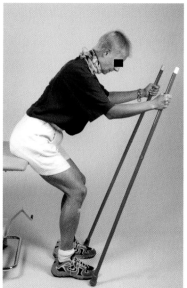
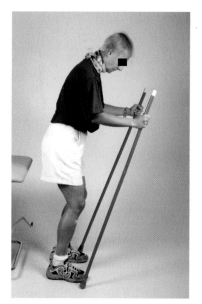

Figs. 6.6–6.8. Rising from a chair

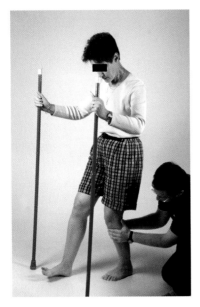
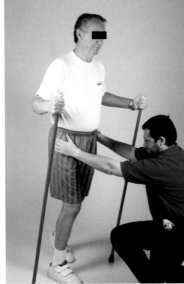
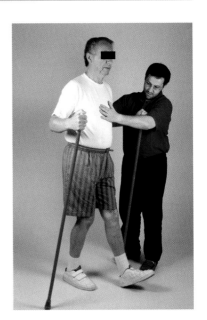

Figs. 6.9–6.11. Level walking

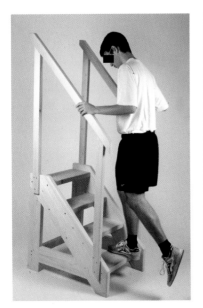
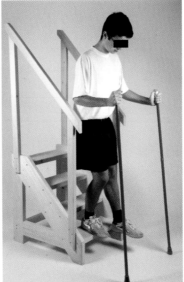
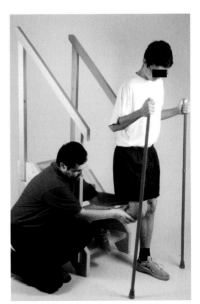

Figs. 6.12–6.14. Managing stairs

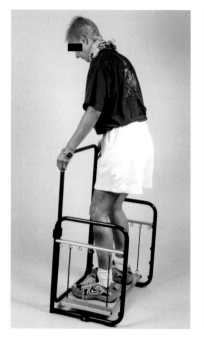
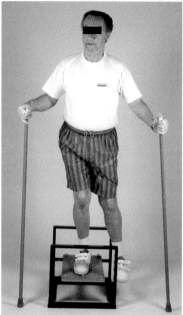
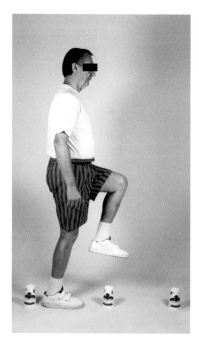

Figs. 6.15–6.17. Low-reactive activities

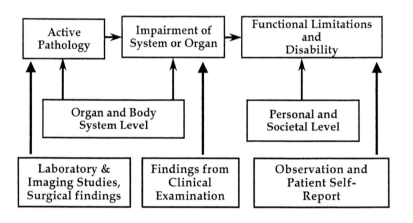

Fig. 6.18. Summary of clinical outcomes in rehabilitation

Rehabilitation Outcomes

Quality assurance and management have been recognized for a systematic approach. Effenberger et al. (2001) stated that problem-oriented documentation will lead to greater effectiveness and improvement of quality of life. Evaluation and quality control in physical therapy and rehabilitation are still lacking definitions and standard procedures. Several aspects of therapeutic interventions (examination, documentation, measurements) differ depending on training, specialization or clinic. Scientific, valid and reliable measurement instruments are required for routine physical therapy and systematic documentation systems. Rehabilitation outcomes can be monitored by pathology, impairment, functional limitation, disability, process outcomes, costs, and patient satisfaction. These data can be used in patient management decisions and to assess clinical performance.

Clinical outcomes must be valid, reliable and responsive and can be categorized as shown in Fig. 6.18. Surgeons document via imaging techniques, clinical examinations, laboratory investigations, surgery reports, and questionnaires. Physiotherapists define functional limitations, observe, analyze, measure, and utilize questionnaires.

Performance-Based Measurements

There is a large spectrum of performance measure instruments. In general a high degree of technical complexity can take psychometric variables into account, such as electronically controlled isokinetic machines (Biodex) and gait analysis systems. This instrumentation requires trained personnel, and is time consuming and financially demanding. A survey (1999) in Switzerland revealed only 220 isokinetic units available in 4,000 clinics. Simpler test measurements increase the likelihood of inaccuracy, validity and reliability. Performance-based measurements evaluate quadriceps strength or electromyographic activation during gait. Andersson et al. (1981) observed changes in gait and clinical status after TKA and concluded that information obtained in a sophisticated gait laboratory is of limited value. Therefore, performance-based measurements in TKA are questionable. The clinician's decision to obtain a particular test should depend on the patient's presentation and goals. When TKA patients have good sensorimotor control and sufficient local and cardiovascular endurance, then more tests are unnecessary. The TKA patient with identical functional outcome and willingness to return to his favorite sport is more likely to benefit from the results of specific tests. Downsides of performance-based measures of function in the clinical setting include the problems of normative data interpretation.

Patient-Reported Measurements

General measures of health status include the Medical Outcome Study short form-36 (SF-36) and the Sickness Impact Profile (SIP). The SF-36 is described in detail in Sect. 5.2. General questionnaires tend to be longer and more difficult to answer, are less responsive than specific measures, and their content may appear to be less relevant for clinicians. Specific measures of knee function include the Lysholm Knee Scale, the Cincinnati Scale, and the Western Ontario and McMaster Universities Osteoarthritis Index (WOMAC), as discussed in Sect. 5.2. The Knee Outcome Survey (KOS) was developed at the University of Pittsburgh by Irrgang et al. (1998) as a patient-reported instrument for measurement of functional limitations commonly experienced by individuals who have various pathological disorders of the knee. The KOS consists of two separate scales: the Activities of Daily Living Scale (ADLS) and the Sport Activities

Scale (SAS). The ADLS includes items related to symptoms and functional limitations experienced during ADL, while the SAS consists of items related to symptoms and functional limitations experienced during sports activities. Symptoms included are pain, stiffness, swelling, instability and weakness. The responses to each item are graduated in terms of the functional limitations that the symptom imposed on the individual during ADL. The responses range from absence of the symptoms to complete loss of function due to the symptom. The functional limitations included in the ADLS are difficulty with regard to walking on level surfaces and stairs, standing, kneeling, squatting, sitting and rising from a sitting position.

In a large study with 397 knee patients, Irrgang et al. (1998) showed that the ADLS is a reliable, valid and responsive instrument for the assessment of functional limitations that result from a wide variety of pathological disorders and impairments of the knee. The KOS-ADLS is short, easy to interpret and easy to score for the patient. Its content is relevant to the patient's knee condition, gives the clinician useful information and represents a good example of common currency in knee rehabilitation outcome measures.

Bibliography

Andersson GB, Andriacchi TP, Galante JO (1981) Correlations between changes in gait and in clinical status after knee arthroplasty. Acta Orthop Scand 52:569–573

Andriacchi TP, Galante JO, Fermier RW (1982) The influence of total knee replacement design on walking and stair-climbing. J Bone Joint Surg 64A:1328–1335

Andriacchi TP, Hurwitz DE (1997) Gait biomechanics and total knee arthroplasty. Am J Knee Surg 10:255–260

Beaupre LA, Davies DM, Jones CA et al (2001) Exercise combined with passive motion or slider board therapy compared with exercise only. A randomized controlled trial of patients following total knee arthroplasty. Phys Ther 81:1029–1037

Bellamy N, Buchanan WW, Goldsmith CH et al (1988) Validation study of WOMAC: a health status instrument for measuring clinically important patient relevant outcomes to antirheumatic drug therapy in patients with osteoarthritis of the hip or knee. J Rheumatol 15:1833–1840

Bergner M, Bobbitt RA, Carter WB et al (1981) The sickness impact profile: development and final revision of a health status measure. Med Care 19:787–805

Berman AT, Bosacco SJ, Israelite C (1991) Evaluation of total knee arthroplasty using isokinetic testing. Clin Orthop 271:106–113

Bizzini M (2000) Sensomotorische Rehabilitation nach Beinverletzungen. Mit Fallbeispielen in allen Heilungsstadien. Thieme, Stuttgart

Bizzini M, Munzinger U (1998) Motion analysis of the squat exercise: influence of the body position on the anterior tibial shear in normal, ACL-deficient and ACL-reconstructed knees. Paper no 28. Abstract book. 8th Congress of the European Society of Sports Traumatology, Knee Surgery and Arthroscopy. Nice, 29 Apr–2 May 1998

Bolanos AA, Colizza WA, McCann PD et al (1998) A comparison of isokinetic strength testing and gait analysis in patients with posterior cruciate-retaining and substituting knee arthroplasties. J Arthroplasty 13:906–915

Boldt JG, Keblish PA, Varma C et al (2001) Patella nonresurfacing in low contact stress (LCS) mobile bearing total knee arthroplasty (TKA): results of 1777 TKA with 2 to 15 years follow up. Paper no 23. Abstract book. 68th AAOS annual meeting. San Francisco, 28 Feb–4 March 2001

Buechel FF Sr, Buechel FF Jr, Pappas MJ et al (2001) Twenty-year evaluation of meniscal bearing and rotating platform knee replacements. Clin Orthop 388:41–50

Canal ST (ed) (1998) Campbell's operative orthopaedics, 9th edn. Mosby, St Louis, p 268

Chao EY, Laughman RK, Stauffer RN (1980) Biomechanical gait evaluation of pre- and postoperative total knee replacement patients. Arch Orthop Trauma Surg 97:309–317

Chiarello CM, Gundersen L, O'Halloran T (1997) The effects of continuous passive motion duration and increment on range of motion in total knee arthroplasty patients. J Orthop Sports Phys Ther 25:119–125

Colwell CW Jr, Morris BA (1992) The influence of continuous passive motion on the results of total knee arthroplasty. Clin Orthop 276:225–228

Coutts RD, Kaita J, Barr R et al (1982) The role of continuous passive motion in the postoperative rehabilitation of total knee replacement. Orthop Translat 6:277–278

Daltroy LH, Morlino CI, Eaton HM et al (1998) Preoperative education for total hip and knee replacement patients. Arthritis Care Res 11:469–478

De Andrade JR, Grant C, Dixon A (1965) Joint distension and reflex muscle inhibition in the knee. J Bone Joint Surg 47A:313–322

DesJardins JD, Walker PS, Haider H et al (2000) The use of a force-controlled dynamic knee simulator to quantify the mechanical performance of total knee replacement design during functional activity. J Biomech 33:1231–1242

Drake BG, Callahan CM, Dittus RS et al (1994) Global rating systems used in assessing knee arthroplasty outcomes. J Arthroplasty 9:409–417

Effenberger H, Mechtler R, Jerosch J et al (2001) Qualitaetsmanagement in der Hueft- und Knieendoprothetik. Orthopaede 30:332–344

Ellenbecker TS, Davies GJ (2001) Closed kinetic chain exercise. A comprehensive guide to multiple-joint exercise. Human Kinetics, Champaign

Enloe LJ, Shields RK, Smith K et al (1996) Total hip and knee replacements treatment programs: a report using consensus. J Orthop Sports Phys Ther 23:3–11

Finch E, Walsh M, Thomas SG et al (1998) Functional ability perceived by individuals following total knee arthroplasty compared to age-matched individuals without knee disability. J Orthop Sports Phys Ther 27:255–263

Fuchs S, Thorwersten L, Niewerth S et al (1997) Proprioceptive capacities of the knee joint with and without endoprothesis. Z Orthop Ihre Grenzgeb 135:335–340

Gatti LA, Bourbon B, Scott CM (1996) The effects of a preoperative educational and exercise program on postoperative mobility in total hip arthroplasty patients. Abstract book. APTA Combined Meeting. Atlanta, 13–18 Febr 1996

Gillquist J (1996) Knee ligaments and proprioception. Guest editorial. Acta Orthop Scand 67:533–535

Grace DL, Cracchiolo A, Dorey FJ (1986) The effect of early weight-bearing in total knee arthroplasty. Clin Orthop 207:178–185

Gresalmer RP, Klein JR (1998) The biomechanics of the patellofemoral joint. J Orthop Sports Phys Ther 28:286–298

Grood ES, Suntay WJ, Noyes FR et al (1984) Biomechanics of the knee extension exercise. Effects of cutting the anterior cruciate ligament. J Bone Joint Surg 66A:725–734

Healy WL, Iorio R, Lemos MJ (2000) Athletic activity after total knee arthroplasty. Clin Orthop 380:65–71

Hefti F, Muller W, Jakob RP et al (1993) Evaluation of knee ligament injuries with the IKDC form. Knee Surg Sports Traumatol Arthroscopy 1:226–234

Huang CH, Cheng CK, Lee YT et al (1996) Muscle strength after successful total knee replacement. Clin Orthop 328:147–154

Inman VT, Ralston HJ, Todd F (1984) Human walking. Williams and Wilkins, Baltimore

Insall J, Ranawat CS, Aglietti P et al (1976) A comparison of four models of total knee replacement prostheses. J Bone Joint Surg 58A:754

Insall J, Dorr LD, Scott RD et al (1989) Rationale for the Knee Society clinical rating system. Clin Orthop 248:13–14

Irrgang JJ, Snyder-Mackler L, Wainner RS et al (1998) Development of a patient-reported measure of function of the knee. J Bone Joint Surg 80A:1132–1145

Irrgang JJ (1999) Outcome management in orthopaedic physical therapy. Personal communication. Schulthess Clinic, Zurich

Jevsevar DS, Riley PO, Hodge WA et al (1993) Knee kinematics and kinetics during locomotor activities of daily living in subjects with knee arthroplasty and in healthy control subjects. Phys Ther 73:229–239

Johnson DP, Eastwood DM (1992) Beneficial effects of continuous passive motion after total condylar knee arthroplasty. Ann R Coll Surg Engl 74:412–416

Johnson DP (1990) The effects of continuous passive motion on wound healing and joint mobility after knee arthroplasty. J Bone Joint Surg 72A:421–426

Jones CA, Voaklander DC, Johnston WC et al (2000) Health related quality of life outcomes after total hip and knee arthroplasties in a community based population. J Rheumatol 27:1745–1752

Jordan LR, Siegal JL, Olivo JL (1995) Early flexion routine: an alternative method of continuous passive motion. Clin Orthop 315:231–233

Kramers-de Quervain IA, Stussi E, Muller R et al (1997) Quantitative gait analysis after bilateral total knee arthroplasty with two different systems within each subject. J Arthroplasty 12:168–179

Kreiblich DN, Vaz M, Bourne RB et al (1996) What is the best way of assessing outcome after total knee replacement? Clin Orthop 331:221–225

Kumar PJ, McPherson EJ, Dorr LD et al (1996) Rehabilitation after total knee arthroplasty: a comparison of 2 rehabilitation techniques. Clin Orthop 331:93–101

Kuster MS, Wood GA, Stachowiak GW et al (1997) Joint load considerations in total knee replacement. J Bone Joint Surg 79B:109–113

Kuster MS, Spalinger E, Blanksby BA et al (2000) Endurance sports after total knee replacement: a biomechanical investigation. Med Sci Sports Exerc 32:721

Lachiewicz PF (2000) The role of continuous passive motion after total knee arthroplasty. Clin Orthop 380:144–150

Larsson L, Grimby G, Karlsson J (1978) Muscle strength and speed of movement in relation to age and muscle morphology. J Appl Physiol 46:451

Lattanzio PJ, Chess DG, MacDermid JC (1998) Effect of the posterior cruciate ligament in knee joint proprioception in total knee arthroplasty. J Arthroplasty 13:580–585

Lephart SM, Riemann BL, Fu FH (2001) Introduction to the sensorimotor system. In: Lephart SM, Fu FH (eds) Proprioception and neuromuscular control in joint stability. Human Kinetics, Champaign

Lorentzen JS, Petersen MM, Brot C et al (1999) Early changes in muscle strength after total knee arthroplasty. A 6-month follow-up of 30 knees. Acta Orthop Scand 70:176–179

MacDonald SJ, Bourne RB, Rorabeck CH et al (2000) Prospective randomized clinical trial of continuous passive motion after total knee arthroplasty. Clin Orthop 380:30–45

Maloney WJ, Schurman DJ, Hangen D et al (1990) The influence of continuous passive motion on outcome in total knee arthroplasty. Clin Orthop 256:162–168

Martin SD, Scott RD, Thornhill TS (1998) Current concepts in total knee arthroplasty. J Orthop Sports Phys Ther 28:252–261

Martin TP, Gundersen LA, Blevins FT et al (1991) The influence of functional electrical stimulation on the properties of vastus lateralis fibers following total knee arthroplasty. Scand J Rehab Med 23:207

Matsuda S, Ishinishi T, White SE et al (1997) Patellofemoral joint after total knee arthroplasty. Effect on contact area and contact stress. J Arthroplasty 12:790

McGinty G, Irrgang JJ, Pezzullo D (2000) Biomechanical considerations for rehabilitation of the knee. A review paper. Clin Biomech 15:160–166

McGuigan FX, Hozach WJ, Moriarty L et al (1995) Predicting quality-of-life outcomes following total joint arthroplasty. J Arthroplasty 10:742–747

McHorney CA, Ware JE, Lu JF et al (1994) The MOS 36-item short form health survey (SF-36) III. Tests of data quality, scaling assumptions and reliability across diverse patient groups. Med Care 32:40–66

McInnes J, Larson MG, Daltroy LH et al (1992) A controlled evaluation of continuous passive motion in patients undergoing total knee arthroplasty. JAMA 268:1423–1428

Michelsen CB, Askanazi J, Grump FE et al (1979) Changes in metabolism and muscle composition associated with total hip replacement. J Trauma 19:29

Mulder T (1991) A process-oriented model of human motor behavior: toward a theory-based rehabilitation approach. Movement science series. Phys Ther 71:157–164

Nadler SF, Malanga GA, Zimmerman JR (1993) Continuous passive motion in the rehabilitation setting: a retrospective study. Am J Phys Med Rehabil 72:162–165

Nagi SZ (1991) Disability concepts revisited: implications for prevention. In: Pope AM, Tarlov AR (eds) Disability in America. Toward a national agenda for prevention. Appendix A. National Academy Press, Washington DC, pp 309–327

Noyes FR, McGinnis GH, Mooar LA (1984) Functional disability in the anterior cruciate insufficient knee syndrome. Review of knee rating systems and projected risk factors in determining treatment. Sports Med 1:278–302

Noyes FR, Barber SD, Mangine RE et al (1991) Abnormal lower limb symmetry determined by function hop tests after anterior cruciate ligament rupture. Am J Sports Med 19:513–518

Palmitier RA, An KN, Scott SG et al (1991) Kinetic chain exercise in knee rehabilitation. Sports Med 11:402–413

Pope RO, Corocoran S, McCaul K et al (1997) Continuous passive motion after primary total knee arthroplasty: does it offer any benefits? J Bone Joint Surg 79B:914–917

Ritter MA, Albohm MJ, Keating M et al (1995) Comparative outcomes of total joint arthroplasty. J Arthroplasty 10:7737–7741

Robinson RP, Simonian T, McCann KJ (1994) Rehabilitation following total knee arthroplasty. In: Fu FH, Harner CD, Vince KG (eds) Knee surgery. Williams and Wilkins, Baltimore

Romness DW, Rand JA (1988) The role of continuous passive motion following total knee arthroplasty. Clin Orthop 226:34–37

Sapega AA (1990) Muscle performance evaluation in orthopaedic practice. Current concepts review. J Bone Joint Surg 72A:1562–1574

Schenk RK (1995) Osseointegration. In: Morscher EW (ed) Endoprosthetics. Springer, Berlin Heidelberg New York

Schmidt RA, Lee TD (1999) Motor control and learning. A behavioral emphasis, 3rd edn. Human Kinetics, Champaign, Ill.

Shelbourne KD, Nitz P (1990) Accelerated rehabilitation after anterior cruciate ligament reconstruction. Am J Sports Med 18:292–299

Simmons S, Lephart S, Rubash H et al (1996) Proprioception following total knee arthroplasty with and without the posterior cruciate ligament. J Arthroplasty 11:763–768

Steindler A (1955) Kinesiology of the human body under normal and pathological conditions. Thomas, Springfield

Su FC, Lai KA, Hong WH (1998) Rising from a chair after total knee arthroplasty. Clin Biomech 13:176–181

Swanik CB, Rubash HE, Barrack RL et al (2000) The role of proprioception in patients with DJD and following total knee arthroplasty. In: Lephart SM, Fu FH (eds) Proprioception and neuromuscular control in joint stability. Human Kinetics, Champaign

Swanik CB, Lephart SM, Rubash HE (2001) Effects of cruciate retaining versus posterior stabilized TKA on proprioception, balance and quadriceps EMG. A prospective randomized study. Paper no 182. Abstract book. 68th AAOS annual meeting. San Francisco, 28 Febr–4 Mar 2001

Taylor SJ, Walker PS (2001) Forces and moments telemetered from two distal femoral replacements during various activities. J Biomech 34:839–848

Taylor SJ, Walker PS, Perry JS et al (1998) The forces in the distal femur and the knee during walking and other activities measured by telemetry. J Arthroplasty 13:428–437

Tegner Y, Lysholm J (1985) Rating systems in the evaluation of knee ligament injuries. Clin Orthop 198:43–49

Van den Berg F (1999) Angewandte Physiologie, vol 1. Das Bindegewebe des Bewegungsapparates verstehen und beeinflussen. Thieme, Stuttgart

Van der Wal JC (1998) The organization of the substrate of proprioception in the elbow region of the rat. Thesis. Rijksuniversiteit Limburg, Maastricht, Holland

Ververeli PA, Sutton DC, Hearn SL et al (1995) Continuous passive motion after total knee arthroplasty: analysis of costs and benefits. Clin Orthop 321:208–215

Walsh M, Woodhouse LJ, Thomas SG et al (1998) Physical impairments and functional limitations: a comparison of individuals 1 year after total knee arthroplasty with control subjects. Phys Ther 78:248–258

Ware JE (1997) SF-36 health survey. Manual and interpretation guide. The Health Institute, New England Medical Center. Nimrod, Boston

Weiler HT, Pap G, Awiszus F (2000) The role of joint afferents in sensory processing in osteoarthritic knees. Rheumatology 39:850–856

Wilk KE, Andrews JR (1992) Current concepts in the treatment of anterior cruciate ligament disruption. J Orthop Sports Phys Ther 15:279–293

Wilk KE, Escamilla RF, Fleisig GS et al (1996) Comparison of the tibiofemoral joint forces and electromyographic activity during open and closed kinetic chain exercises. Am J Sports Med 24:518–527

Wilk KE, Zheng N, Fleisig GS et al (1997) Kinetic chain exercise: implications for the anterior cruciate ligament patient. J Sport Rehab 6:49–54

Wilson SA, McCann PD, Gotlin RS et al (1996) Comprehensive gait analysis in posterior-stabilized knee arthroplasty. J Arthroplasty 11:359–367

Worland RL, Arredondo J, Angles F et al (1998) Home continuous passive motion versus professional physical therapy following total knee replacement. J Arthroplasty 13:784–787

Yashar AA, Venn-Watson E, Welsh T et al (1997) Continuous passive motion with accelerated flexion after total knee arthroplasty. Clin Orthop 345:38–43

CHAPTER 7

Jens G. Boldt · P. Thümler · Peter A. Keblish · M. Vogt

Complications

7.1 Anterior Knee Pain Following Total Knee Arthroplasty

Jens G. Boldt, P. Thümler

Anterior knee pain following total knee arthroplasty (TKA) represents a common and challenging complication. It is frustrating for both the patient and the surgeon. Commonly a specific cause for this pain or discomfort is not present. Differential diagnoses are multiple and include biomechanical patellofemoral problems (maltracking), soft tissue, synovial and prosthetic impingements, component malpositioning, wound problems, skin neuroma, effusion, and infection. Finding the right diagnostic tool is difficult, as are treatment options. This chapter focuses on the clinical approach, suggested investigations, and a treatment algorithm in patients presenting with anterior knee pain after TKA. Our conclusions are supported by personal experience and studies, literature research, as well as data from 27 specific cases in one major joint replacement center. The challenging fact in this problematic subgroup is that a significant number of patients fail to present with a pathology or do not improvement despite specific management. Successful therapy may range from physiotherapy, or simple subcutaneous infiltration of local anesthetics, to complex revision surgery with exchange of all components.

Inclusion criteria in this study were all primary TKA seen at 1-year follow-up with anterior knee pain plus a moderate or poor clinical outcome using the Knee Society Score. Reduced mobility, pain, and patella problems were most frequent in this group. Infection and trauma were exclusion criteria. Two different mobile bearing knee systems were utilized, the low contact stress (LCS; DePuy Int, Leeds, UK) and the MBK (Zimmer, Warsaw, USA). From more than 200 LCS and 70 MBK prostheses, 27 cases entered the study, all of which underwent routine blood screening (erythrocyte sedimentation rate (ESR), leucocytes, C-reactive protein (CRP)) and x-ray examination. Radiographic analysis was focused on patella track-ing, congruency, and patella tilt with comparable pre- and postoperative skyline radiographs. Patella tracking was based on alignment of the femoral trochlear sulcus and the crown of the patella and measured in millimeters of lateral deviation on comparable pre- and postoperative skyline views.

Spiral computed tomography (CT) investigation was used for evaluation of tibial and femoral component rotational alignment. All data for femoral component rotational positioning were analyzed using a helical CT scanner. Femoral component rotational alignment was calculated by referencing the two posterior condyles to the transepicondylar axis (TEA), which was a line drawn between the spike of the lateral epicondyle and the sulcus of the medial epicondyle, as recently recommended by Yoshino et al. (2001) (Fig. 7.1). One case was excluded because of inability to identify the medial sulcus despite 2 mm cuts. Angles were calculated utilizing sophisticated helical CT-implemented software. Midflexion instability was tested under fluoroscopy. When aseptic loosening or infection was ruled out, Tc99 and/or gallium scintigraphy was performed, as well as arthrography (Fig. 7.2).

Hoffa Fat Pad Impingement Associated with Anteroposterior Glide Prostheses (22%)

The LCS anteroposterior (AP) glide mobile bearing TKA has theoretical advantages in that it promises a logical synthesis of combined AP translation and rotation ability, both of which are limited by surrounding soft tissues only. Predominant advantages were considered to be reduced polyethylene wear and preservation of the posterior cruciate ligament (PCL). However, clinical downsides were observed in various European centers and included early occurrence of Hoffa fat pad impingement associated with anterior knee pain. In flexion the PCL "pushes" the bearing anteriorly (Fig. 7.3). This was observed in all AP glide cases that presented with circumscript anterior knee pain. There was an unusually high overall

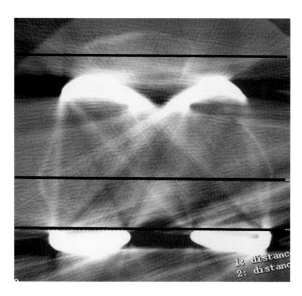

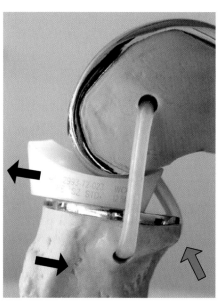

Fig. 7.1. Transverse CT scans are a practical method for accurate determination of femoral component rotational positioning in TKA. Example of a well-aligned femoral component parallel to the TEA. The TEA is best referenced from the apex of the lateral epicondyle to the sulcus of the medial epicondyle. The rotation angle is measured from that TEA line to the posterior femoral resection line (interface). Femoral component alignment parallel to TEA ensures optimum patellofemoral tracking

Fig. 7.3. Knee model showing possible mechanism for anterior bearing translation in flexion due to PCL forward "push" or laxity

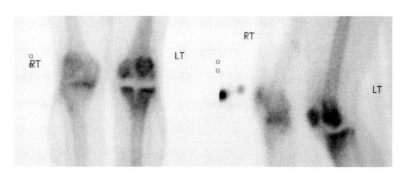

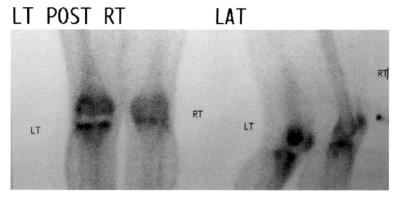

Fig. 7.2. Gallium three-phase bone scan demonstrating increased peripatellar and interface activity. Interface activity can be active for as long as 5 years, but patellar and synovial activity is more sensitive and specific

Fig. 7.4 a, b. Lateral radiographs with enhanced soft tissue technique may reveal Hoffa fat pad footprint impingement by the bearing

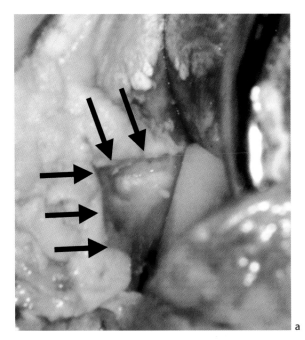

a

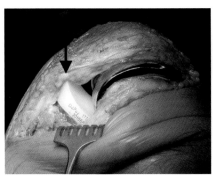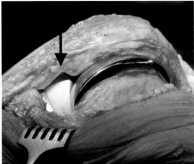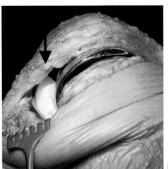

b

incidence of anterior knee pain in AP glide TKA compared with excellent results utilizing the rotating only platform TKA from the same manufacturer.

Diagnostic evaluation included clinical examination in terms of firm digital pain revealing pressure over the patella tendon, a positive local anesthetic test, soft tissue enhanced lateral radiographs, arthroscopic evaluation, and gallium scintigraphy. Six of 27 (22%) anterior knee pain cases presented with Hoffa fat pad impingement, all of which were considered to be related to surgical technique. Gallium scans as well as diagnostic arthroscopy prior to revision surgery revealed increased uptake correlated with intraoperative findings of fat pad fibrosis and/or necrosis. Another regular observation was a footprint of the bearing into the fat pad (Fig. 7.4), which in retrospect was visible as a soft tissue shadow on lateral radiographs (Fig. 7.5). Revision surgery revealed evidence of increased anterior bearing shift (push by

PCL) causing fat pad impingement. Five of seven cases improved significantly after fat pad excision, bearing exchange, denervation and PCL sacrifice, but two cases did not (Figs. 7.6, 7.7). Histopathologic investigations revealed partly necrotic and partly sclerosed scar tissues. All AP mobile bearings were simply exchanged to rotating mobile bearings only during surgery.

Because of these experiences, the use of AP glide bearings has been discontinued and rotating only mobile bearings are now implanted. Excessive resection and denervation of the Hoffa fat pad is recommended when AP glide bearing are used. Reports from surgeons using this device in Asian populations are comparable with those of the rotating only platform. Hoffa fat pad and intraoperative impingement tests should be established, when AP glide prostheses are desired. However, even then, anterior knee pain cannot be totally excluded.

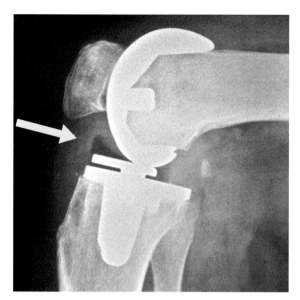

Fig.7.5. Hoffa fat pad footprints due to repetitive mechanical impingement

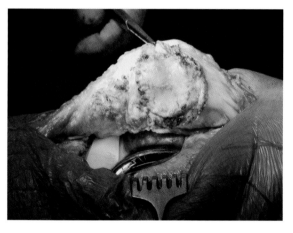

Fig.7.7. The remaining "shaved" fat pad is denervated via cautery

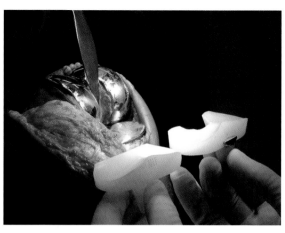

Fig.7.6. Surgical example of fat pad resection and bearing exchange to rotating platform only

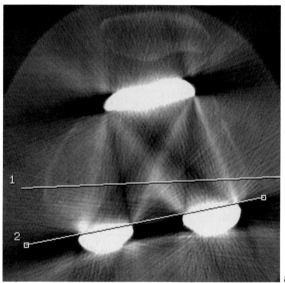

Fig.7.8a,b. CT scan example of 8 degrees excessive internal malrotation of the femoral component and the intraoperative situs demonstrating malresection

Fig. 7.9 a,b. Midflexion instability when varus and valgus stresses are employed

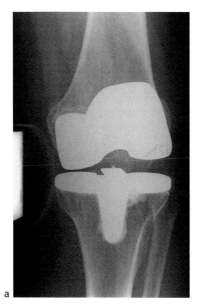
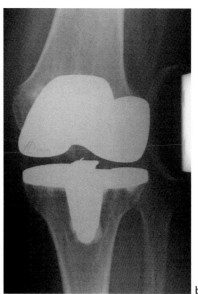

Femoral Component Internal Malrotation and Arthrofibrosis (30%)

The most common technical error observed was a significantly increased incidence of femoral component internal rotation in this group with anterior knee pain (Fig. 7.8). Eight of 27 cases had femoral component internal malrotation with a mean internal rotation of 4.2 degrees (0–8) in relation to the TEA (normal femoral component rotation equals zero degrees = parallel to TEA). All 12 cases were associated with some degree of reduction in their knee joint range of motion, including lack of extension and flexion under 60 degrees. Femoral component rotational alignment is dependent on technique and instruments, and influences patella tracking, gap balance, and soft tissue kinematics. Deviation into internal rotation results in poor patellofemoral tracking and clinical outcomes. Potential complications, such as painful and/or stiff TKA (arthrofibrosis), have been shown to correlate with significant internal rotation of the femoral component in other studies (Sect. 7.3). Four femoral components were revised. Three knees improved, one did not.

We, therefore, recommend CT evaluation of component alignment in clinically painful knees. Cases that present with internal malrotation should be considered for revision surgery with the view to revise the femoral component when internal malrotation of more than 5 degrees in combination with midflexion instability (Fig. 7.9), arthrofibrosis, or other biomechanical dysfunction is confirmed. Prevention of patellofemoral problems is possible with any method that provides perfect femoral rotational alignment.

Isolated Patellofemoral Subluxation (11%)

Patellofemoral subluxation with proper femoral component alignment was encountered in three of 27 (11%) cases. All preoperative radiographs revealed significant lateral patella subluxation in combination with varus (two cases) and valgus (one case) deformity (Fig. 7.10). This fact stresses the importance of perfect and unimpeded patella tracking during surgery. Patellae that track laterally preoperatively show a high tendency to do the same post-TKA. Therefore, existing lateral patella drift, proper component positioning, extensive lateral releases, patelloplasty with lateral facet contouring, congruent contact throughout full range of motion and appreciation of active vastus lateralis forces must be encountered during surgery in order to avoid these complications. All three patients were treated with arthroscopic lateral releases (in to out) and partial denervation: two improved, one did not.

Overstuffed Patellofemoral Compartment (7%)

When comparing pre- and postoperative CT scans, two of 27 cases demonstrated significantly enlarged and increased anterior (unresurfaced) patella compartment. The actual height was measured on CT

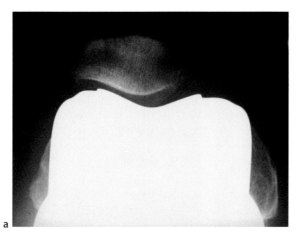

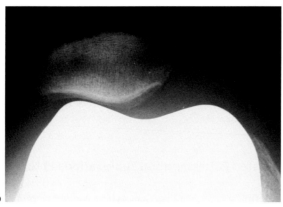

Fig. 7.10. **a** Isolated lateral patella subluxation and **b** combined with femoral internal malrotation

scans taking the TEA into account in the non-operated and TKA knee. Clinical appearance also revealed a more proud and tender patella with a positive Zohlen sign. Both patients were advised conservative measures. We have no clinical experience for ultimate patella contouring and there is no information in the current literature; however, we would be inclined to offer this treatment when the patient's pain threshold rises above the tolerable level.

Skin Neuroma and Contact Allergy (11 %)

In two cases, anterior knee pain was caused by surgically compromised cutaneous nerves that developed a painful skin neuroma in the lateral and distal aspect of the midline incision. An area of approximately 4 by 8 cm was affected with paresthesia and sharp local skin pain. There was deep pain and increased discomfort during full range of motion; managing stairs was impossible. All other investigations, including clinical examination, radiographs, CT scans, and

blood screening, were negative. Both patients were successfully treated with repetitive local anesthetic injections (plus non-crystalloid glucocorticoids) near the operating scar and oral vitamin complexes for 6 weeks (Fig. 7.11). The third case, which did not respond to this treatment, presented with additional skin efflorescence and was ultimately diagnosed a proven PMMA cement contact allergy. She underwent successful isolated tibial component revision because of non-responding conservative therapy and increasing radiolytic lines at the tibial cement–bone interface (Fig. 7.12).

Intra-articular Bacterial Infection (4 %)

In one patient, bacterial intra-articular infection was identified (beta hemolysing *Staphylococcus aureus*). Additional arthrofibrosis, internal malrotation of the femoral component (5 degrees) and patella subluxation was present. However, she refused excision arthroplasty at that time and was treated with arthroscopic lavage, but strongly advised for a radical two-stage revision procedure.

Anterior Knee Pain without Specific Findings (15 %)

In four of 27 (15 %) cases no obvious pathology could be identified. All possible tests including infection screening were negative. This subgroup was treated conservatively with intense physiotherapy, proprioceptive training, non-steroidal anti-inflammatory drugs and pain relief. They are under close supervision and regularly followed up. None of these conservative measures has led to significant improvements. Although one is tempted to consider these cases as having reflex sympathetic dystrophy (RSD) or complex regional pain syndrome (CRPS), we are not convinced that this is the case. However, unexplainable anterior knee pain following TKA is a frustrating finding and highly dissatisfying, and is discussed in more detail in Sect. 7.6 – "The unhappy knee".

Discussion

Successful clinical outcomes after TKA are dependent upon multifactorial issues, the most important of which are patella treatment and femoral component rotational alignment. Prosthetic design and implantation of femorotibial components vary with dif-

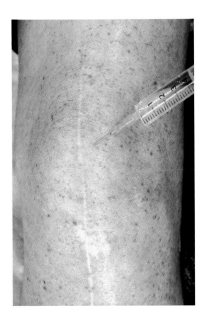

Fig. 7.11. Operating scar cutaneous nerve neuroma, which was treated successfully with local anesthetic injections

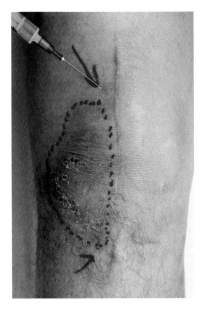

Fig. 7.12. Clinically tested PMMA cement contact allergy leading to secondary efflorescences. The cement was removed and converted to a cementless tibial component

ferent total knee systems. The surgeon must evaluate and address variables that include varus–valgus alignment, extra-articular deformities, soft tissue contractions, exaggerated Q-angle, patella position, size, and shape, as well as femorotibial rotation. Intraoperative variables include surgical approach, femo-

rotibial stability, soft tissue management, extensor mechanism and patella treatment, prosthetic selection and positioning. Femoral component rotational alignment has gained more attention in recent literature, as component malpositioning "negatively" influences knee kinematics, including patellofemoral tracking and range of motion. Internal malrotation often leads to flexion instability, poor biomechanics, and patellofemoral tracking problems with lateral subluxation. It is also associated with painful knees.

Rotational malpositioning creates a trapezoidal rather than rectangular flexion gap with an altered patellofemoral articulation and unbalanced femorotibial kinematics. Instability in flexion with a tighter medial and more lax lateral compartment occurs when the femoral component is internally malrotated. This is frequently combined with lateral patellofemoral subluxation and instability (lift off) of the lateral compartment in flexion. In most TKA systems, for a given amount of tibial resection, an appropriate amount of posterior condylar resection is required to create a symmetric flexion gap. Tibial rotation position, an important consideration in fixed bearing designs, is also a factor that affects gap balance and the patellofemoral joint. Tibial rotational positioning is of lesser concern in mobile bearing TKA because of the ability (of the bearing) to adapt to tibiofemoral rotation in flexion and extension.

The results of our personal observations focussed on possible causes for problematic and painful TKA. Reduced mobility, pain, and patella problems were most frequent in this group. There was an increased incidence of femoral component internal rotation in this group with poor outcome. Mean internal rotation was 4.2 degrees (0–8) in relation to the TEA. Lateral subluxation as demonstrated in two examples may be caused by femoral internal malrotation or passive and active patella soft tissue attachments. We recommend CT evaluation of component alignment in clinically painful knees. Cases that present with internal malrotation should be considered for revision surgery with the view to revise the femoral and/or tibial component.

In summary, anterior knee pain following TKA represents a challenging problem. Specific diagnoses are difficult to establish, particularly in cases with normal radiographic features. Appreciation of further available investigations is crucial in identifying and pinpointing this complex problem. An algorithmic approach is recommended when anterior knee pain is detected during routine TKA follow-up, including:

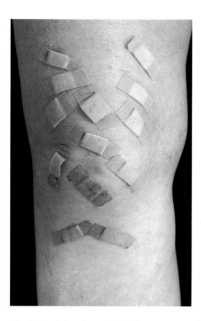

Fig. 7.13. Infection of TKA after conservative local infiltration therapy for anterior knee pain. Iatrogenic effects cannot be excluded

1. Exclusion of neurological, spine or hip problems
2. Clinical examination for neuroma, instability, patella subluxation, fat pad impingement, hip and spine problems
3. Radiographic evaluation for component and bearing alignment, mechanical axes, patella tracking, interface situation, bone appearance and response, loose bodies, osteophytes
4. Routine blood investigation for leucocytes, ESR, CRP, and joint fluid aspiration
5. CT scan for femoral and tibial component rotational alignment
6. Tc99 and gallium scintigraphies.

All non-invasive investigations should be performed first. However, even after full-spectrum investigation, some knees offer no specific cause for anterior knee pain. In these cases, patients should be advised to wait for pain improvement in the first 12–18 months after surgery. Silent infection and chondrolysis may be other causes of discomfort. There is little evidence that "convenient" diagnoses such as RSD or CRPS can be made responsible. Further details of this interesting problem are discussed in Sect. 7.6 – "The unhappy knee" (Fig. 7.13).

Bibliography

Akagi M, Matsusue Y, Mata T, Asada Y, Horiguchi M, Iida H, Nakamura T (1999) Effect of rotational alignment on patellar tracking in total knee arthroplasty. Clin Orthop 366:155–163

Arima J, Whiteside LA, McCarthy DS, White SE (1995) Femoral rotational alignment, based on the anteroposterior axis, in total knee arthroplasty in a valgus knee. A technical note. J Bone Joint Surg Am 77:1331–1334

Berger RA, Rubash HE, Seel MJ, Thompson WH, Crossett LS (1993) Determining the rotational alignment of the femoral component in total knee arthroplasty using the epicondylar axis. Clin Orthop 286:40–47

Berger RA, Crossett LS, Jacobs JJ, Rubash HE (1998) Rotation causing patellofemoral complications after total knee arthroplasty. Clin Orthop 356:144–153

Buechel FF (1982) A simplified evaluation system for the rating of the knee function. Orthop Rev 11:97–101

Churchill DL, Incavo SJ, Johnson CC, Beynnon BD (1998) The transepicondylar axis approximates the optimal flexion axis of the knee. Clin Orthop 356:111–118

Dennis DA, Komistek RD, Walker SA, Cheal EJ, Stiehl JB (2001) Femoral condylar lift-off in vivo in total knee arthroplasty. J Bone Joint Surg Br 83:33–39

Eckhoff DG, Piatt BE, Gnadinger CA, Blaschke RC (1995) Assessing rotational alignment in total knee arthroplasty. Clin Orthop 318:176–181

Engh GA (2000) Orienting the femoral component at total knee arthroplasty. Am J Knee Surg 133:162–165

Fehring TK (2000) Rotational malalignment of the femoral component in total knee arthroplasty. Clin Orthop 380:72–79

Griffin FM, Insall JN, Scuderi GR (1998) The posterior condylar angle in osteoarthritic knees. J Arthroplasty 13:812–815

Griffin FM, Insall JN, Scuderi GR (2000) Accuracy of soft tissue balancing in total knee arthroplasty. J Arthroplasty 15:970–973

Hungerford DS (1995) Alignment in total knee replacement. Instr Course Lect 44:455–468

Katz MA, Beck TD, Silber JS, Seldes RM, Lotke PA (2001) Determining femoral rotational alignment in total knee arthroplasty: reliability of techniques. J Arthroplasty 16:301–305

Lonner JH, Siliski JM, Scott RD (1999) Prodromes of failure in total knee arthroplasty. J Arthroplasty 14:488–492

Mantas JP, Bloebaum RD, Skedros JG, Hofmann AA (1992) Implications of reference axes used for rotational alignment of the femoral component in primary and revision knee arthroplasty. J Arthroplasty 7:531–535

Nagamine R, Miura H, Inoue Y, Urabe K, Matsuda S, Okamoto Y, Nishizawa M, Iwamoto Y (1998) Reliability of the anteroposterior axis and the posterior condylar axis for determining rotational alignment of the femoral component in total knee arthroplasty. J Orthop Sci 3:194–198

Nagamine R, Miura H, Bravo CV, Urabe K, Matsuda S, Miyanishi K, Hirata G, Iwamoto Y (2000) Anatomic variations should be considered in total knee arthroplasty. J Orthop Sci 5:232–237

Olcott CW, Scott RD (1999) The Ranawat Award. Femoral component rotation during total knee arthroplasty. Clin Orthop 367:39–42

Olcott CW, Scott RD (2000) A comparison of 4 intraoperative methods to determine femoral component rotation during total knee arthroplasty. J Arthroplasty 15:22–26

Poilvache PL, Insall JN, Scuderi GR, Font-Rodriguez DE (1996) Rotational landmarks and sizing of the distal femur in total knee arthroplasty. Clin Orthop 331:35–46

Scuderi GR, Insall JN, Scott NW (1994) Patellofemoral pain after total knee arthroplasty. J Am Acad Orthop Surg 2:239–246

Stiehl JB, Abbott BD (1995) Morphology of the transepicondylar axis and its application in primary and revision total knee arthroplasty. J Arthroplasty 10:785–789

Stiehl JB, Cherveny PM (1996) Femoral rotational alignment using the tibial shaft axis in total knee arthroplasty. Clin Orthop 331:47–55

Stiehl JB, Dennis DA, Komistek RD, Keblish PA (1997) In vivo kinematic analysis of a mobile bearing total knee prosthesis. Clin Orthop 345:60–66

Stiehl JB, Dennis DA, Komistek RD, Crane HS (1999) In vivo determination of condylar lift-off and screw-home in a mobile-bearing total knee. J Arthroplasty 14:293–299

Whiteside LA, Arima J (1995) The anteroposterior axis for femoral rotational alignment in valgus total knee arthroplasty. Clin Orthop 321:168–172

Yamada K, Imaizumi T (2000) Assessment of relative rotational alignment in total knee arthroplasty: usefulness of the modified Eckhoff method. J Orthop Sci 5:100–103

Yoshino N, Takai S, Ohtsuki Y, Hirasawa Y (2001) Computed tomography measurement of the surgical and clinical transepicondylar axis of the distal femur in osteoarthritic knees. J Arthroplasty 16:493–497

7.2 Wear, Periprosthetic Osteolysis and Loosening

Peter A. Keblish

Factors influencing wear, fixation, function and pain of total knee arthroplasty (TKA) are multifactorial and include prosthetic design, kinematics, implant technique, patella management, materials (past and present), patient issues (compliance, possible genetic predisposition) as well as repetitive trauma, the ageing process and osteoporosis. Many of these factors are addressed in other chapters in this book. Recent improvements in material science, sterilization processing and precision of implantation utilizing navigation systems may eliminate some current problems – but long-term evaluations are not available at this time. Therefore, current and recent past experiences need to be acknowledged in order to appreciate and hopefully solve the problems related to issues of wear in TKA.

Initial experience with TKA problems related to issues of patella failure and fixation (cement failure,

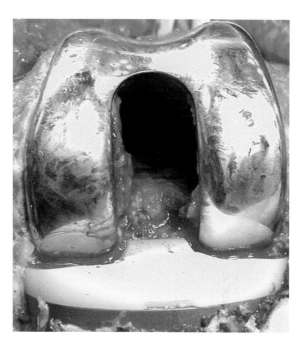

Fig. 7.14. Clinical example of severe distal femoral osteolysis at 7 years

cement disease). Patella pain with non-resurfaced patella lead to the development of patella resurfacing. Initially, an all-polyethylene patella component was utilized. Subsequently, metal-backed patella and modular fixed bearing resurfacing became common practice. Patella problems re-emerged as the most common reason for re-operation in TKA in the 1980s. The reality of mechanical, technical, and materials failure became more apparent with the addition of modularity in most systems. Most designs ignored or did not recognize the weakness of ultra-high molecular weight polyethylene (UHMWPE) when used with the incongruent contact and high stresses seen in many prosthetic designs (Fig. 7.14). Therefore, "cement disease" has proven to be a lesser problem than "poly wear disease", which has become the local cancer and main cause of total joint failure – to date more severe and extensive in total hip arthropathy than in TKA. Subsequent research has shown that sub-microscopic particles induce more severe osteolysis than initially noted in TKA; however, similar osteolysis is now a recognized problem in TKA (Fig. 7.14). Documented retrievals (Collier) revealed evidence of articulating and non-articulating backside wear leading to failure; this became a common cause of failure in the 1980s and early 1990s (Fig. 7.15).

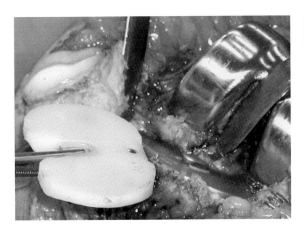

Fig. 7.15. Wear and cement intrusion that prevented perfect seating of modular polyethylene insert. Severe femoral osteolysis was present

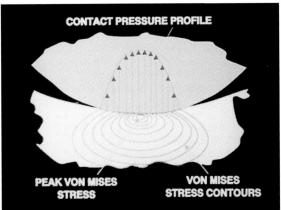

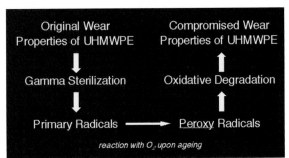

Fig. 7.16. a Cross-section of polyethylene failure in contact stress designs, showing maximum pressure in the sub-surface zone. b Algorithm of polyethylene failure influenced by sterilization, radicals, oxygen, and mechanical stress

Ultra-High Molecular Weight Polyethylene

Studies of polyethylene related to quality, shelf life, thickness, conformity, etc. led to the realization that UHMWPE was the weak link in longevity of metal-polyethylene articulations. Additional studies by Collier et al. described the so-called "white line" of oxidative surface degradation in aged and/or radiation in air sterilized UHMWPE (Fig. 7.16). These intrinsic material deficits, coupled with problems of high contact stress designs, less than optimum technique, and patient-specific factors, have resulted in a large number of failures and/or impending failures in the total knee population at the time of this publication. Examples of these failures are most significant in thin polyethylenes with high contact stress (incongruent bearing designs), leading to wear, osteolysis and at times baseplate fractures (Fig. 7.17).

Periprosthetic Osteolysis

Periprosthetic osteolysis (PPO) is the process of bone resorption and is most commonly related to UHMWPE microscopic wear. It involves "turning on" activation of enzyme systems, which lead to osteolytic bone resorption. Wear induces synovitis via a cascade of cellular activity (Fig. 7.18), which leads initially to a mechanical and chemical synovial response. Larger UHMWPE particles, especially from edge fracture, lead to a granulomatous entrapment often seen at revision surgery. Small and sub-microscopic particles induce an altered response that leads to secondary synovial effusion, which appears to be handled individually with different patients. Pain and ultimate total joint failure are consequences of the process, which often begins in an incipient way.

Diagnosis and treatment of the symptomatic TKA secondary to polyethylene wear involves the early recognition of subtle radiographic changes, which will direct the medical or surgical intervention as indicated. Medical drug research has discovered that agents such as Fosamax (Rubash, Schmalzried et al. 1997) may be of some benefit, but clinical results are not convincing at this time. Hopefully, drug therapy will become an option (early) when the problem is recognized. Therefore, early surgical intervention (bearing exchange) with allograft impaction if needed is now recommended before severe changes with bone defects and/or metallosis occur (Fig. 7.19). Treatment with strut and/or cancellous allografts (radiographic changes) has proven successful when performed prior to metal-to-metal contact (Fig. 7.20). Newer polyethylene components with improved sterilization techniques and short shelf life, in addition to bone graft fill of osteolytic areas, should be recommended when signs of PPO are confirmed.

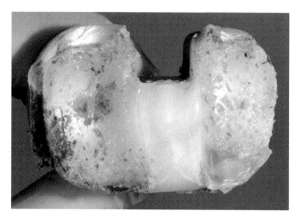

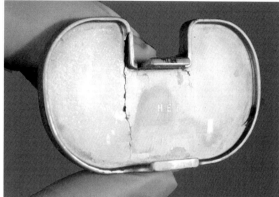

Fig. 7.17. Severe articulating surface, backside abrasion, and fracture of tibial baseplate in posterior cruciate ligament retaining flat-on-flat design at 3 years

Fig. 7.18. a Schematic of steps involved in osteolytic process. b Histologic section of a macrophage (giant cell) engulfing a microscopic particle of UHMWPE

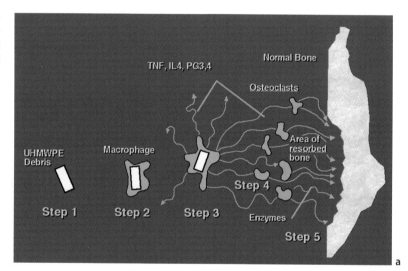

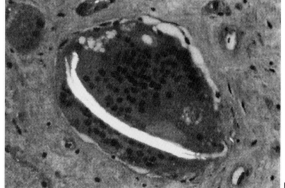

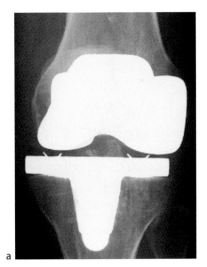
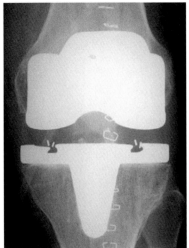

a   b

Fig. 7.19. a Considerable meniscal bearing wear with minimal tibial osteolysis. Note stable cementless interfaces at 15 years. b Treatment with bearing exchange only

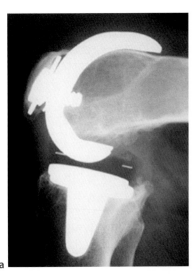
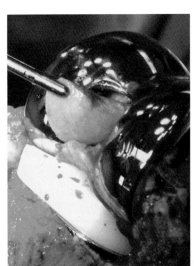

a   b

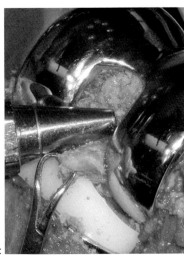
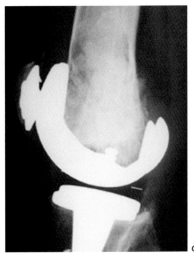

c   d

Fig. 7.20. a Minimal bearing wear, but significant femoral periprosthetic osteolysis at 9 years. b Allograft technique with use of fibular strut and freeze-dried cancellous impaction grafting. c Completion of allograft technique performed prior to final bearing exchange. d Two-year follow-up with incorporation of graft. Bearing exchange has established articular stability and congruity

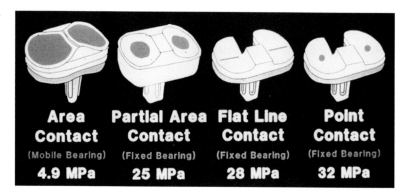

Fig. 7.21. Wear of UHMWPE in different designs over time

Wear: Diagnosis and Treatment

Wear and consequences of wear from a clinical standpoint represent the most significant challenge to the total knee surgeon and designing engineers. Many clinical and basic research studies (Greenwald et al. 2001, Schmalzried et al. 1997, Wimmer et al. 1998) have addressed the problem areas. The knowledge that polyethylene thickness (Bartels, Oishi et al. 1996) and conformity (Greenwald et al. 2001) improve long-term wear has directed most current designs to a more conforming, anatomic, lower contact stress philosophy. The low contact stress (LCS) design concept was ahead of its time in the 1970s in recognizing that contact stresses under 10 MPa loads were important in long-term viability of prosthetic surface interfaces (Pappas, Buechel et al. 1991) in order to achieve larger area contact and low contact stress. Movements at the non-articulating interface utilizing mobile bearings are a requirement if these criteria are to be met (Fig. 7.21). Kinematic compromises and subsequent multidirectional surface stresses also lead to increased wear (Stiehl et al. 2001, Komistek et al. 1998, Dennis et al. 1998). Additional negative factors such as "less than optimal" alignment, patella tilt and/or gap imbalance will further increase wear and potential failure.

The knowledgeable total knee surgeon must appreciate the consequences of wear and recognize early signs such as pain, effusion, instabilities, and suspicious lytic areas in the periprosthetic bone. Prospective awareness of potential clinical problems needs to be communicated to patients. This is a challenge, as it poses a negative connotation to a seemingly excellent result in a patient who is clinically asymptomatic. The surgeon must discuss early radiographic findings with the patient and explain the problem and need for follow-up radiographs on a more frequent basis. Early symptoms such as effusion or a feeling of instability may occur without pain and patients need

to be informed that these symptoms are usually signs of wear. Although it is difficult to recommend repeat surgery in minimally symptomatic patients, an aggressive approach is advised, as most problems can be solved with simple bearing exchange using newer UHMWPE – which can theoretically last a lifetime provided that a proper balanced TKA is restored.

Aseptic loosening of prosthetic components is multifactorial, as are all areas of TKA, and has been covered in other chapters. The relationship of osteolysis to aseptic loosening and/or impending loosening secondary to structural collapse is the most common situation presenting at the time of writing. As previously noted, aseptic loosening appears to be similar in some cemented and cementless TKAs of proven designs (LCS, Whiteside, Hoffman, Insall), but more common in many cementless designs. Factors that relate to aseptic loosening include cementing technique, bone preparation, alignment, contact stresses, contact area, bone quality, and synovial fluid mechanics.

Fluid Mechanics

An understanding of fluid mechanics and the so-called "fluid pump" (Schmalzried et al. 1997) has been incited as a key factor in aseptic loosening secondary to osteolysis. This process was initially noted in total hip arthroplasty shaft osteolysis in apparently well-fixed components. Subsequent review and evaluation discovered that "patch coated" or less than circumferential coated prostheses allow a pumping of the synovial fluid into any interface of low resistance. This phenomenon is also observed in other biological models such as inflammatory arthritis with excessive synovial response (rheumatoid arthritis, hemophilia) where ligamentous erosion exposed areas of less resistance reflect the earliest pathology. The findings of periarticular cysts in non-operated arthritic joints are explained by the synovial pump theory. Regarding TKA, cemented and cementless components need to be implanted in a manner that provides optimum seal of the interfaces. Virtually all modern cementless designs avoid patch coating because of these findings. However, weak areas or small voids may be present despite excellent technique, and open cancellous bone (common at the femoral side) is susceptible to synovial infiltration. Distal femoral osteolysis is noted more commonly and most likely presents open posterior condyles, larger intercondylar surface area and mediolateral gutters, where ligament attachments (often less than normal) allow ingress via the synovial pump with subsequent osteoclastic and enzymatic activity.

Radiologically, many patients demonstrate extensive wear with little to no osteolysis, while others demonstrate minimal radiographic wear (hips and knees) and extensive osteolysis. The exact reasons for this discrepancy are not known, but related factors include genetic make-up (Goodman 1996, Goater et al. 2002, Ulrich-Vinther et al. 2002), immune response, and reports that particulate volume is time related to development of osteolysis. Medical treatment to address osteoclastic or osteolytic activity is a possibility for the future, but current evidence is not available (Schmalzried et al. 1997).

Wear issues remain the primary challenge in total joint arthroplasty. Recent improvements in materials are encouraging. Wear osteolysis and aseptic loosening should not represent a major problem in TKA if several issues are addressed:

1. Consistency of precise implantation alignment. Evolving navigation techniques are practical and may become of significant benefit in the near future.
2. Soft tissue integrity is maintained, even in severe deformities when more constrained devices are being used.
3. Optimum kinematics are achieved in the chosen implant.
4. Patella-friendly femoral designs are utilized.
5. Prosthetic devices with proper polyethylene thickness and conformity are utilized. Mobile bearing prostheses have a proven 25-year track record and allow for all-important rotation, which is present in normal knee kinematics.
6. Medical grade polyethylene of richest quality control is utilized and improved over time.
7. Cementless implantation is performed with exacting technique, use of autograft augmentation, and only in designs with proven results.

Bibliography

Aglietti P, Buzzi R (1988) Posteriorly stabilised total-condylar knee replacement. Three to eight years' follow-up of 85 knees. J Bone Joint Surg Br 70:211–216

Beaule PE, Campbell PA, Walker PS, Schmalzried TP, Dorey FJ, Blunn GW, Bell CJ, Yahia L, Amstutz HC (2002) Polyethylene wear characteristics in vivo and in a knee stimulator. J Biomed Mater Res 60:411–419

Benjamin J, Szivek J, Dersam G, Persselin S, Johnson R (2001) Linear and volumetric wear of tibial inserts in posterior cruciate-retaining knee arthroplasties. Clin Orthop 392:131–138

Benson LC, DesJardins JD, LaBerge M (2001) Effects of in vitro wear of machined and molded UHMWPE tibial inserts on TKR kinematics. J Biomed Mater Res 58:496–504

Bohl JR, Bohl WR, Postak PD, Greenwald AS (1999) The Coventry Award. The effects of shelf life on clinical outcome for gamma sterilized polyethylene tibial components. Clin Orthop 367:28–38

Buechel FF, Pappas MJ, Greenwald AS (1991) Use of survivorship and contact stress analyses to predict the long-term efficacy of new generation joint replacement designs. A model for FDA device evaluation. Orthop Rev 20:50–55

Dennis DA, Komistek RD, Colwell CE Jr, Ranawat CS, Scott RD, Thornhill TS, Lapp MA (1998) In vivo anteroposterior femorotibial translation of total knee arthroplasty: a multicenter analysis. Clin Orthop 356:47–57

Dennis DA, Komistek RD, Stiehl JB, Walker SA, Dennis KN (1998) Range of motion after total knee arthroplasty: the effect of implant design and weight-bearing conditions. J Arthroplasty 13:748–752

Dennis DA, Komistek RD, Walker SA, Cheal EJ, Stiehl JB (2001) Femoral condylar lift-off in vivo in total knee arthroplasty. J Bone Joint Surg Br 83:33–39

Goater JJ, O'Keefe RJ, Rosier RN, Puzas JE, Schwarz EM (2002) Efficacy of ex vivo OPG gene therapy in preventing wear debris induced osteolysis. J Orthop Res 20:169–173

Goodman SB (1996) Does the immune system play a role in loosening and osteolysis of total joint replacements? J Long Term Eff Med Implants 6:91–101

Greenwald AS, Bauer TW, Ries MD (2001) Committee on Biomedical Engineering, Committee on Hip and Knee Arthritis. New polys for old: contribution or caveat? J Bone Joint Surg Am 83A (Suppl 2):27–31

Haas BD, Komistek RD, Dennis DA (2002) In vivo kinematics of the low contact stress rotating platform total knee. Orthopedics 25 (Suppl 2):s219–s226

Harman MK, Banks SA, Hodge WA (2001) Polyethylene damage and knee kinematics after total knee arthroplasty. Clin Orthop 392:383–393

Heim CS, Postak PD, Plaxton NA, Greenwald AS (2001) Classification of mobile-bearing knee designs: mobility and constraint. J Bone Joint Surg Am 83A (Suppl 2):32–37

Hirakawa K, Bauer TW, Yamaguchi M, Stulberg BN, Wilde AH (1999) Relationship between wear debris particles and polyethylene surface damage in primary total knee arthroplasty. J Arthroplasty 14:165–171

Hoff WA, Komistek RD, Dennis DA, Gabriel SM, Walker SA (1998) Three-dimensional determination of femoral-tibial contact positions under in vivo conditions using fluoroscopy. Clin Biomech 13:455–472

Insall JN, Scuderi GR, Komistek RD, Math K, Dennis DA, Anderson DT (2002) Correlation between condylar lift-off and femoral component alignment. Clin Orthop 403:143–152

Jones VC, Barton DC, Fitzpatrick DP, Auger DD, Stone MH, Fisher J (1999) An experimental model of tibial counterface polyethylene wear in mobile bearing knees: the influence of design and kinematics. Biomed Mater Eng 9:189–196

Jones VC, Williams IR, Auger DD, Walsh W, Barton DC, Stone MH, Fisher J (2001) Quantification of third body damage to the tibial counterface in mobile bearing knees. Proc Inst Mech Eng (H) 215:171–179

Jones VC, Barton DC, Auger DD, Hardaker C, Stone MH, Fisher J (2001) Simulation of tibial counterface wear in mobile bearing knees with uncoated and ADLC coated surfaces. Biomed Mater Eng 11:105–115

Kadoya Y, Kobayashi A, Ohashi H (1998) Wear and osteolysis in total joint replacements. Acta Orthop Scand Suppl 278:1–16

Keblish PA, Varma AK, Greenwald AS (1994) Patellar resurfacing or retention in total knee arthroplasty. A prospective study of patients with bilateral replacements. J Bone Joint Surg Br 76:930–937

Komistek RD, Dennis DA, Mabe JA (1998) In vivo determination of patello-femoral separation and linear impulse forces. Orthopade 27:612–618

Komistek RD, Stiehl JB, Dennis DA, Paxson RD, Soutas-Little RW (1998) Mathematical model of the lower extremity joint reaction forces using Kane's method of dynamics. J Biomech 31:185–189

Komistek RD, Dennis DA, Mabe JA, Walker SA (2000) An in vivo determination of patellofemoral contact positions. Clin Biomech (Bristol, Avon) 15:29–36

Kuster MS, Stachowiak GW (2002) Factors affecting polyethylene wear in total knee arthroplasty. Orthopedics 25 (Suppl 2):s235–s242

Lavernia CJ, Sierra RJ, Hungerford DS, Krackow K (2001) Activity level and wear in total knee arthroplasty: a study of autopsy retrieved specimens. J Arthroplasty 16:446–453

Mahoney OM, McClung CD, de la Rosa MA, Schmalzried TP (2002) The effect of total knee arthroplasty design on extensor mechanism function. J Arthroplasty 17:416–421

Majewski M, Weining G, Friederich NF (2002) Posterior femoral impingement causing polyethylene failure in total knee arthroplasty. J Arthroplasty 17:524–526

McClung CD, Zahiri CA, Higa JK, Amstutz HC, Schmalzried TP (2000) Relationship between body mass index and activity in hip or knee arthroplasty patients. J Orthop Res 18:35–39

McClung CD, Martell J, Moreland JR, Amstutz HC (2000) The John Charnley Award. Wear is a function of use, not time. Clin Orthop 381:36–46

Mochida Y, Bauer TW, Koshino T, Hirakawa K, Saito T (2002) Histologic and quantitative wear particle analyses of tissue around cementless ceramic total knee prostheses. J Arthroplasty 17:121–128

Oishi CS, Kaufman KR, Irby SE, Colwell CW Jr (1996) Effects of patellar thickness on compression and shear forces in total knee arthroplasty. Clin Orthop 331:283–290

Puertolas JA, Larrea A, Gomez-Barrena E (2001) Fracture behavior of UHMWPE in non-implanted, shelf-aged knee prostheses after gamma irradiation in air. Biomaterials 22:2107–2114

Puloski SK, McCalden RW, MacDonald SJ, Rorabeck CH, Bourne RB (2001) Tibial post wear in posterior stabilized TKA. An unrecognized source of polyethylene debris. J Bone Joint Surg Am 83A:390–397

Sathasivam S, Walker PS, Campbell PA, Rayner K (2001) The effect of contact area on wear in relation to fixed bearing and mobile bearing knee replacements. J Biomed Mater Res 58:282–290

Schmalzried TP, Akizuki KH, Fedenko AN, Mirra J (1997) The role of access of joint fluid to bone in periarticular osteolysis. A report of four cases. J Bone Joint Surg Am 79:447–452

Schmalzried TP, Campbell P, Schmitt AK, Brown IC, Amstutz HC (1997) Shapes and dimensional characteristics of polyethylene wear particles generated in vivo by total knee replacements compared to total hip replacements. J Biomed Mater Res 38:203–210

Schmalzried TP, Shepherd EF, Dorey FJ, Jackson WO, de la Rosa M, Fa'vae F, McKellop HA, Stiehl JB, Dennis DA, Komistek RD, Keblish PA (2000) In vivo kinematic comparison of posterior cruciate ligament retention or sacrifice with a mobile bearing total knee arthroplasty. Am J Knee Surg 13:13–18

Stiehl JB, Dennis DA, Komistek RD, Keblish PA (1997) In vivo kinematic analysis of a mobile bearing total knee prosthesis. Clin Orthop 345:60–66

Stiehl JB, Komistek RD, Dennis DA (1999) Detrimental kinematics of a flat on flat total condylar knee arthroplasty. Clin Orthop 365:139–148

Stiehl JB, Dennis DA, Komistek RD, Crane HS (1999) In vivo determination of condylar lift-off and screw-home in a mobile-bearing total knee arthroplasty. J Arthroplasty 14:293–299

Stiehl JB, Komistek RD, Haas B, Dennis DA (2001) Frontal plane kinematics after mobile-bearing total knee arthroplasty. Clin Orthop 392:56–61

Stiehl JB, Komistek RD, Dennis DA, Keblish PA (2001) Kinematics of the patellofemoral joint in total knee arthroplasty. J Arthroplasty 16:706–714

Ulrich-Vinther M, Carmody EE, Goater JJ, Sballe K, O'Keefe RJ, Schwarz EM (2002) Recombinant adeno-associated virus-mediated osteoprotegerin gene therapy inhibits wear debris-induced osteolysis. J Bone Joint Surg Am 84A:1405–1412

Walker PS, Blunn GW, Lilley PA (1996) Wear testing of materials and surfaces for total knee replacement. J Biomed Mater Res 33:159–175

Walker PS, Komistek RD, Barrett DS, Anderson D, Dennis DA, Sampson M (2002) Motion of a mobile bearing knee allowing translation and rotation. J Arthroplasty 17:11–19

Wasielewski RC, Galante JO, Leighty RM, Natarajan RN, Rosenberg AG (1994) Wear patterns on retrieved polyethylene tibial inserts and their relationship to technical considerations during total knee arthroplasty. Clin Orthop 299:31–43

Weaver JK, Derkash RS, Greenwald AS (1993) Difficulties with bearing dislocation and breakage using a movable bearing total knee replacement system. Clin Orthop 290:244–252

White SE, Paxson RD, Tanner MG, Whiteside LA (1996) Effects of sterilization on wear in total knee arthroplasty. Clin Orthop 331:164–171

Wimmer MA, Andriacchi TP (1997) Tractive forces during rolling motion of the knee: implications for wear in total knee replacement. J Biomech 30:131–137

Wimmer MA, Andriacchi TP, Natarajan RN, Loos J, Karlhuber M, Petermann J, Schneider E, Rosenberg AG (1998) A striated pattern of wear in ultrahigh-molecular-weight polyethylene components of Miller-Galante total knee arthroplasty. J Arthroplasty 13:8–16

7.3 Arthrofibrosis Following Total Knee Arthroplasty

Jens G. Boldt

Painful knees with reduced range of motion (ROM) in total knee arthroplasty (TKA) are a frustrating complication for both the patient and the surgeon. Arthrofibrosis is an ill-defined entity that results in functional impairment following TKA and ligament reconstructive surgery. Treatment options vary from physiotherapy, long-term peridural anesthesia, closed manipulation, arthroscopic debridement and open procedures including revision surgery with exchange of prosthetic components. The results of these procedures are often limited and unsatisfactory. The prevalence of arthrofibrosis in mobile bearing TKA ranges from 1% to 2%, up to 17% as an indication for revision surgery. The etiology and specific pathogenesis of arthrofibrosis have not been clearly identified and hypotheses include biochemical as well as immunological factors, predisposition, reflex sympathetic dystrophy (RSD), complex regional pain syndrome (CRPS), metal allergies, low-grade infection, villonodular synovitis and mechanical factors. Histopathological analyses of fibrotic tissue frequently found in arthrofibrotic knee joints revealed massive connective tissue proliferation with deposition of disordered matrix proteins and increased expression of collagen type VI subsynovially as well as around the capillary walls. These histological findings are comparable with those in lung fibrosis and superficial fibromatosis. The most common associated clinical symptoms in patients who develop arthrofibrosis in TKA, in increasing order of frequency, are: reduced ROM, swelling and pain, all of which require some form of treatment but with limited success.

From our clinical observations, arthrofibrosis appeared to be associated with femoral component internal malrotation. Internal malpositioning of the femoral component with reference to the transepicondylar axis (TEA) creates a trapezoidal rather than rectangular flexion gap with poor patellofemoral articulation and unbalanced knee kinematics particularly in flexion (Fig. 7.22). Repetitive microtrauma of the knee joint following unsuccessful reconstructive ligament surgery is an established model causing local arthrofibrosis within the knee joint (cyclops syndrome). We hypothesized that arthrofibrosis in TKA may equally be triggered by repetitive microtrauma that occurs when the TKA is not balanced during each walking cycle due to internal malrotation of the femoral component.

From a cohort of 3,058 mobile bearing low contact stress (LCS, DePuy Int, Leeds, UK) TKAs performed in one center since 1988, 49 (1.6%) cases were diagnosed with arthrofibrosis. The femoral component design of the LCS prosthesis has remained unchanged for the past 26 years. The surgical technique of the LCS system defines femoral component rotational positioning using the tibial (mechanical) axis and a balanced rectangular flexion gap as reference without using anatomical landmarks. Postoperative rehabilitation consisted of immediate automatic continuous passive motion that was applied in the recovery room followed by an extensive physiotherapy program and early weight bearing within 48 h after surgery.

All patients with arthrofibrosis were contacted by telephone. Five patients were deceased at the time of investigation, leaving 44 patients who entered the study. Six patients could not be motivated to attend our clinic for further investigation. Of this group only one patient underwent revision surgery of the prosthesis elsewhere, two refused further attendance for personal reasons, two lived too far away and one did not feel well enough for transport. We were able to recruit 38 of 44 (86%) patients for clinical examination and helical computed tomography (CT) investigation to determine femoral component rotation referencing from the TEA.

Mean age was 65 years (49–76). All TKA patients in this center underwent routine clinical examination and follow-up radiographs at 1 week, 6 weeks, 6 months, 1 year, 5 years or when complications occurred. Inclusion criteria of the arthrofibrosis group were reduced ROM of less than 90 degrees or with an extension deficit of more than 10 degrees regardless of preoperative diagnosis. ROM in the arthrofibrosis group ranged from 40 to 90 degrees with a mean of 70 degrees. Exclusion criteria were infection, late hemarthrosis or thromboembolic events. All 38 arthrofibrosis cases underwent one or more manipulations under anesthesia (mean 1.9), 26 (71%) underwent open debridement, 15 (40%) arthroscopic debridement, six (16%) were revised for bearing exchange, four (11%) for tibial component revision, three (8%) underwent resurfacing of a primarily unresurfaced patella, three (8%) underwent repositioning of the tibial tubercle and one (3%) had the patella removed. None of the patients included in our study had undergone femoral component revision (Table 7.1).

Fig. 7.22. When femoral component rotation is referenced to the posterior condyles (a), this leads to internally malrotated femoral resection lines (*black line*). Femoral anteroposterior resection parallel to the transepicondylar axis (*white line*) is widely accepted as the best reference for femoral component rotational alignment (b)

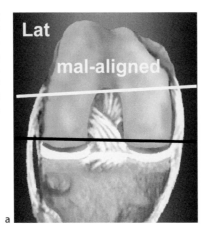
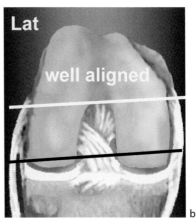

Fig. 7.23 a, b. Transverse CT views are a practical method for accurate determination of femoral component rotational positioning in TKA best referenced to the transepicondylar axis (*TEA*). Example of internal malrotation with the patella parallel to the TEA (a) and a well-aligned femoral component parallel to the TEA (b)

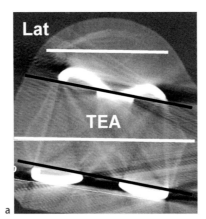
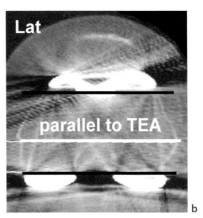

Table 7.1. Frequency of treatment in the arthrofibrosis group in percentages. Knee motion in this group was not effectively improved by any of these procedures. Note that no femoral component has been revised at the time of revision surgery in the last 11 years

Manipulations (mean 1.9, range 1–3)	100%
Open debridement	71%
Arthroscopic debridement	40%
Bearing exchange	16%
Tibial component revision	11%
Secondary patella resurfacing	8%
Alteration of tibial tubercle	8%
Removal of patella component	3%
Oversizing	3%

A control group of 38 patients with well-functioning LCS TKAs was matched and underwent identical evaluation. Mean age was 67 years (range 54–77). Inclusion criteria for the control group were ROM of over 100 degrees, lack of per- or postoperative complications and excellent or good clinical results according to a modified Hospital for Special Surgery (HSS) score. ROM in the control group ranged from 100 to 135 degrees with a mean of 115 degrees.

CT Scan Evaluation

All data for femoral component rotational positioning were performed using a helical CT scanner by two independent consultant radiologists, who were not aware of whether the patient belonged to the arthrofibrosis or the control group (single blind) (Fig. 7.23). For determination of femoral component rotational alignment, the two metallic posterior condyles were referenced to the TEA, which was drawn between the spike of the lateral epicondyle and the sulcus of the medial epicondyle, as recently recommended by Yoshino et al. (2001). One patient had to be excluded because of inability to identify an appropriate anatomical landmark (medial sulcus) on CT scans. All angles were calculated using CT scan implemented software and a hard copy was made.

Statistical Analyses

All data were analyzed by an independent statistician. The angles in each group showed a normal distribution (one-sample Kolmogorov-Smirnov test). As such, parametric statistical analyses were employed. Differences between groups for the parameter femoral rotation were examined using the unpaired Student's t-test. Significance was accepted at the 5% level. Over a period of 8 months all patients who were scheduled for 1-, 5- or 10-year routine follow-up were invited to participate in the control group until the appropriate number of the matched group was obtained. Of this group all patients had excellent or good clinical results and no patient refused participation.

Clinical Results

Thirty-eight patients with arthrofibrosis entered the study and were compared with a matched group of 38 TKA cases who served as controls. Age, gender, body mass index, diagnosis and type of prosthesis were the same in both groups. There was a significant trend ($p<0.05$) for a high proportion of high tibial correcting osteotomies in the arthrofibrosis group prior to TKA surgery, with eight (18%) patients in the arthrofibrosis group versus one (3%) in the control group. Three of 38 cases in the arthrofibrosis group had poliomyelitis affecting the lower limbs compared with no case in the control group. A further three cases in the arthrofibrosis group underwent open reduction and internal fixation of a previous intra-articular knee joint fracture compared with no fracture in the control group. There were no rheumatoid cases in the arthrofibrosis group, but two rheumatoid cases in the control group. Nine cases underwent asthroscopic meniscal surgery prior to TKA in both groups; this is, therefore, not associated with arthrofibrosis.

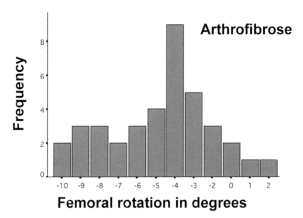

Fig. 7.24. Normal distribution of femoral component rotational alignment in the arthrofibrosis group. Mean internal malrotation of the arthrofibrosis group was 4.7 degrees, ranging from 10 degrees IR to 1 degree ER. The difference was highly significant ($p<0.00001$); therefore, arthrofibrosis is highly significantly associated with internal malrotation of the femoral component in reference to the TEA

CT Results

All angles were normally distributed in both groups using the one-sample Kolmogorov-Smirnov test. Femoral alignment in the arthrofibrosis group was significantly internally malrotated with a mean of 4.7 degrees, ranging from 10 degrees internal rotation (IR) to 1 degree external rotation (ER). Standard deviation in the arthrofibrosis group was 2.9 and standard error 0.5 (Fig. 7.24). Femoral alignment in the control group was parallel (mean of 0.3 degrees IR) to the TEA, ranging from 4 degrees IR to 5 degrees ER. Standard deviation was 2.2 and standard error 0.4 (Fig. 7.25). The difference in femoral rotational alignment between the groups was highly significant ($p<0.00001$).

The scientific pathogenesis of arthrofibrosis in TKA is not fully understood in the recent literature, but represents a serious complication with a poor prognosis following TKA surgery. The prevalence of arthrofibrosis is relatively low, at 1–2%, but is an indication for revision surgery in up to 17%. A stiff total knee replacement represents a serious functional impairment and considerable dissatisfaction to those patients who suffer from it (Figs. 7.26, 7.27). No obvious reason for this type of complication could be identified either in the literature or in our series, which makes this a frustrating complication for both the patient and the surgeon. The etiology and pathogenesis of arthrofibrosis are not well understood and include a broad spectrum of factors such as biochemical, immunological and mechanical. Differential

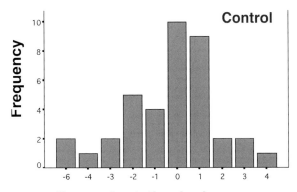

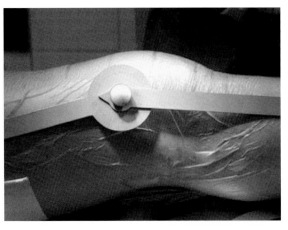

a

Fig. 7.25. Normal distribution of femoral component rotational alignment in the control group. Mean rotation of the femoral component in the control group was parallel (0.3 degrees) to the transepicondylar axis. The control group demonstrates that correct femoral component rotational alignment can be reliably achieved utilizing the tibial axis method and balanced flexion tension gap without anatomical landmark identification intraoperatively

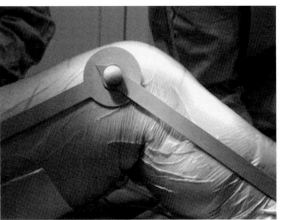

b

Fig. 7.27. Arthrofibrotic TKA in full flexion to 40 degrees (a) and full extension with 10 degrees deficit (b) at revision surgery. Total range of motion equals 30 degrees

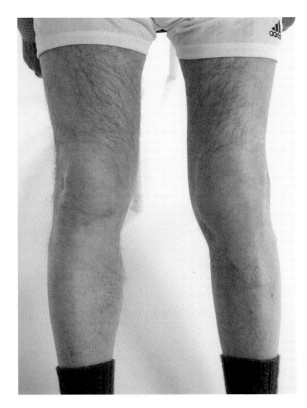

Fig. 7.26. Clinical appearance of an arthrofibrotic TKA 4 years postoperatively showing diffuse swelling. On examination, the swelling is firm and not fluctuating

diagnoses are RSD, CRPS, predisposition and low-grade infection; however, specific clinical differentiation appears difficult. None of these diagnoses could be directly associated or correlated with arthrofibrosis, neither could a single factor causing arthrofibrosis be identified.

Localized and often sphere-shaped arthrofibrosis within the Hoffa fat pad, commonly described as cyclops syndrome, is a recognized complication in ligament reconstructive surgery most likely caused by mechanical repetitive trauma in cases with malpositioned and tight cruciate ligament grafts. We, therefore, hypothesized that internal malrotation of the femoral component in reference to the TEA would cause repetitive trauma and/or a too tight medial compartment that could trigger increased fibrotic activity within the synovial tissues as a biological response to non-physiological knee kinematics. Tibial rotational positioning is of lesser concern in this study because all prostheses were mobile bearing

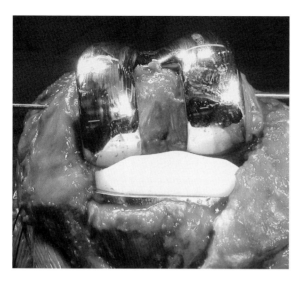

Fig. 7.28. Intraoperative image of an internally malrotated femoral component. Kirschner wires mark both lateral and medial femoral epicondyles. *Black arrow* indicates lateral lift off

devices with the ability to adapt automatically to tibiofemoral rotation in both flexion and extension. However, instability in flexion with a tighter medial and more lax lateral compartment occurs when the femoral component is internally malrotated. This is frequently combined with lateral patellofemoral subluxation and instability (lift off) of the lateral compartment in flexion (Fig. 7.28). The natural knee has a tighter medial and looser lateral compartment in order to accommodate physiological kinematics with a higher translation laterally than medially. A situation in which the surgeon places the femoral component in internal rotation could create a balanced lateral, but a relatively tight medial compartment. A TKA that is tight in flexion will certainly stretch repetitively the medial collateral ligament complex in each walking cycle, causing pain and/or discomfort. These disturbed knee kinematics are considered a possible source not only for chronic pain, but also for synovial fibrotic activity. It remains impossible, though, to determine whether the tighter medial or the laxer lateral compartment or both trigger arthrofibrosis.

The TEA is a generally accepted anatomical landmark for best femoral component alignment compared with the Whiteside line and the posterior condyle line. However, the angle between the TEA and the posterior condylar line shows natural variation of up to 6 degrees. Rotationally deformed femurs, hip pathologies, valgus or varus knee deformities and previous fractures/operations play a further role in the orientation of the TEA.

There are different opinions of surgical approach regarding soft tissue releases, tibia first or femoral first bone cuts as well as the femoral rotation resection. The most common method of tibial resection is perpendicular to the mechanical axis with some degree of posterior inclination. For a given amount of tibial resection, an appropriate amount of posterior condylar resection is required to create a symmetric flexion gap. Established methods of determining femoral rotational positioning in TKA are: Whiteside's line, TEA and 3 degrees of external rotation from the posterior condyles. Olcott and Scott (2000) have recently reported that these three most accepted methods were most consistent in yielding a symmetric, balanced flexion gap within 3 degrees. However, the TEA did not yield flexion gap symmetry in 10% of neutral varus TKA and in 14% of valgus TKA, with discrepancies varying from 9 degrees too little to 6 degrees too much, which would be unacceptable. The authors practise a combination of these methods to avoid these potential discrepancies and malresections.

Clinical studies by Stiehl and Cherveny (1996) comparing the tibial axis method with the posterior condylar method for determining femoral rotation in four different fixed bearing knee systems utilizing a femoral-first approach reported the following numbers: 72% requirement of lateral release, 7% patella fractures and 4–5 degrees of external rotation when the posterior condyle method was used. In comparison there were 28% lateral release, no patella fracture and 0–1 degrees of external rotation to the TEA when the tibial shaft axis method was used. In a cadaver study of eight knees involving three surgeons, Katz et al. (2001) showed that determination of femoral component rotational positioning was more reliable using a balanced flexion gap and the anteroposterior axis.

In our study, the method used to define femoral rotation depended on a tibial resection perpendicular to both the tibial and mechanical axes and a symmetrical (rectangular) flexion gap, which automatically defines femoral rotation positioning without the need for anatomical landmarks. The tibial axis method eliminates these errors by prospectively establishing the soft tissue flexion tension, therefore setting the appropriate femoral rotation position independent of arbitrary landmarks. The control group in this study with well-functioning TKA had a mean femoral component alignment that was parallel (0.3 degrees) to the TEA. These data demonstrate that correct femoral component rotational alignment can be achieved on average with the tibial axis method, which does not depend on anatomical landmark identification. There were, however, patients in the control group with well-functioning TKA despite having an internally rotated femoral component of 5 or 6 degrees. This shows that the etiology of arthrofibrosis is likely to be multifactorial and certainly not triggered by femoral component rotational positioning alone. TKA may still provide excellent mobility with an internally rotated femoral component, probably because the flexion–extension gaps remain balanced throughout the entire range of motion.

Femoral rotation malresection is an accepted cause of patella maltracking in TKA, but has not yet been associated with arthrofibrosis. Femoral rotation alignment is technique and instrument dependent and influences patella tracking, flexion gap balance, and soft tissue kinematics. In addition, the current study suggests that there is an association between arthrofibrosis and internal malrotation of the femoral component. Arthrofibrotic TKA in our center responded poorly to treatment that included intensive and early physiotherapy, long-term peridural anesthesia, closed manipulation, arthroscopic debridement and open procedures including revision surgery with exchange of prosthetic components.

The data of our observations show that arthrofibrosis in TKA is highly significantly associated with femoral component internal malrotation. However, a specific etiological factor causing arthrofibrosis could not be identified. On the basis of these results it was hypothesized that non-physiological kinematics (lift off, tight medial compartment) in TKA with malaligned femoral components influence or trigger arthrofibrosis in TKA. When arthrofibrosis is associated with femoral component internal malrotation of more than 4 degrees in conjunction with no other pathology, we recommend rebalancing the flexion gap and realigning the femoral component. An anecdotal 12 cases in two centers underwent femoral component revision with a 75% chance of significant clinical improvement.

Bibliography

Arima J, Whiteside LA, McCarthy DS, White SE (1995) Femoral rotational alignment, based on the anteroposterior axis, in total knee arthroplasty in a valgus knee. A technical note. J Bone Joint Surg Am 77:1331–1334

Bain AM (1966) Treatment of paralytic flexion contracture of the knee following poliomyelitis. Physiotherapy 52:274–276

Berger RA, Rubash HE, Seel MJ, Thompson WH, Crossett LS (1993) Determining the rotational alignment of the femoral component in total knee arthroplasty using the epicondylar axis. Clin Orthop Jan;286:40–47

Berger RA, Crossett LS, Jacobs JJ, Rubash HE (1998) Malrotation causing patellofemoral complications after total knee arthroplasty. Clin Orthop 356:144–153

Buechel FF (1982) A simplified evaluation system for the rating of the knee function. Orthop Rev 11:9

Churchill DL, Incavo SJ, Johnson CC, Beynnon BD (1998) The transepicondylar axis approximates the optimal flexion axis of the knee. Clin Orthop 356:111–118

Court C, Gauliard C, Nordin JY (1999) Technical aspects of arthroscopic arthrolysis after total knee replacement (in French). Rev Chir Orthop Reparatrice Appar Mot 85:404– 410

Delcogliano A, Franzese S, Branca A, Magi M, Fabbriciani C (1996) Light and scan electron microscopic analysis of cyclops syndrome: etiopathogenic hypothesis and technical solutions. Knee Surg Sports Traumatol Arthrosc 4:194–199

Dennis DA, Komistek RD, Walker SA, Cheal EJ, Stiehl JB (2001) Femoral condylar lift-off in vivo in total knee arthroplasty. J Bone Joint Surg Br 83:33–39

Engh GA (2000) Orienting the femoral component at total knee arthroplasty. Am J Knee Surg 13:162–165

Fehring TK (2000) Rotational malalignment of the femoral component in total knee arthroplasty. Clin Orthop 380:72–79

Griffin FM, Insall JN, Scuderi GR (1998) The posterior condylar angle in osteoarthritic knees. J Arthroplasty 13:812–815

Kaper BP, Smith PN, Bourne RB, Rorabeck CH, Robertson D (1999) Medium-term results of a mobile bearing total knee replacement. Clin Orthop 367:201–209

Katz MA, Beck TD, Siler JS, Seldes RM, Lotke PA (2001) Determining femoral rotational alignment in total knee arthroplasty: reliability of techniques. J Arthroplasty 16:301–305

Lilleas FG, Stiris M (1999) Tidsskr. Villonodular synovitis – a rare cause of knee joint locking. Nor Laegeforen 119:1648

Lindenfeld TN, Wojtys EM, Husain A (2000) Surgical treatment of arthrofibrosis of the knee. Instr Course Lect 49:211–221

Lonner JH, Siliski JM, Scott RD (1999) Prodromes of failure in total knee arthroplasty. J Arthroplasty 14:488–492

Mantas JP, Bloebaum RD, Skedros JG, Hofmann AA (1992) Implications of reference axes used for rotational alignment of the femoral component in primary and revision knee arthroplasty. J Arthroplasty 7:531–535

Millett PJ, Williams RJ, Wickiewicz TL (1999) Open debridement and soft tissue release as a salvage procedure for the severely arthrofibrotic knee. Am J Sports Med 27:552–561

Nagamine R, White SE, McCarthy DS, Whiteside LA (1995) Effect of rotational malposition of the femoral component on knee stability kinematics after total knee arthroplasty. J Arthroplasty 10:265–270

Nagamine R, Miura H, Inoue Y, Urabe K, Matsuda S, Okamoto Y, Nishizawa M, Iwamoto Y (1998) Reliability of the anteroposterior axis and the posterior condylar axis for determining rotational alignment of the femoral component in total knee arthroplasty. J Orthop Sci 3:194–198

Noyes FR, Berrios-Torres S, Barber-Westin SD, Heckmann TP (2000) Knee. Prevention of permanent arthrofibrosis after anterior cruciate ligament reconstruction alone or combined with associated procedures: a prospective study in 443 knees. Surg Sports Traumatol Arthrosc 8:196–206

Olcott CW, Scott RD (1999) The Ranawat Award. Femoral component rotation during total knee arthroplasty. Clin Orthop 367:39–42

Olcott CW, Scott RD (2000) A comparison of 4 intraoperative methods to determine femoral component rotation during total knee arthroplasty. J Arthroplasty 15:22–26

Poilvache PL, Insall JN, Scuderi GR, Font-Rodriguez DE (1996) Rotational landmarks and sizing of the distal femur in total knee arthroplasty. Clin Orthop 331:35–46

Ries MD, Badalamente M (2000) Arthrofibrosis after total knee arthroplasty. Clin Orthop 380:177–183

Rillmann P, Berbig R (1998) Long-term peridural anesthesia and minimally invasive therapy of arthrofibrosis of the knee joint (in German). Swiss Surg 4:187–192

Romanos G, Schroter-Kermani C, Hinz N, Bernimoulin JP (1991) Immunohistochemical distribution of the collagen types IV, V, VI and glycoprotein laminin in the healthy rat, marmoset (callithrix jacchus) and human gingivae. Matrix 11:125–132

Romero J, Duronio JF, Alexander N, Sohrabi A, Hungerford DS (1995) Knee kinematics in TKA: the impact of classical versus anatomic alignment of femoral component malrotation. Trans Orthop Res Soc 20:742–748

Romero J, Duronio JF, Sohrabi A, Alexander N, MacWilliams BA, Jones LC, Hungerford DS (2001) Varus and valgus flexion laxity of total knee alignment methods in loaded cadaveric knees. Clin Orthop 390

Shelbourne KD, Patel DV (1999) Treatment of limited motion after anterior cruciate ligament reconstruction. Knee Surg Sports Traumatol Arthrosc 7:85–92

Sprague NF (1987) 3D Motion-limiting arthrofibrosis of the knee: the role of arthroscopic management. Clin Sports Med 6:537–549

Stiehl JB, Abbott BD (1995) Morphology of the transepicondylar axis and its application in primary and revision total knee arthroplasty. J Arthroplasty 10:785–789

Stiehl JB, Cherveny PM (1996) Femoral rotational alignment using the tibial shaft axis in total knee arthroplasty. Clin Orthop 331:47–55

Stiehl JB, Dennis DA, Komistek RD, Keblish PA (1997) In vivo kinematic analysis of a mobile bearing total knee prosthesis. Clin Orthop 345:60–66

Stiehl JB, Dennis DA, Komistek RD, Crane HS (1999) In vivo determination of condylar lift-off and screw-home in a mobile-bearing total knee. J Arthroplasty 14:293–299

Whiteside LA, Arima J (1995) The anteroposterior axis for femoral rotational alignment in valgus total knee arthroplasty. Clin Orthop 321:168–172

Yoshino N, Takai S, Ohtsuki Y, Hirasawa Y (2001) Computed tomography measurement of the surgical and clinical transepicondylar axis of the distal femur in osteoarthritic knees. J Arthroplasty 16:493–497

Zeichen J, van Griensven M, Albers I, Lobenhoffer P, Bosch U (1999) Immuno histochemical localization of collagen VI in arthrofibrosis. Arch Orthop Trauma Surg 119:315–318

7.4 Surgical Management of Infected Total Knee Arthroplasty

Jens G. Boldt

Infection in total knee arthroplasty (TKA) is the most serious complication of all. The potentially catastrophic risks involved with infection include medical implications such as increased risk of thromboembolic events, osteomyelitis, hematosepsis, and life-threatening multiorgan failure, as well as orthopedic drawbacks such as removal of all implants, arthrodesis, or limb amputation. The incidence of infection in TKA ranges from 1 to 23% (Ranawat, Riley, Hungerford, Insall), but has decreased in the past two decades with the introduction of increased awareness of sterile behavior, air-flow operating theatres, improved cementing techniques loaded with powder antibiotics, shorter operating times and more awareness of gentle soft tissue handling. Recent figures for infection post TKA average less than 5%. The identification of infection in TKA is the most difficult step in this complex complication. Treatment options are multiple depending on the aggressiveness of the bio-organism, the patient's health/immune response, time after surgery, osteolysis, bone defects or implant loosening. Management algorithms include debridement with implant salvage in the very early stage, one-stage revision, two-stage reimplantation, long-term spacer, and arthrodesis. In this chapter I shall discuss all options that are available in the literature, providing personal preferences as well.

Diagnosis of Infected TKA

Any given TKA that presents with effusion, pain, instability, inflammation and/or wound-healing problems within 3 months postoperatively should be considered an infection until proven otherwise. Confirmation of knee infection is challenging at times because of the inability to identify a specific organism. This is the case in at least 20% of our own cases despite in-depth investigations that include laboratory examination of knee joint aspirate plus synovial tissue specimens, elevation of less specific serum markers such as erythrocyte sedimentation rate (ESR) and C-reactive protein (CRP), technetium-99m labeled bone scans, and other radioactively marked leukocyte scans. When in doubt, any suspicion of infection following TKA has to be treated sooner rather than later as a positive case. The sensitivity and specificity of joint aspirations, gram staining, clinical signs, white blood cell (WBC) count, CRP levels, radiographic analysis, bone scans, and leukocyte scans, vary considerably. However, they are important tools that help to approximate the likelihood of an infection. Therefore no current test can unequivocally exclude infection. The surgeon has to embellish and assemble all individual data that are available in order to plan further treatment, which may include several substantial revision procedures with all consequences. However, when in doubt, open exploration, radical debridement, pulsatile lavage and obtaining supplementary tissue samples are recommended.

Unspecific Symptoms and Investigations of Infection

Unspecific symptoms and investigations of infection include: (1) clinical appearances presenting as swelling, inflammation, effusion, and pain of the knee joint; (2) biochemical parameters such as WBC, ESR, and CRP; (3) rapid development of radiolucent lines in all zones, particularly at the tibial interface; (4) bone scan, indium 111 leukocyte scans, polymerase chain reaction (PCR), fluorine-18 fluorodesoxyglucose positron emission tomography (FDG-PET), Tc99m hexamethylpropylene amine oxime WBC scintigraphy and Tc99m labeled monoclonal anti-NCA-90 granulocytes antibody Fab' fragment (MN3 Fab'). These more sophisticated (and expensive) tests may not necessarily increase the accuracy of the diagnosis and are, therefore, restricted to use in clinical research institutes and universities rather than being of practical use for average orthopedic centers. There are both false positive and negative results in all listed investigations. Specificity for leukocyte scans is reported as 85% (Rand and Brown 1990), MN3 Fab' antibodies 58% (Ivaneeviae et al. 2002), and FDG-PET 53% (Van Acker et al. 2001).

Specific Investigations with Highest Sensitivity

Specific investigations with the highest sensitivity are positive cultures of synovial fluid and synovial membrane. Usually one or mixed bacterial (or fungal) organisms prove infection. Most infectious disease laboratories provide a culture of the identified organism plus resistance and sensitivity listing of effective antibiotic drugs.

The organism identified (and its sensitivity to antibiotics) dictates further surgical management of the infected TKA. For instance, early infection within 6 weeks, without radiographic bone involvement, and (gram positive) staphylococci that are suitable for local and systemic antibiotic treatment, may be successfully treated with an open debridement, pusatile lavage, synovectomy and systemic antibiotics. On the other hand, late infection with signs of aseptic loosening, and an aggressive organism unsuitable for antibiotic treatment, is best treated with a two-stage procedure.

Grading and Staging of Infected TKA

Infection in TKA is divided into early or late occurrence and varies depending on identification of specific organisms and sensitivities in acute, low-grade, or occult grades. All combinations and their clinical implications will be discussed.

Early Acute Infection

This represents the most straightforward group to diagnose and treat, where signs of infection such as swelling, inflammation, effusion, redness, pain, and sometimes wound breakdown accompanied with secretion occur within the first 6 weeks postoperatively. Blood chemistry investigations are positive with elevated ESR, WBC, and CRP, as well as culture proof of bacterial organisms with sensitivities.

Treatment of early acute infection with sensitive organisms has a high success rate, when done early and aggressively with open procedures. Any closed procedure or arthroscopically guided washout, drainage, or synovectomy is highly unlikely to eliminate infection in TKA and is not recommended. Treatment of an infected TKA varies depending on the type of organism and the time frame between onset and diagnosis.

In cases that are radiographically free of radiolucent lines with gram-positive staphylococci that are highly sensitive to antibiotics, revision surgery should consist of an open debridement, synovectomy, and pulsatile lavage with antiseptic agents (10 liters or more) to remove bacterial slime and debris. All-polyethylene bearings are exchanged and stable component fixation is confirmed at the same time. Non-damaged or scratched cemented implants with a well-fixed cement–bone interface may be removed, sterilized and reimplanted into the old cement shell. Treatment includes continuous parenteral antibiotics for a fortnight followed by a 6- to 12-week oral antibiotic regimen, suction drainage for 2–4 days and early protected mobilization (after 5 days of bed rest). The local knee and wound status, as well as ESR, WBC, and CRP must be observed weekly. If the above attributes improve, the patient should be reviewed every 3 months for at least 1 year, or if symptoms reoccur. Data from the Schulthess Clinic in Zurich, Switzerland indicate a success rate of over 80% when treated with this algorithm. The patient should be informed about the advantages and disadvantages of this procedure, risk factors regarding function, potential problems, and statistical reoccurrence.

A two-stage procedure is the treatment of choice in all other early and acute infections, particularly in cases with mixed, gram-negative, or multiply resistant organisms, bone involvement at the fixation interface, signs of septic loosening, poor patient status, or organisms spreading diseases. Complete removal of all components including cement (if used), extensive debridement, and pulsatile lavage as described above are recommended. The surgeon may decide on the preferred type of temporary spacer. We recommend a double gentamycin-loaded molded cement block (with a thickness of the tibial component plus bearing insert) and reimplantation of the sterilized femoral component into a new cement bed. Postoperative follow-up is identical to that of the one-stage procedure, with reimplantation of new prosthetic components after a period of usually 6–12 weeks, depending on inflammation parameters.

Early Low-Grade Infection

This category represents a diagnostic dilemma, because infection causes minimal clinical implications, with slow progress. Culture specimens are often positive on one occasion and associated with bacteria commonly found in the physiological flora. Classic inflammatory parameters may be normal, including CRP, WBC, and ESR. Therefore, management of these types of knees (and patients) is challenging. Close observation is required and any sign of deterioration should be taken seriously. Whenever in doubt, open debridement, lavage and pulsatile lavage with antiseptic agents in an antibiotic-free period should include reinvestigation of synovial and (prosthetic) polyethylene slime specimens for culture and sensitivity. Early occurrence of and progressing radiolucent lines at the implant- or cement–bone interface are the most likely signs of infection. This category of patient may benefit from sophisticated bone, leukocyte, or FDG-PET scans, or modern genetic investiga-

tions including PCR or MN3 Fab' antibody screening. Intraoperative gram staining is recommended for confirmation of infection. Soft tissue (frozen section) biopsy with findings of ten or more WBC per high-power histologic field correlates with infection.

Early Occult Infection

The diagnosis of an occult infection is paradox, as it represents a painful TKA, in which all cultures have been negative. Therefore, differential diagnoses for painful TKA (see Sect. 7.1) have to be excluded first, before consideration of an open procedure. Common factors that may contribute to a painful and/or swollen TKA are either mechanical (instability, malposition of components, etc.), vegetative (reflex sympathetic dystrophy, complex regional pain syndrome), or idiopathic. Careful exclusion of all listed parameters is necessary before revision surgery is considered. If revised, intraoperative gram staining and WBC high-power examination are recommended for detection of infection. Antibiotic cement is recommended if a one-stage procedure is considered (Freeman, Buechel).

Late Acute Infection

Infected TKA with verified organisms is best treated on an urgent basis with a two-stage procedure, a method well described and supported by the literature (Insall, Ranawat, Rand, Drobny, Munzinger). The time interval between reimplantation, however, may be extended. Long-term outcome has significantly inferior results when infection is detected and treated late (Wang et al. 2002). If an acute septic arthritis from a known source with sensitive bacteria is treated immediately, debridement with bearing exchange or one-stage revision may be considered, especially in the elderly debilitated patient.

Late Low-Grade Infection

As with early low-grade infection, late onset of infection after months or years seems to be associated with classic elevation of inflammatory parameters, positive bone or leukocyte scans and polyethylene wear debris. Data from the Schulthess Clinic were interesting in that there was an association of late low-grade infections with failed constrained knee prostheses after a mean of about 10 years. In all cases, knees tested positive for organisms and polyethylene damage was massive (wear disease), often combined with considerable periprosthetic osteolysis (PPO) and/or metallosis. A TKA that falls into this category should be treated as an aseptic loose prosthesis with special consideration to debridement, lavage, gentamycin-enhanced cement and postoperative antibiotic regimen. Petrie et al. (1998) reported a significantly increased risk of developing infection in TKA associated with considerable wear osteolysis and metallosis. This fact explains the increased prevalence and late onset of infection in TKA older than 10 years.

Late Occult Infection

Late low-grade infection can be mimicked in cases with extensive PPO, significant bone loss and prosthetic loosening. Therefore, the surgeon may consider a one-stage revision surgery with cautious consideration of soft tissue clearance and antibiotics.

Infection of total joint replacement is without doubt the most severe complication. The incidence of infection as the cause of revision surgery post TKA is reported to be up to 38% (Fehring et al. 2001, Weng et al. 2002). Despite being treated immediately with a successful two-stage revision, long-term results are significantly inferior (Barrack et al. 2000). Better outcome is expected with aggressive management rather than a more conservative approach (Wang et al. 2002). Reported success rates of early two-stage revisions in (gram positive) infected TKA range from 64% (Walker and Schurman 1984), 80% (Wilde and Ruth 1988), 82% (Gacon et al. 1997), 90% (Petty 1995), 97% (Brandt et al.1999), up to 100% (Rosenberg et al. 1988). Early and aggressive management is favored in recent publications, when infection is confirmed. Delay in superficial site wound healing is a significant risk factor for developing deep wound infections; therefore, early and aggressive debridement and salvage are recommended to prevent prosthetic infection (Saleh et al. 2002, Dennis 1997, Simmons and Stern 1996). Furthermore, postoperative hemarthosis and hematoma place the prosthesis at risk (Weiss and Krackow 1993, Saleh et al. 2002).

There is general consensus that gram-negative and other non-gram-positive organisms have a significantly worse prognosis (Jacobs et al. 1989, Virolainen et al. 2002), particularly infections caused by anaerobic bacteria (*Clostridium perfringens*) (Wilde et al. 1988) or fungi such as Candida (Yang et al. 2001). Patients who are at higher risk because of diabetes mellitus or poor general health require more careful management and observation regarding infection. Chiu et al. (2001) reported a significant prevalence of infection in diabetic patients. Therefore, he recommends adding antibiotics (cefuroxime) to the cement in primary TKA.

Both diagnosis and management are difficult and require clinical experience as well as an optimal logistical background, including professional laboratory analysis and infectious disease specialists. There is a trend towards the so-called two-stage prosthesis-conserving procedure, early rehabilitation, and reduced hospitalization. Closed management such as drainage or arthroscopic wash-out has a very high failure rate in eradicating infection. The other extreme is excision arthroplasty with or without external or internal arthrodesis, an unsatisfactory management for both the patient and the surgeon. Temporary implantation of a "spacer prosthesis", which allows mobility and load capacity, is a newer concept, which allows more functional rehabilitation in the interim period between reimplantation.

Risk Factors for Developing Infection in Joint Arthroplasty

There are multiple factors increasing the risk of infection, which may be divided into three groups: (1) iatrogenic and environmental, (2) coexisting diseases, and (3) immune suppressive medical treatment (Table 7.2). There are no hard data available in the literature stating which factor is more likely to increase the risk for infection, although some are considered as potentially higher risk. In accordance with clinical observations, we regard both a disciplined environment and appreciation of soft tissues, in addition to a short operating time, to be the most influential factors for preventing infection. Antibiotics should be administered at induction or prior to anesthesia. Antibiotic saturation in the lower limb takes at least 5 minutes (Friedman et al. 1990), therefore the tourniquet should not be inflated prior to this time frame. The total joint surgeon should pay careful attention to high-flow clean-air operating rooms, space suits, short operating time, meticulous soft tissue handling and hemostasis.

Further factors that are influential include previous knee surgeries, the patient's status, body mass index, teeth status and oral hygiene, which also need to be addressed during the consent interview. Disease conditions, particularly type I and type II diabetes mellitus, cardiovascular disease with impaired arterial perfusion of the lower limb, thromboembolic

Table 7.2. Risk factors for developing infection in TKA

Environmental/surgeon	Coexisting disease	Immune suppression
Clean-air operating room	Previous knee surgery	Chronic infections
Space suits	Body mass index	Urogenital focus
Disciplined staff	Oral hygiene	Digestive focus
Operating time	Diabetes mellitus	Hepatitis B, C
Soft tissue handling	Vascular impairment	Cytomegalovirus, human immunodeficiency virus
Hemostasis	Thromboembolic	Drugs
Drainage	Hematosepsis	Wear disease
	Hemophilia	Metallosis

events and postoperative prevention treatment further increase the risk of infection. Additional sources of articular infection are chronic infections of the urogenital or digestive system, and hematosepsis. Patients who suffer from hemophilia viral hepatitis or other infectious diseases (TBC, cytomegalovirus, human immunodeficiency virus, etc.) have altered immune systems, which reduce the healing response. Every medical treatment that is immune suppressive enhances the probability of infection in TKA.

Arthrodesis in infected TKA has gained less popularity, as the results appear to be inferior to a two-stage revision (Jorgensen and Torholm 1995, David, Incavo et al. 2000, Manzotti et al. 2001). Above-the-knee amputation should be the last resort, but may become necessary in cases with life-threatening hematosepsis caused by infected TKA. Takedown of an arthrodesed knee and conversion to TKA is a very challenging procedure with a poor success rate, as discussed in Sect. 4.14.

The surgeon and the patient must be continuously aware of infection and every effort is required to help reduce this dramatically jeopardizing complication in one of the most successful operations in orthopedic surgery.

Bibliography

Barrack RL, Engh G, Rorabeck C, Sawhney J, Woolfrey M (2000) Patient satisfaction and outcome after septic versus aseptic revision total knee arthroplasty. J Arthroplasty 15: 990–993

Bohler M, Danielczyk I, Kasparek M, Knahr K (2000) Gonarthrosis and empyema in geriatric patients. Combined synovectomy and KTEP implantation procedure. Z Orthop 138:69–73

Brandt CM, Duffy MC, Berbari EF, Hanssen AD, Steckelberg JM, Osmon DR (1999) Staphylococcus aureus prosthetic joint infection treated with prosthesis removal and delayed reimplantation arthroplasty. Mayo Clin Proc 74:553–558

Burger RR, Basch T, Hopson CN (1991) Implant salvage in infected total knee arthroplasty. Clin Orthop 273:105–112

Chiu FY, Lin CF, Chen CM, Lo WH, Chaung TY (2001) Cefuroxime-impregnated cement at primary total knee arthroplasty in diabetes mellitus. A prospective, randomised study. JBJS Br 83:691–695

Dennis DA (1997) Wound complications in total knee arthroplasty. Orthopedics 20:837–840

Fehring TK, Odum S, Griffin WL, Mason JB, Nadaud M (2001) Early failures in total knee arthroplasty. Clin Orthop 392:315–318

Friedman RJ, Friedrich LV, White RL, Kays MB, Brundage DM, Graham J (1990) Antibiotic prophylaxis and tourniquet inflation in total knee arthroplasty. Clin Orthop 260:17–23

Gacon G, Laurencon M, van de Velde D, Giudicelli DP (1997) Two stages reimplantation for infection after knee arthroplasty. Apropos of a series of 29 cases. Rev Chir Orthop Reparatrice Appar Mot 83:313–323

Henkel TR, Boldt JG, Drobny TK, Munzinger UK (2001) TKA after formal knee fusion using unconstrained and semi-constrained components: a report of 7 cases. J Arthroplasty 16:768–776

Incavo SJ, Lilly JW, Bartlett CS, Churchill DL (2000) Arthrodesis of the knee: experience with intramedullary nailing. J Arthroplasty 15:871–876

Insall JN, Thompson FM, Brause BD (1983) Two stage reimplantation for the salvage of the infected TKA. J Bone Joint Surg Am 65:1087–1098

Ivaneeviae V, Perka C, Hasart O, Sandrock D, Munz DL (2002) Imaging of low-grade bone infection with a technetium-99m labelled monoclonal anti-NCA-90 Fab' fragment in patients with previous joint surgery. Eur J Nucl Med Mol Imaging 29:547–551

Jacobs MA, Hungerford DS, Krackow KA, Lennox DW (1989) Revision of septic total knee arthroplasty. Clin Orthop 238: 159–166

Jorgensen PS, Torholm C (1995) Arthrodesis after infected knee arthroplasty using long arthrodesis nail. A report of five cases. Am J Knee Surg 8:110–113

Lewis PL, Brewster NT, Graves SE (1998) The pathogenesis of bone loss following total knee arthroplasty. Orthop Clin North Am 29:187–197

Manzotti A, Pullen C, Deromedis B, Catagni MA (2001) Knee arthrodesis after infected total knee arthroplasty using the Ilizarov method. Clin Orthop 389:143–149

Petrie RS, Hanssen AD, Osmon DR, Ilstrup D (1998) Metal-backed patellar component failure in total knee arthroplasty: a possible risk for late infection. Am J Orthop 27:172–176

Petty W (1995) Operative management of the infected knee. Orthopedics 18:927–929

Rand JA, Brown ML (1990) The value of indium 111 leukocyte scanning in the evaluation of painful or infected total knee arthroplasties. Clin Orthop 259:179–182

Rosenberg AG, Haas B, Barden R, Marquez D, Landon GC, Galante JO (1988) Salvage of infected total knee arthroplasty. Clin Orthop 226:29–33

Saleh K, Olson M, Resig S, Bershadsky B, Kuskowski M, Gioe T, Robinson H, Schmidt R, McElfresh E (2002) Predictors of wound infection in hip and knee joint replacement: results from a 20 year surveillance program. J Orthop Res 20:506–515

Scott SJ, Hennessey MS, Parkinson RW, Molloy AP (2001) Long-term outcome of the 'Beefburger' procedure in patients unsuitable for two-stage revision following infected TKR. Knee 8:281–286

Simmons TD, Stern SH (1996) Diagnosis and management of the infected total knee arthroplasty. Am J Knee Surg 9:99–106

Van Acker F, Nuyts J, Maes A, Vanquickenborne B, Stuyck J, Bellemans J, Vleugels S, Bormans G, Mortelmans L (2001) FDG-PET, 99mtc-HMPAO white blood cell SPET and bone scintigraphy in the evaluation of painful total knee arthroplasties. Eur J Nucl Med 28:1496–1504

Virolainen P, Lahteenmaki H, Hiltunen A, Sipola E, Meurman O, Nelimarkka O (2002) The reliability of diagnosis of infection during revision arthroplasties. Scand J Surg 91:178–181

Walker RH, Schurman DJ (1984) Management of infected total knee arthroplasties. Clin Orthop 186:81–89

Wang CJ, Huang TW, Wang JW, Chen HS (2002) The often poor clinical outcome of infected total knee arthroplasty. J Arthroplasty 17:608–614

Weiss AP, Krackow KA (1993) Persistent wound drainage after primary total knee arthroplasty. J Arthroplasty 8:285–289

Weng X, Li L, Qiu G, Li J, Tian Y, Hen J, Wang Y, Jin J, Ye Q, Zhao H (2002) Treatment of infected total knee arthroplasty. Zhonghua Wai Ke Za Zhi 40:669–672

Wilde AH, Ruth JT (1988) Two-stage reimplantation in infected total knee arthroplasty. Clin Orthop 236:23–35

Wilde AH, Sweeney RS, Borden LS (1988) Hematogenously acquired infection of a total knee arthroplasty by Clostridium perfringens. Clin Orthop 229:228–231

Windsor RE, Bono JV Infected total knee replacement. J Am Acad Orth Surg 2:44–53

Yang SH, Pao JL, Hang YS (2001) Staged reimplantation of total knee arthroplasty after Candida infection. J Arthroplasty 16:529–532

7.5 Infectious Disease Management in Total Knee Arthroplasty

M. Vogt

After knee prosthesis implantation the bacteria "race to the artificial surface" begins. Adhesions, such as fibronectin, induce attachment of staphylococci and other bacteria. Phagocytosis is severely hampered due to the artificial surface (frustrated phagocytosis). Bacteria and a hydrated matrix of polysaccharides and proteins form a biofilm, the so-called slime. Within that slime bacteria undergo complex genetic changes and become up to 1,000-fold more resistant to antibiotics than free-floating "planktonic" forms. Slime bacteria grow slowly and are, therefore, less likely to become a target for conventional antibiotics. Free-floating bacteria are continuously shed from that biofilm and may cause symptoms of infection. New data indicate that antibiotics penetrate rapidly into the biofilm but may be inactivated in that environment by various mechanisms. Conventional methods of resistance development are not primarily seen in biofilms.

Planktonic bacteria are killed in vivo by antibiotics, possibly suppressing clinically apparent infections. When therapy is discontinued, biofilm bacteria may initiate infection by shedding off new planktonic bacteria from the slime. This fact causes infections to smolder for months or years with subtle clinical symptoms. Therefore it seems logical that such chronic infections may be cured by removing the responsible biofilm only (Stewart and Costerton 2001). This straightforward approach is difficult to accomplish; therefore, supporting therapies are needed for biofilm infections in internal medicine (cystic fibrosis, continuous ambulatory peritoneal dialysis catheters) and surgery (artificial heart valves, orthopedic implants).

Antibiotic Strategies of Infected Orthopedic Implants

Possible algorithms have been elucidated to choose optimal management of infected total knee arthroplasty (TKA). Infections in TKA occur relatively seldom and large multicenter trials are not available. Therefore, development of internationally accepted guidelines for diagnosis and treatment of infected TKA is difficult. Orthopedic surgeons, microbiologists and infectious disease physicians should work in a dedicated interdisciplinary team for optimal management of infected TKA.

Table 7.3. Essential criteria to select patients suitable for conservative treatment of orthopedic device-related infections (adapted from Widmer 2001)

Acute device-related infection with symptoms of less than 14–28 days
Implant stable, no signs of loosening
Microbiological etiology established, single organism, multiple samplings positive
Pathogen susceptible to oral antibiotics (long-term therapy planned)
Antibiotic with proven effectiveness in humans (see Table 7.4)
Strict adherence to long-term treatment (>6 months) possible

Early postoperative infections post surgery are commonly wound infections caused by *Staphylococcus aureus* or coagulase-negative staphylococci (CNS).

Delayed infection occurs between 3 months and 2 years and is commonly caused by exogenous or hematogenous bacteria such as CNS, propioni bacterium species, anaerobes and *S. aureus*.

Late infections occur after 2 years and begin suddenly in asymptomatic knees and patients. They often present with severe clinical signs and are caused by streptococci, *S. aureus*, and gram-negative bacteria (Berbari et al. 1998, Widmer 2001). In the window before results of microbiological identification become available, empiric treatment has thus to cover bacteria depending on the stage of infection (Bose et al. 1995, Widmer 2001). Infections that occur around 10 years after surgery are often associated with increased wear, which causes decreased immune response in the knee joint.

From the infectious disease perspective, early postoperative infections usually respond well to rapid debridement and long-term antibiotic therapy. Success rates are lower in delayed or late infections. Table 7.3 (from Widmer 2001) lists required criteria for possible implant salvage.

Device Removal

One-stage replacement is often used for early infections not qualifying for the "device retention approach" with low-virulent organisms or for chronic infections with loose prostheses and intact soft tissue. It is of utmost importance not to begin antibiotic treatment before adequate microbiologic samples have been obtained. There is no justification to treat patients empirically with oral antibiotic for suspected prosthetic infection without a clear therapeutic strategy and without team communication.

Orthopedic Device-Related Infections

To allow identification of bacterial growth in culture, antibiotic treatment should be discontinued 2–4 days prior to revision surgery under stable general health conditions. At least five biopsy specimens from periprosthetic tissues must be obtained to reach adequate diagnostic sensitivity (Atkins et al. 1998). The antibiotic regimen may begin immediately after sampling. As perioperative prophylaxis should also cover gram-negative organisms, we recommend 2 g ceftriaxone i.v. as a single dose intraoperatively in the starting regimen.

Table 7.4 summarizes current recommendations for antibiotic selection (adapted from Widmer 2001). Treatment should continue for at least 6 months. As an integral part of the procedure, irrigation and suction drainage is recommended for approximately 3 days, during which the patient needs monitoring for direct or indirect recurrence of infection, including: knee joint, wound, C-reactive protein (CRP), erythrocyte sedimentation rate (ESR), and white blood cells (WBC). If CRP levels fail to decrease, treatment should be prolonged for up to 12 months. Side effects and interactions of rifampin in particular should be monitored closely. Monotherapy with rifampin is not recommended because of potential development of resistance.

Two-stage Procedure

Management with temporary excision arthroplasty is performed in delayed or late infections presenting with: loosened components, necrotic soft tissues, sinus, abscess, extensive bone defects, and if the responsible microorganism is either unknown or virulent, such as methicillin-resistant *Staphylococcus aureus* or *Pseudomonas*. Microbiologic sampling should be performed without concurrent antibiotic therapy. Thereafter, intraoperative antibiotic treatment is commenced (Table 7.4). Implants are removed, soft tissues are radically debrided, an antibiotic-carrying spacer is implanted, and irrigation–suction drainage is applied for 2–3 days. Antibiotic therapy is recommended for at least 2 weeks, although longer treatment of 6 weeks is preferred prior to reimplantation.

Table 7.4. Antimicrobial agents for acute orthopedic device-related infections (adapted from Widmer 2001)

Pathogen	Initial treatment[b]	Time	Subsequent oral treatment (min. 6 months)
Empiric treatment[a,c]	Vancomycin[c] 2×1 g iv plus Rifampin 2×450 mg iv, po		
S. aureus, CNS, methicillin sensitive	Flucloxacillin 4×2 g iv plus Rifampin 2×450 mg iv, po	2–4 weeks	Ciprofloxacin 2×750 mg, po plus Rifampin 2×450 mg, po
S. aureus, CNS, methicillin resistant	Vancomycin 2×1 g iv plus Rifampin 2×450 mg iv, po		4–6 weeks od Ciprofloxacin 2×750 mg, po
			Cotrimoxazole 20/100 mg/kg per day, po
			Fusidic acid od 3×500 mg, po
			Teicoplanin od 400 mg/day iv or im
			Plus rifampin 2×450 mg, po
Streptococci	Amoxicillin 4×2 g iv plus Gentamicin 3×1 mg/kg iv	4–6 weeks 2 weeks	Amoxicillin 3×750–1,000 mg, po
Pseudomonas aeruginosa	Ceftazidime 3×2 g iv or	4–6 weeks	Ciprofloxacin 2×750 mg
	Cefepime 3×2 g iv plus Tobramycin 5 mg/kg per day iv single dose		
Other gram-negatives	Ciprofloxacin 2×400 mg iv	2 weeks	Ciprofloxacin 2×750 mg
Anaerobes	Clindamycin 3×600 mg iv	2–4 weeks	Clindamycin 3×600 mg

[a] Treatment should be changed as soon as responsible microorganism is detected

[b] Dose adjustments necessary in patients with obesity, impaired renal function, old age, liver disease

[c] If gram-negative pathogens are possible on the basis of clinical symptoms (urinary tract infection), gram-negative coverage is necessary (ciprofloxacin or ceftriaxone) until culture results become available

For index revision surgery, the following factors need careful attention: significant improvement or normalization of CRP and ESR values, afebrile temperatures, complete wound healing, healthy soft tissue appearance with a patient in good general health condition.

Prior to reimplantation, antibiotics should be withheld for approximately 4 days to optimize yield of intraoperative culturing. After appropriate sampling of five tissue biopsies, antibiotic treatment is recommenced. Rifampin is an integral part of antibiotic regimens if S. aureus and CNS are responsible for the initial infection. To cover potential gram-negative pathogens in the perioperative period, a single dose of ceftriaxone after microbiologic sampling should be added. Culture results will guide further treatment. Negative cultures suggest successful treatment. With uneventful postoperative recovery, antibiotics should be given for only approximately 14 days. If this proposed algorithm is followed closely, positive cul-

tures after reimplantation (recurrence of infection) will be rare. In case of positive cultures, antibiotic treatment should be continued for at least 6 months.

Debridement with Retention of the Infected Device

Zimmerli, Widmer and colleagues first evaluated combination chemotherapy with rifampin in animal models and later in a randomized controlled clinical trial where staphylococcal implant infections were treated (Widmer et al. 1992, Zimmerli et al. 1998). Cure of infection without removing the implant was achieved in the majority (80–100%) of properly selected patients (Table 7.3), while other approaches without rifampin co-therapy led to disappointing results (Brandt et al. 1997). As mentioned earlier, only a small subset of patients with orthopedic device-related infections benefit from conservative approaches.

Patients with delayed infections have less favorable outcomes (Tattevin et al. 1999). Best results were obtained if debridement and antibiotic treatment were started very early; treatment was unsuccessful when started after 1 or 2 weeks (Keating and Steckelberg 1999). Patients with suspected acute infection should be evaluated on an emergency basis and the pathogen identified by all means. In patients with classic signs of local and systemic infection, blood culture samples and debridement without antibiotic pretreatment are recommended. After obtaining multiple samples for culture, antibiotics are started without delay. Preoperative aspiration gives initial information on the expected pathogen, but careful intraoperative sampling will deliver definite answers in a situation where long-term treatment needs a firm basis for both the physician and the patient.

Exact therapy depends on the nature of the pathogen and its sensitivity to tested antibiotics. As soon as sensitivity data are available, empiric therapy should be discontinued in favor of recommended treatment, despite the fact that the empiric approach may have been clinically successful. Intravenous therapy can be changed to oral regimens after 2–4 weeks if clinical signs, CRP, WBC and ESR show a favorable development. Careful evaluation of clinical signs may indicate recurrence of infection earlier than serial measurements of WBC, CRP and ESR. Local pain in conjunction with a rise in CRP values may show failure of the conservative approach.

In infected TKA, duration of conservative treatment is scheduled for at least 6 months. In compliant patients, treatment is recommended for another 1–3 months. After stopping antibiotics, the patient is advised to report new pain or fever at any time. CRP values are measured once weekly in the first month, every second week in the next month and then once a month for up to 6 months.

Suppressive antibiotic therapy can be considered in patients who are unsuitable for surgery. Although chances for cure are small, individual case reports show that very selected patients may ultimately benefit from this approach. In one case a dual infection with *Peptostreptococcus micros* and *Propionibacterium acnes* was cured with needle aspiration, irrigation, and antibiotic therapy for 26 months. Infection continued to be absent at 55 months follow-up (Stoll et al. 1996).

Bibliography

Atkins BL, Athanasou N, Deeks JJ et al (1998) Prospective evaluation of criteria for microbiological diagnosis of prosthetic-joint infection at revision arthroplasty. J Clin Microbiol 36:2932–2939

Berbari EF, Hanssen AD, Duffy MC et al (1998) Risk for prosthetic joint infection: case control study. Clin Infect Dis 27:1247–1254

Bose WJ, Gearen PF, Randall JC, Petty W (1995) Long-term outcome of 42 knees with chronic infection after total knee arthroplasty. Clin Orthop Relat Res 319:285–296

Brandt CM, Sistrunk WW, Duffy MC et al (1997) *Staphylococcus aureus* prosthetic joint infection treated with debridement and prosthesis retention. Clin Infect Dis 24:914–919

Keating MR, Steckelberg JM (1999) Orthopedic prosthesis salvage. Clin Infect Dis 29:296–297

Stewart PS, Costerton JW (2001) Antibiotic resistance of bacteria in biofilms. Lancet 358:135–138

Stoll T, Stucki G, Brühlmann P, Vogt M, Gchwend N, Michel BA (1996) Infection of a total knee joint prosthesis by *Peptostreptococcus micros* and *Propionibacterium acnes* in an elderly RA patient: implant salvage with long-term antibiotics and needle aspiration/irrigation. Clin Rheumatol 15:399–402

Tattevin P, Crémieux A-C, Pottier P, Huten D, Carbon C (1999) Prosthetic joint infection: when can prosthesis salvage be considered? Clin Infect Dis 29:292–295

Widmer AF, Gaechter A, Ochsner PE, Zimmerli W (1992) Antimicrobial treatment of orthopedic implant-related infections with rifampin combinations. Clin Infect Dis 14:1251–1253

Widmer AF (2001) New developments in diagnosis and treatment of infection in orthopedic implants. Clin Infect Dis 33 [Suppl 2]:S94–S106

Zimmerli W, Widmer AF, Blatter M, Frei R, Ochsner PE (1998) Role of rifampin for treatment of orthopedic implant-related staphylococcal infections. JAMA 279:1537–1541

7.6 The Unhappy Knee
Peter A. Keblish, Jens G. Boldt

The unhappy knee after total knee arthroplasty (TKA) represents a subset of patients who inflict stress and discomfort on the operating surgeon and doctor–patient relationship. Subjective and objective findings are present in variable degrees and must be addressed in a more intense and empathic manner. Review of radiographs, pertinent studies, treatment options (medical, physical treatment program), and reasonable expectations at various times must be discussed with the patient. Treatment options are more difficult to recommend if there are no obvious or suspected mechanical reasons for the unsatisfactory result. This chapter will review the potential reasons and management options for an unhappy knee arthroplasty patient from the preoperative evaluation, to the decision to recommend surgery, to the projected final outcome. Time-related symptoms related to the index operation may direct a given treatment approach differently at different postoperative intervals. The goal of treatment is to convert an unhappy TKA patient into a satisfied, albeit not perfectly happy, patient.

Preoperative evaluation and recommendation for TKA is clear-cut in a high percentage of patients. Clinical and radiographic correlation, patient motivation and understanding of risk factors are appropriate, and early results are good or excellent in 90–95% in most series. The unhappy knee represents less than 5% of cases, but occupies 95% of surgeon challenge and stress. The majority of patients with an unhappy knee will improve with time – often taking as long as 18–24 months (personal observation) – if the operating surgeon remains focused, empathic and caring. However, a small percentage of TKA patients remain unhappy and may not reflect a poor functional result as measured by scoring systems, the most common way of communicating outcomes.

What can we learn, retrospectively, from the unhappy TKA patient, which can be applied to understanding and treatment? How can we apply this understanding to future avoidance of similar factors that continue to face the surgeon? How can we learn from our mistakes, if they are contributory to unhappy knees?

Risk Factors

In the preoperative assessment, generally accepted risk factors include:
1. The multiply operated knee
2. History of fibromyalgia, generalized unexplained pain
3. Patient with unreasonable expectations
4. Work-related injuries superimposed on pre-existing arthritic knees

Subtle, less recognized risk factors include:
1. The underinformed patient, who starts questioning why "all factors of knee replacement were not discussed", usually after any postoperative symptoms occur.
2. Presence of normal flexion (>120 degrees) in an active patient who is not aware that loss of terminal flexion is likely post TKA. A patient with preoperative flexion of 140 degrees and postoperative range of motion of 100–110 degrees is frequently an unhappy patient.

3. Failure to achieve full extension, which may be related to prosthetic design, operative technique, gap balance, and/or poor patient compliance, i.e. the passive, less aggressive patient, with poor pain tolerance and rehabilitation potential.
4. Unrecognized psychological problems and/or unrealistic family expectations and/or comparison with patients who have excellent results.
5. Slight physiological valgus in patients with familial hereditary varus preoperatively and/or in short obese females, who have difficulties clearing medial soft tissues. The lesson is to leave these people in physiological varus with a proven prosthetic design.

The majority of the preoperative assessment factors are easy to ignore rather than recognize as potential problems, as TKA is very successful. Previously, treatment for the arthritic knee was less predictable, and expectations were more reasonable and appropriate. Currently, expectation is high and at times surgery recommended without careful patient evaluation. It is suggested that conservative management be tried, especially when the patient is seen for the first time. It is not uncommon for patients and/or family members to overstate pain, which is important, as pain is the main cause of the unhappy knee. Therefore, it is important to document the specifics of pain, such as location, pattern, time, rest versus ambulatory, response to medication, etc. at any given time.

The Early Unhappy Knee

Pain and stiffness are the most common reasons for development of the less than ideal (always expected) result in TKA. The issue can be addressed in many ways and the number of publications on the subject is increasing. The unhappy TKA patient can usually be identified in the early postoperative period. Early identification of the potential problem is important and includes recognition of (1) postoperative pain that extends beyond normal, (2) hemarthrosis/effusion related to factors such as over-anticoagulation, poor drainage, etc., (3) need for extensive surgical releases, and (4) poor patient compliance/low pain tolerance. Reports of stiffness requiring manipulation have varied from 8 to 60% in the past. However, with modern prostheses and improved technique, the problem should now be in the 5–10% range. Knee manipulation is somewhat controversial and must be evaluated on an individual basis. When performed early (within 6–8 weeks), personal experience and literature support the value of the procedure. The techniques include aspiration, volume injection of marcaine and epinephrine (with or without steroids) in an operating room setting. Spinal epidural anesthesia with management of continuous passive motion is recommended in extreme cases. If performed after 12 weeks, arthroscopic evaluation or miniarthrotomy (lateral-suprapatellar) for lysis of adhesions should be considered. Manipulation must be performed carefully with the weight of the leg and gentle pressure at the level of the upper tibia providing the necessary force to break adhesions. Gentle massage of the patella and lateral gutter in difficult cases is also effective. Fracture with manipulation is a potential risk and can be avoided by careful technique.

Provided there are no major technical (surgical) blocks to flexion, the procedure can correct a potential "unhappy knee" into a pain-free happy patient. The problem is identification and follow-up, especially as hospital stays are shorter and different physical therapists from many areas (and individual teaching) work with the patients. Communication with patients/therapists and family will identify the patient at risk and encourage earlier postoperative visits. The majority of patients may be happy with a pain-free 90 degrees flexion (some people's goal) in the early postoperative period, but very disappointed with 90 degrees as the final result. The surgeon needs to evaluate patients' expectations, which vary constantly. Long-term unhappy TKA patients relate to functional limitations; many of these patients need the extra attention. The operating surgeon must make the patient understand the long-term issues and the need to achieve the optimum range of motion in the first 6–12 weeks. Some patients will improve motion (up to 2 years) but the vast majority will not. An aggressive positive approach is required at all times.

The Intermediate-Term Unhappy Knee

The unhappy TKA in the intermediate postoperative period (6 weeks to 6 months) is often related to periarticular as well as intra-articular inflammation (synovitis, bursitis, enthisitis). Hemarthrosis or synovial effusion to some degree is common and usually does not need attention. If persistent and/or significant, aspiration under sterile conditions in the clinic should be considered to rule out infection and provide pain relief. Injection of marcaine with epinephrine is often effective and can reverse a negative to a

positive patient response, leading to improvement in pain, cooperation with rehabilitation and better range of motion. If infection has been ruled out, steroid injection may be considered.

Medical management with use of non-steroidal agents or short courses of steroids, ice, and elastic support stockings and/or a soft brace are other options that can maintain patient confidence. Patients should be seen on a frequent basis and close contact maintained during this period. If infection and mechanical prosthetic reasons for the unhappy knee have been ruled out at this time, proceed with confidence and utilize all accepted methods to reverse the situation. Re-admission with re-manipulations using postoperative epidural analgesia, anti-anxiety medication, lidoderm patches, muscle relaxants, etc. should be considered in more recalcitrant cases to minimize the potential for complex regional pain syndrome (CRPS) or reflex sympathetic dystrophy (RSD) of the knee, which is a controversial subject and very rare in pure form compared with post-traumatic ankle/foot or wrist/hand problems. Much has been written about Sudeck, RSD, CRPS and the various treatment options.

The diagnosis of CRPS or RSD, in this author's experience, is less commonly made today than it was in the earlier days of TKA. This observation, and other reports (Boldt et al. 2003) suggest that the diagnosis may be an excuse for non-recognition of technical, mechanical, prosthetic or soft tissue problems related to the surgery. The early or intermediate painful postoperative knee patient, if ignored or untreated, is more likely to develop a CRPS-like syndrome than the patient treated with care and the appropriate measures available today. During the postoperative treatment of this group of patients, other potential causes of knee pain should be considered, including (1) vascular, (2) spine referred, neurogenic, (3) hip arthritis, referred, (4) metabolic, (5) delayed infection, (6) rheumatologic, and (7) centrally induced. This author has personally "cured" several unhappy TKA patients with ipsilateral total hip arthroplasty, spinal facet joint injection or epidural steroid injection and changing a medication (rheumatoid protocol). In addition, a patient with a brain tumor and a perfectly functioning knee with CRPS-like pain improved following tumor surgery. The message is "to explore the obvious and not so obvious" when patients with perfectly placed and well-fixed TKA have pain out of proportion to clinical/radiological signs.

The Late Unhappy Knee

The chronically "unhappy TKA" is one that, arbitrarily, persists beyond the 6 months time frame. At this point, the more subtle mechanical causes of pain and stiffness or instability must be re-evaluated. Careful examination for component malalignment, patella maltracking, mid-flexion instabilities, or femoral or tibial malrotation, which represent the most likely technical errors in TKA, must be excluded. Malalignment may lead to an early "polyethylene wear" synovitis, which is the final common determinator and may begin to appear at the 6 months postoperative period.

Pain, stiffness, and varus from 8 to 12 degrees (Daluga) are the most common reasons cited for the unhappy knee. The five main causes are: (1) polyethylene wear synovitis, (2) patella problems, (3) poor alignment, (4) soft tissue make-up, and (5) prosthetic loosening. Each of these factors can be broken down to subsets from the skin incision to prosthetic implantation, prosthetic position and alignment, and sizing and kinematics of the prosthesis being utilized. A recent study by Scranton (2001) reviewed pain and stiffness in 33 patients with two different fixed bearing designs. Results of manipulation for postoperative stiffness vary between reports; it is usually most effective when performed early (3–12 weeks). Literature reports have shown that Tc99m scans remain "hot" for 1 year plus in cement and cementless designs, and may explain discomfort noted in a higher percentage of patients during the first 18 months.

Cemented versus cementless evaluation is addressed in Sect. 2.2. In evaluating an unhappy cementless TKA (with good alignment, technique, etc.), care must be taken to inform the patient that this is a more biologic procedure and healing "inflammation" may account for some feelings of warmth and aching as the natural healing occurs. This process may take up to 18–24 months and diagnostic studies such as bone scans will remain "hot" for an extended period in cementless TKA. Avoiding premature operations in these cases is critical, unless there is definite aseptic loosening (Hoffman, Corr 1990).

Diagnostic studies recommended in evaluation of the unhappy TKA at any given stage should have a rationale. Assuming infection is unlikely (negative testing: culture, sensitivity, synovial biopsy, leukocyte scans, newer genetic testing, etc.), plain radiographs and serial clinical examinations are most important. If there is suspicion of rotational malalignment, consideration of computed tomography scans is recommended.

Patella pain and/or extensor mechanism dysfunction is an often-cited cause of an unhappy TKA. Evaluation and treatment vary from a more intense rehabilitation (quadriceps strengthening) to reoperation to correct any of the known causes of anterior knee pain. Again, with improved surgery, prostheses and understanding of femoral rotation, patella-related problems can be avoided (with or without patella resurfacing). Preoperative rehabilitation stressing quadriceps function is valuable from an objective and subjective patient awareness standpoint. Non-resurfaced patellae have a reported failure rate of 1.1% in our series with the low contact stress anatomic femoral design (Boldt and Keblish 2001), but other non-conforming prosthetic designs have a higher level of failure. Resurfaced patellae have similar failure rates (Sect. 3.1), often for different reasons. Anterior knee pain that is incapacitating needs to be treated surgically but the majority of early symptoms will improve with the conservative methods outlined. Not all anterior knee pain is patella bone related; it may vary from dermal paresthesia or neuroma (Hardy) to early femoral prosthetic loosening.

The unhappy TKA patient is always a challenge and needs to be addressed in a algorithmic manner, which relates to: (1) the postoperative time frame, (2) patient psychological make-up, pain tolerance, etc., (3) presence or absence of known complications at surgery or in the early postoperative period. If an obvious technical error is discovered, it must be addressed and fixed. Avoiding delay in reoperation for obvious technical errors may convert an early unhappy knee to a very satisfied patient and avoid the chronic problem, which includes persistent pain or stiffness, difficult communication, and legal implications.

With improvements in technique and prosthetic design, and better anesthesia with early pain control, the issue of true CRPS or RSD should present a relatively rare event. There is increasing evidence and personal experience that a cause for the "unhappy TKA" is usually present and treatable. Early recognition and management of the problem, often subtle, can make a major difference in outcomes. The surgeon must look for the obvious as well as non-knee-related diagnoses in a given patient. Patient "informed" consent in the preoperative consultation must identify risk factors in those having a higher likelihood of unhappy knees following TKA.

Bibliography

Boldt JG, Hodler J, Zanetti M, Munzinger UK (2003) Is arthro-fibrosis associated with femoral component internal malro-tation in TKA? AAOS presentation, New Orleans

Buechel FF Sr, Buechel FF Jr, Pappas MJ, Dalessio J (2002) Twenty-year evaluation of the New Jersey LCS rotating plat-form knee replacement. J Knee Surg 15:84–89

Christensen CP, Crawford JJ, Olin MD, Vail TP (2002) Revision of the stiff total knee arthroplasty. J Arthroplasty 17:409–415

Fehring TK, Odum S, Griffin WL, Mason JB, Nadaud M (2001) Early failures in TKA. Clin Orthop 392:315–319

Hartley RC, Barton-Hanson NG, Finley R, Parkinson RW (2002) Early patient outcomes after primary and revision total knee arthroplasty. A prospective study. J Bone Joint Surg Br 84:994–999

Hull JB, Hobbs C, Sidebottom S (1999) Anterior knee pain syn-drome. A review of current concepts and controversies. J R Army Med Corps 145:89–94

Johnson DF, Love DT, Love BR, Lester DK (2000) Dermal hy-poesthesia after total knee arthroplasty. Am J Orthop 29:863–866

Karabatsos B, Mahomed NN, Maistrelli GL (2002) Functional outcome of total knee arthroplasty after high tibial osteot-omy. Can J Surg 45:116–119

Koeter S, Bell CS, Jackson RW (1999) Fabellar pain after total knee arthroplasty. Am J Knee Surg 12:172–174

Laskin RS (1999) The painful knee. Orthopedics 22:869–870

Mahomed NN, Liang MH, Cook EF, Daltroy LH, Fortin PR, Fos-sel AH, Katz JN (2002) The importance of patient expecta-tions in predicting functional outcomes after total joint ar-throplasty. J Rheumatol 29:1273–1279

Milgrom C, Finestone A, Shlamkovitch N, Giladi M, Radin E (1996) Anterior knee pain caused by overactivity: a long term prospective followup. Clin Orthop 331:256–260

Nimon G, Murray D, Sandow M, Goodfellow J (1998) Natural history of anterior knee pain: a 14- to 20-year follow-up of nonoperative management. J Pediatr Orthop 18:118–122

Pap G, Meyer M, Weiler HT, Machner A, Awiszus F (2000) Prop-rioception after total knee arthroplasty: a comparison with clinical outcome. Acta Orthop Scand 71:153–159

Scher DM, Paumier JC, di Cesare PE (1997) Pseudomeniscus following total knee arthroplasty as a cause of persistent knee pain. J Arthroplasty 12:114–118

Schneider U, Breusch SJ, Thomsen M, Wenz W, Graf J, Niethard FU A new concept in the treatment of anterior knee pain: patellar hypertension syndrome

Scranton PE Jr (2001) Management of knee pain and stiffness after total knee arthroplasty. J Arthroplasty 16:428–435

Suter E, Herzog W, Bray RC (1998) Quadriceps inhibition fol-lowing arthroscopy in patients with anterior knee pain. Clin Biomech (Bristol, Avon) 13:314–319

Takahashi M, Miyamoto S, Nagano A (2002) Arthroscopic treatment of soft-tissue impingement under the patella af-ter total knee arthroplasty. Arthroscopy 18:E20

Witonski D (1999) Anterior knee pain syndrome. Int Orthop 23:341–344

Witonski D, Wagrowska-Danielewicz M (1999) Distribution of substance-P nerve fibers in the knee joint in patients with anterior knee pain syndrome. A preliminary report. Knee Surg Sports Traumatol Arthrosc 7:177–183

Subject Index